WQ 140 REI

KU-267-795

# Midwifery: Freedom to practise?

*An international exploration of midwifery practice*

WITHDRAWN

Book No.    05597859

30121 0 05597859

Yet, Freedom! Yet thy banner, torn, but flying,
Streams like the thunder-storm *against* the wind.

Lord Byron, Childe Harolde IV st 98

*For all midwives in the international search for
freedom to practise*

*For Elsevier*

*Commissioning Editor:* Mary Seager
*Development Editor:* Rebecca Nelemans, Fiona Conn
*Project Manager:* Morven Dean
*Designer:* George Ajayi

# Midwifery:
# Freedom to practise?

*An international exploration of
midwifery practice*

*Edited by*
Lindsay Reid

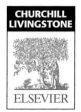

Edinburgh London New York Oxford Philadelphia St Louis Sydney Toronto 2007

## CHURCHILL
## LIVINGSTONE
### ELSEVIER

An imprint of Elsevier Limited

© 2007, Elsevier Limited. All rights reserved.

No part of this publication may be reproduced, stored in a retrieval system, or transmitted in any form or by any means, electronic, mechanical, photocopying, recording or otherwise, without the prior permission of the Publishers. Permissions may be sought directly from Elsevier's Health Sciences Rights Department, 1600 John F. Kennedy Boulevard, Suite 1800, Philadelphia, PA 19103-2899, USA: phone: (+1) 215 239 3804; fax: (+1) 215 239 3805; or, e-mail: *healthpermissions@elsevier.com*. You may also complete your request on-line via the Elsevier homepage (*http://www.elsevier.com*), by selecting 'Support and contact' and then 'Copyright and Permission'.

First published 2007

ISBN-13: 978-0-443-10312-4
ISBN-10: 0-443-10312-7

**British Library Cataloguing in Publication Data**
A catalogue record for this book is available from the British Library

**Library of Congress Cataloging in Publication Data**
A catalog record for this book is available from the Library of Congress

**Notice**
Neither the Publisher nor the Editor assume any responsibility for any loss or injury and/or damage to persons or property arising out of or related to any use of the material contained in this book. It is the responsibility of the treating practitioner, relying on independent expertise and knowledge of the patient, to determine the best treatment and method of application for the patient.

*The Publisher*

## Working together to grow
## libraries in developing countries

www.elsevier.com | www.bookaid.org | www.sabre.org

**ELSEVIER** | BOOK AID International | Sabre Foundation

ELSEVIER

your source for books,
journals and multimedia
in the health sciences

**www.elsevierhealth.com**

The
publisher's
policy is to use
**paper manufactured
from sustainable forests**

Printed in China

# CONTENTS

# CONTRIBUTORS

**Rudīte Brūvere** DipMid, Licence to Practise, CertIndPract
*Licensed independent midwife; Midwife, Family Health Center 'The Stork's Nest', Riga; Midwifery issues teacher, Health Promotion State Agency, Riga; Managing Director of NGO 'The Family Cradle', Latvia*

**Rea Daellenbach** PhD
*Lecturer, School of Midwifery, Christchurch Polytechnic Institute of Technology, New Zealand*

**Polly Ferguson** RN, RM, ADM, PGCEA, MSc
*Nursing Officer for Women's Reproductive Health, Welsh Assembly Government, Wales, UK*

**Jenny Gamble** DipAppScNurseEd, BN, MHlth (Research), PhD
*Lecturer, Convenor, Master of Midwifery Program, School of Nursing and Midwifery, Griffith Health, Griffith University, Meadowbrook, Queensland, Australia*

**Mary Higgins** RM, MComm
*Clinical Midwifery Manager, Unified Maternity Services, Cork, Ireland*

**Julia Hussein** MBBCh, MRCOG, MScPHDC
*International Technical Partner Leader, IMMPACT (Initiative for Maternal Mortality Programme Assessment), University of Aberdeen, Scotland, UK*

**Sandy Kirkman** RN, RM, DipAdultEd, MTD, BA, MTh, PhD
*Principal Lecturer/Postgraduate tutor, School of Care Sciences, University of Glamorgan, Wales, UK*

**Barbara Kuypers** RN, RM, ADM, MSc
*Professional Advisor for Midwifery, Nursing and Midwifery Council, UK*

**Elaine Madden** DipSocSci, BS(Hons), MSc Midwifery Studies, RFN, RGN, RM, Dip Prof Studies Midwifery
*Maternity Services Lead Midwife at Ulster Hospital, Belfast, Northern Ireland, UK*

**Rosemary Mander** MSc, PhD, RGN, SCM, MTD
*Professor of Midwifery, School of Health in Social Science, University of Edinburgh, Scotland, UK*

**Cheryl Nikodem** DCur, MCur, BACur, DipMid, DipNurse
*Associate Professor, School of Nursing, University of the Western Cape, South Africa*

**Mary Nolan** MA, BA (Hons), PhD, RGN
*Senior Tutor, National Childbirth Trust, UK*

**Tamunosa Okiwelu** BSc (Hons), MSc, PhD, RN, RM, RNAdmin
*Independent Consultant (Women's Health) California, USA*

**Ann Matekwe-Phoya** BSc, MSc, PhD RN, RM
*Director of Health Sector Wide Approach (SWAP), Malawi*

**Lindsay Reid** PhD, BA, Educational Studies, Dip Education, Midwife, ADM
*Midwife writer and researcher, Fife, Scotland, UK*

**Liz Stephens** BSc (Hons), MA, PGDip, RGN, RM
*Consultant midwife, St George's Hospital, London, England, UK*

**Juliet Thorpe** RN, RM, MMid
*Home birth midwife, member Home Birth Midwives' Practice, Christchurch; Expert Advisor New Zealand College of Midwives*

**Janet Ansong Tornui** BA(Hons), DipHealthEd, MSc, RM, RPHN
*Chief Research Assistant, IMMPACT Project, Noguchi Memorial Institute of Medical Research, Legon, Ghana*

**Barbara Vernon** BA (Hons), PhD
*Executive Officer, Australian College of Midwives, Australia*

# PREFACE

*Midwifery: Freedom to practise?* has had a long gestation – perhaps for the whole of my time in midwifery in Wales, England and Scotland. It has developed through incidents in practice, in teaching, through historical research about midwives and their practice (from both archival sources and oral testimonies), and from observing behaviour of midwives, medical practitioners and others who work with women and their infants during pregnancy, labour and the postnatal period. So, the feeling has been there, poorly formed and articulated: just a feeling of dissatisfaction that things in the world of childbearing, maternity care and midwifery were not quite right.

In some parts of the world the birthing life is very much more than 'not quite right'. In the poorest countries of the world 1 in 10 women die of maternal causes (Camm 2005; see also Chapters 5 and 15).

In the twentieth century circumstances improved for many. Mortality rates, both maternal and infant, fell in many countries of the world; pain relief in labour developed, became modernised and sophisticated; antibiotics and blood transfusions became commonplace; birth came into hospital. Midwives and mothers through legislation, culture and custom became accustomed to a medical model of childbirth.

So that's all right then. Or is it?

Why might it not be all right to use a medical model of childbirth to the exclusion of the midwifery or social model? For a start, it removes choice from women; it perpetuates a 'we know best' type of thinking which negates the ability and intelligence of women to articulate what they want; and, if allowed to go unchecked, women would have no knowledge of any other way of giving birth. Thus, women would not learn the whole truth of what could be possible and the idea that women are not able to birth normally would be perpetuated. In addition, within constraints of the medical model, a midwife, qualified and legally permitted to practise is not free to practise and make considered decisions with a woman about her care.

Most pregnant women have the potential to have a normal and safe pregnancy and give birth without medical intervention. Midwives who have freedom to practise and the courage and confidence to use their freedom to help women who are able to labour and give birth within the bounds of normality will be using the holistic midwifery/social model. At the same time, those midwives will have the freedom to make decisions about their practice with the women for whom they are caring in a partnership situation. This might mean that in the interests of the woman or baby a decision might be made to call medical help, move to a situation that requires a shift to a more medical model of care. However, the mother's interests may lie in allowing a normal birth to remain normal and within the midwifery model. The point is that the midwife within her freedom to practise, or autonomy in practice, will have the confidence to take the responsibility to make the decision. Mothers will benefit from access where necessary to both models of care.

The issue of midwives and whether or not they have freedom to practise is an important one. Government initiatives, local or national protocols, and, actions of personalities frequently impose restrictions of varying degrees on midwives and their ability to practise as they might wish to. Linked with this is the notion of 'best practice'. How does current practice measure against 'best practice'? And, indeed, what is 'best practice'? An exploration of the realities of everyday midwifery practice always with the idea of the benchmark of 'best practice' in mind and using examples from an international perspective demonstrates how those who are free to practise midwifery reflect best practice both individually and collectively. Surely future freedoms within the international issues, arguments and controversies of midwifery should rest with midwives themselves: by highlighting the issues facing them and offering suggestions on how to attain a goal of freedom to practise.

In this book, we aim to provide a wide look at the realities facing midwives today as they struggle to provide 'woman-centred care' in their own environments. We also aim to engender among student midwives and midwives a knowledge and enthusiasm for the concept of freedom to practise midwifery. This has been done by an exploration and examination of midwifery practice on an international scale. In each country there is a different tempo – there are varying issues, arguments and controversies. Under the over-arching domain of freedom to practise we demonstrate issues in international perspectives of midwifery. The authors have responded to the invitation to contribute to the book and each author or group of authors has grasped the opportunity to take up the overall theme of 'freedom to practise' but with a particular subject or issue relevant to each situation and chosen country as a preferred topic. Thus the chapters of this multi-contributed book tackle different, yet linked issues in midwifery. The overall sphere of influence of freedom to practise is the dynamic which links the chapters and provides a universal learning tool for midwives. In accordance with the primary aim, the wider purpose of the book will show how midwives in different countries of the world are making progress towards the goal of 'freedom to practise'. Please note that all website URLs are correct at time of going to press.

*Lindsay Reid, 2006*

**Reference**
Camm J 2005 The women the world forgot. Midwives 8(10):406

# ACKNOWLEDGEMENTS

## Book editor's acknowledgements

I should like to offer a big thank you to all who have had an input into this book. The list of names ranges far and wide. While it is difficult to mention everyone, I acknowledge with gratitude all who have listened to me on the subject of this book and thank you for your patience and help.

I would like to highlight some who made a particular contribution: Dr Margaret McGuire, for her initial energetic brainstorming discussion and never-ending encouragement; Professor Rosemary Mander for always being ready to suggest lunch and offer support and advice; all staff at Elsevier but with particular thanks to Mary Seager, Senior Commissioning Editor (now retired) for her help and encouragement from the outset of this project; Dame Lorna Muirhead for much investigating on my behalf and valued support; Dr Anne Cameron, always ready to check references and find books; Elizabeth Mansion and Carol Curran of the Scottish Multiprofessional Maternity Development Group, for long-term listening, continued interest and help; Vivienne Riddoch, Managing Editor of *The Practising Midwife*, for her help with the cover; all the contributors to this book for their chapters, their willingness to work with me and their help in drawing the book together.

And, of course, David: what would I do without you? Thank you.

## Contributors' acknowledgements

### Chapter 3

Jenny Gamble and Barbara Vernon would like to acknowledge Bruce Teakle, President, Maternity Coalition – Queensland.

### Chapter 4

Elaine Madden would like to acknowledge the following midwives for their constructive criticism and advice during the writing of this chapter: Helen Wallace, Lesley Barrowman, Breedagh Hughes, Ruth Clarke, Marlene Sinclair and Lindsay Reid.

## Chapter 7

Rosemary Mander would like to acknowledge the financial support of the British Academy in undertaking the research project on which this chapter is based. She is very grateful for the support of the Department of Nursing Science in the University of Turku, particularly Dr Hanna-Leena Melender. She would also like to express her sincere thanks to Kaisa Hakala of Aktiivinen Synnytys Ry for all her help. She really appreciates the help of all of the women and healthcare staff who spent time sharing their ideas with her. Finally, she would like to thank Iain Abbot for preparing the illustration.

## Chapter 9

Barbara Kuypers would like to acknowledge and thank all persons who assisted in providing information and data for the Review which has informed this chapter. Special thanks to MOET and in particular to Cara Macnab, for the invitation to join the deployment and to individual members of the faculty who facilitated access to midwives, theatre nurses, obstetricians and anaesthetists for the duration of the MOET training courses.

Particular thanks also go to: the Iraqi midwives who travelled to the Shaibah Logbase so that interviews and discussions could take place and to the physicians who assisted with interpretation; Jane Wilshaw (DFID Health Advisor) and Lieutenant Colonel Carine Horsburgh (UK Medical Group stationed with the CPA) who provided a number of opportunities for discussions and also forwarded a number of written reports that have made very useful appendices for this Review.

Finally, she wishes to thank the Lewisham Hospital NHS Trust for enabling her to make this visit during a particularly busy time for the hospital.

## Chapter 10

Mary Higgins would like to acknowledge Rhona O'Connell and Déirdre Daly.

# CHAPTER ONE

# Introduction

LINDSAY REID

Midwives who are free to practise and make decisions are free to embrace the World Health Organisation's (WHO) principles of perinatal care and free to use current evidence for the promotion of normal birth (Sandall 2005). It appears strange that words and phrases such as 'freedom to practise' and 'autonomy' and 'free to make decisions' are still being discussed when in many countries midwifery practice is legislated for. Fraser and Cooper go into some detail about the definition and capabilities of the midwife, fitness for practise, award and purpose, and autonomous midwifery practice (Fraser and Cooper 2003). The latest Nursing and Midwifery Council (NMC) publication on midwives rules and standards also reproduces the definition of a midwife that is recognised by the WHO and the International Federation of Gynaecologists and Obstetricians (FIGO):

A midwife is a person who, having been regularly admitted to a midwifery education programme, duly recognised in the country in which it is located, has successfully completed the prescribed course of studies in midwifery and has acquired the requisite qualifications to be registered and/or legally licensed to practise midwifery.

She must be able to give the necessary supervision, care and advice to women during pregnancy, labour and the postpartum period, to conduct deliveries on her own responsibility and to care for the newborn and the infant. This care includes preventative measures, the detection of abnormal conditions in mother and child, the procurement of medical assistance and the execution of emergency measures in the absence of medical help. She has an important task within the family and the community. The work should involve antenatal education and preparation for parenthood and extends to certain areas of gynaecology, family planning and childcare. She may practise in hospitals, clinics, health units, domiciliary conditions or in any other service.

*NMC (2004:36)*

As far as freedom to practise is concerned, this definition appears unequivocal. Yet, currently, the way in which midwives are practising in different countries varies: some are free to practise in their own right; some are doctors' helpers; and others are somewhere on a continuum in between. Some midwives are prevented from practising freely by local or national policies and protocols, and personalities, either their own or those of others. In this book we show how midwives in different countries of the world are acknowledging the problems of freedom to practise and are making progress towards the goal of freedom to practise. However, we also show how some midwives have real problems in even viewing this goal.

There are many unresolved issues for midwives regarding their level of freedom to practise and confidence in practice. We explore these issues from a worldwide aspect, highlighting what has gone before, particularly to give a snapshot of, and subsequent discussion on, early twenty-first century aspects of midwifery practice, attitudes of midwives and opinions on further professional development of midwives. This will enlighten midwives and others in many countries about how midwifery practices, attitudes and legislation differ from country to country. We also show how change and progress differs across the world in the ability of midwives: to achieve freedom to practise; to make decisions about practice and education; and to develop professionally. Thus, we hope that the chapters of the book will encourage those student midwives and midwives who are hoping for greater decision-making powers; who may see recent change in legislation in, for instance New Zealand and some Canadian provinces as a springboard to greater freedom; who may indeed have legislative freedom to practise normal midwifery but who still come up against barriers when they attempt to do so; and, who, for whatever reason, have stopped trying to stand on their own feet.

What do we mean by 'freedom to practise' in the context of midwifery? When this book was at the proposal stage I tended to use the word 'autonomous' instead. But the words 'autonomous' and 'autonomy' if used without explanation might imply the taking up of an isolationist stance and we would not want to do this or to say that midwives should do this. As stated in Chapter 14 p 266:

> The autonomous nature of midwifery does not mean that midwives can practise any way they want. Midwifery practice is shaped by the organisation of maternity services, the midwives' own personal situations and the decisions made by their clients.

Midwifery can no more be totally independent than can the medical profession, nor any other group who would work with others within a team framework. The words 'autonomous' and 'autonomy' can indicate independence but also indicate a freedom, which in this case is the freedom of midwives to determine their own actions or behaviour when practising normal midwifery, and the freedom of the profession to make its own decisions over, for instance, education and practice. This is an autonomy which enables one professional group to co-operate with others on an equal basis. This is freedom to practise. Through it parity and respect for the opinions and practice of others within the framework can be maintained.

Freedom to practise midwifery must reflect best practice. But the very notion of 'best practice' is an argument in itself. For this reason after this introduction, the book moves to a discussion chapter on the notion of best practice, its aims and realities. This chapter does not pretend to give any hard and fast answers to 'What is best practice?' On the other hand, it tries to open out the argument, to demonstrate that best practice:

- can be individual or collective
- may be governed by feelings, policies, protocols
- will change as new research changes the evidence base
- will change with history, culture, the geographical situation and the wishes of women and pressure groups.

Therefore underpinning the chapters is the philosophy of best midwifery practice particularly that which is evidence based.

All midwives, from the most to the least experienced, should have a part to play in promulgating best practice. Legislation, restriction, protocol and policy exist at both governmental and local levels. These should be midwifery led. In this way freedom to practise midwifery must reflect best practice, both individual and collective. And future freedoms within the international issues, arguments and controversies of midwifery should rest with midwives themselves: by highlighting the issues facing them and offering suggestions on how to attain a goal of freedom to practise.

Each writer or group of writers has brought her own style of writing to the book. In addition each chapter deals with a differing aspect of midwifery with issues pertinent to the country under discussion. I have been impressed by the differences in the issues portrayed, the varying attitudes both positive and negative, of others to midwives, and the different ways in which the quest for freedom to practise for midwives is being taken forward. At the same time there is a similarity in the attitudes of the writers: the ever-present thread linking the chapters is the desire for freedom to practise midwifery; writers and readers will compare and contrast situations in different countries, recognise and empathise with problems elsewhere, and learn from possible solutions; and all want the best for women and their babies. Through it all there is a desire to give women the benefit of best practice through midwifery freedom.

Following the discussion in Chapter 2 on best practice, in Chapter 3 attention focuses on midwifery in Australia. This chapter describes the context of midwifery care in Australia, explains the main barriers to midwives assuming their full role and highlights some of the recent developments that give hope for the future of the midwifery profession and maternity care in Australia. Thus, despite a midwifery profession still in 'transition' and barriers to freedom of midwives' practice, the future looks bright with a growing recognition of the role and significance of midwifery by all involved. Not least of those involved, midwives themselves are examining themselves, coming to see their roles differently and to agitate for greater freedom to practise.

Halfway across the world in Northern Ireland midwives are also aspiring to autonomy within a multi-professional partnership. This is addressed in Chapter 4. Progress towards midwifery autonomy in Northern Ireland has been hindered by high intervention rates and a medicalised model of care coupled with concerns about demography, health and social factors, practice roles, education of midwives, leadership in midwifery and women's choices. Not least of these concerns is the fact that for the final decades of the twentieth century Northern Ireland was beset by civil disturbance, conflict and political unrest. These have all played a part in the development of midwifery practice. This chapter acknowledges the problems, looks for solutions and concludes that there is a strong desire to establish and promote the role of the midwife and redress the imbalance of power between the medical and midwifery models.

Chapter 5 examines influences of the health system on midwifery practice in two sub-Saharan African countries, Ghana and Malawi. It explores the realities of how the health system affects the practice of midwives in Ghana and Malawi and asks what strategies can be used to pave the way forward for the future. We see how on one hand the foundation of the professionalisation of midwives in Ghana and Malawi has provided a strong basis for the health systems of these countries. On the other hand, midwives depend on the health system to provide a functional environment which supports the provision of high-quality care. The chapter looks at the challenges and problems of being a midwife in Ghana and Malawi. It stresses the need for an outlook which extends beyond the boundaries of single nation states to consider also the effects and consequences of key global issues, in particular the movement to reduce maternal and infant mortality and morbidity.

Does being a principality with an assembly government help midwives in Wales to be free to practise? This question has been used as the title for Chapter 6. Here, with an eye to this main question, the authors examine influences on midwives in Wales and their freedom to practise. To do this they explored the effects of documents, both those exclusively Welsh and those from further afield, but in particular the *All Wales Normal Labour Pathway* (NLP) (2003) and the work and influence of the NLP on maternity care in Wales. The introduction of the NLP has had an impact on midwifery care all over Wales and helps to provide the answer to the initial question: being a principality with self-determination has made a positive difference in midwives' freedom to practise.

Chapter 7 examines the situation of the Finnish midwife and although it acknowledges that similarities exist between midwives in Finland and those in other countries, there are certain crucial issues of history, demography, geography and current change which have a bearing on Finnish midwives' freedom to practise. This chapter is one of two in this book (see Chapter 12) in which some midwives admit to practising according to the mother's wishes, but in secret, and against an authority born of a colonial past and a present dominated by others. Here is evidence of midwives choosing freedom to give what they saw as best practice.

Chapter 8, which suggests that we are most likely to achieve freedom to practise by positioning ourselves alongside women, explores what we mean by midwifery-led care and whether or not it gives us freedom to practise. The chapter identifies ways for promoting midwifery-led and woman-centred care; highlights ways in which the use of this philosophy of care might reveal problems in practice; and questions whether or not midwives in England have the freedom to practise midwifery-led care within the constraints of the modern day National Health Service (NHS). The chapter challenges midwives to be childbirth activists, to fight for normality and midwifery-led units, to demand and question and work together for services that support normality, and, to stand alongside, with and for, women.

Chapter 9 tackles the problems of midwifery practice in Iraq, recently at war and still in the midst of conflict. It outlines a series of issues that have affected and continue to impinge on the delivery of care for childbearing women. This adds context to the culture of pregnancy and birth and the profession of midwifery in Iraq. The chapter also demonstrates how conflict impacts on the infrastructure of a country's healthcare provision and how this influences the choices that clinical practitioners have regarding their practice in both public and private sectors. Freedom to practise demands challenges. Some professionals will wish to extend their scope of practice and expertise. At the same time they have to cope with pioneering new services against a backdrop of civil unrest and personal danger. For some practitioners, all of their professional lives have been during times of war or constraint on practice. The need to make a living and stay safe is an important one. Thus, freedom to practise one's profession has to be put into the context of the history of the country.

Chapter 10 reviews the recent history of Irish midwifery which illustrates factors that contribute to the limited freedom to practise experienced by midwives at the beginning of the twenty-first century. These aspects comprise the work of the Government including legislation, and attitudes of bodies appointed by Government. Through acknowledging the history we begin to see why midwives in Ireland today are not free to practise as the International Confederation of Midwives (ICM 1992) has described. There remains a lack of understanding and communication between Government and the profession of midwifery which has contributed to the limitation of professional development of midwives in Ireland. To examine this more closely, the chapter also looks at midwifery in Ireland today and current factors that affect midwifery.

Chapter 11 examines the situation of midwifery in South Africa and discusses some of the issues that have an impact on South African midwives and their freedom to practise midwifery. Documentation of practice of midwives (*geswore vroemoere*) in South Africa goes back to 1652 (Nolte 1998) and included some certified midwives as well as traditional midwives. Today, traditional midwives still practise and there is talk of making their role more official. Registered midwives work within the bounds of regulation, public and private practice and an environment which is culturally diverse and burdened with disease. Many women are human immunodeficiency virus (HIV) positive. It is clear that the HIV/acquired immune deficiency syndrome (AIDS) epidemic has had a severe impact on midwives and their practice from both personal and professional aspects. More governmental acknowledgement, effort and resources would go some way towards recognising the crucial role midwives play in saving the lives of mothers and babies and enabling them to enjoy the freedom to practise.

Midwifery in Latvia changed in the twentieth century. As the old holistic ideas of working in harmony with soul and body were set aside with the onset of the communist regime, midwives became unhappy in their work, women were dissatisfied and frustrated by their birth experience and perinatal outcomes were poor. Chapter 12 examines how midwives have coped and are coping now, as Latvia came under communist rule and then became independent again in 1991. Change has come slowly. However, since 1991, midwives in Latvia have been going through a process of acceptance: of themselves, of one another, and, that they are once again free to practise midwifery. Women can now once again give birth at home in Latvia. In the post-1991 years, as in Finland (Chapter 7) some midwives helped mothers who wanted a home birth in secret. Now, choice of the place of birth in Latvia is gradually becoming more flexible and midwives who help mothers birth their babies at home are no longer breaking the law. This chapter describes aspects of how the changes are taking place.

Chapter 13 explores the question of normality in childbirth in Scotland today, its links with a social/midwifery model of maternity care and freedom of midwives to practise. An overview of the historical narrative of twentieth-century midwifery in Scotland regarding childbirth and intrapartum care reveals the increasingly medicalised care of childbearing women (Reid 2003). The chapter explores issues which seem to influence normality in childbirth in Scotland today both positively and negatively: policy, both local and governmental; aspects of the geography and demography of Scotland; place of birth; the culture of medical dominance of maternity services in Scotland; and progress in multi-professional partnership and understanding.

Midwifery in New Zealand has gone through a renaissance over the past 15 years. Chapter 14 examines some aspects of midwifery care in New Zealand where, following legislation introduced in 1990, registered midwives provide maternity care independently of medical practitioners. They now have the choice whether they work in the community providing continuity of care to women or take up employment within maternity facilities. This chapter focuses on what 'freedom to practise' means for caseloading midwives; traces the development of the contemporary social, professional and legal expectations of midwifery; tells a story about how one group of midwives who offer home births in a major urban centre put autonomy into practice; and investigates the historical background to legislative changes of New Zealand's regulatory framework for midwives. The framework positions partnership between midwives and women at its centre and since its inception, midwifery as a profession in New Zealand has flourished.

Chapter 15 looks at the ways in which childbirth organisations the world over have contributed to the understanding and development of best practice in midwifery. It explains how the voices of childbearing women have been heard in different countries, and how consumer organisations have worked alongside midwives to shape services that are truly responsive to the physical, emotional, social and spiritual needs of women. Campaigning groups have many differing questions to face about the success of childbirth organisations, their support from midwives and what women want from their childbirthing experience. Although the pace of change is slow, the chapter highlights how childbirth organisations can and do make a difference to women's experience, birth outcomes, midwives' freedom to practise, and the use and commonsense of a midwifery model of childbirth for women for whom this is appropriate.

To assist with deeper examination of the issues included in this book, each chapter ends with some relevant reflective questions.

We have written *Midwifery: freedom to practise?* to encourage others involved to appreciate that freedom to practise midwifery is achievable. We show how midwives who are free to practise are able to offer normality in childbirth where and when this is appropriate. They have the confidence to acknowledge the presence and value of different models of care for childbearing women. They will also have the confidence, in the interests of best practice, to help women to decide what is the best and most appropriate way of care for them.

We hope that the contents of this book will act as a conduit for students of midwifery and midwives to implement as fully as possible, freedom to practise.

## References

Fraser DM, Cooper MA 2003 The Midwife. In: Fraser DM and Cooper MA (eds) Myles' textbook for midwives. Edinburgh and London, Churchill Livingstone, pp 3–11

ICM 1992 Definition of the midwife. Ref 90/1/PP, ICM, London

National Assembly for Wales 2003 The All Wales Normal Labour Pathway (HOWIS access). National Assembly for Wales, Cardiff

Nolte AGW 1998 A Textbook for Midwives. Van Schaik, Pretoria

NMC 2004 Midwives Rules. NMC, London p 36

Reid L 2003 Scottish midwives 1916–1983: The Central Midwives Board and practising midwives. Unpublished PhD thesis, University of Glasgow

Sandall J 2005 Promoting normal birth: weighing the evidence. In: Downe S (ed) Normal Childbirth. Elsevier, Edinburgh, pp 161–171

# CHAPTER TWO

# Best practice: aims and realities

LINDSAY REID

One of the terms frequently used in midwifery is 'best practice'. This almost abstract notion is something to which all midwives aspire, whether or not they have total freedom within their practice. It therefore appears appropriate to explore briefly the concept of best practice with the idea of attempting to bring some light into what is meant by this term. For that reason, before we venture into the differing aspects and politics of midwifery practice in the varying countries chosen for exploration, it is relevant to examine best practice in midwifery.

This chapter will attempt to unravel some of the thinking behind 'best practice', and some of the ideas that may come within this concept, which is based on shifting sands of varying circumstances of where, when, how and with whom we are practising. Because of all the differences, best practice is a difficult idea to evaluate and this chapter will consider if it is possible to do this. And, we should acknowledge that although people do what they perceive to be their best, it may not always be what collectively is considered to be best practice: this makes any analysis of best practice more complicated. It may also create barriers between thinking and doing. An individual's idea of what constitutes best practice may not coincide with the collective idea or protocol of what is best.

The notion of best practice can be said to be the best way of doing things. The word 'model' is used frequently to give an example of a specific philosophy of style. Hunt (1997) discusses models of change, and to acknowledge and activate change in practice where necessary, accords with the idea of models in childbirth on a continuum of practice. This continuum need not necessarily be fixed, but may, to a certain extent, fluctuate within different circumstances. This chapter will explore the ideas of models of childbirth, in particular medical and social. What do we mean by the term model? How can the two models be compared and contrasted? Can the two models work together, or at least, be mutually compatible? As midwives, general practitioners (GPs) and obstetricians are part of the same team it seems reasonable for them to try to find ways of exercising tolerance towards each other in negotiating everyday practice and discussing ideas for long-term policy making.

Linked with the best way of doing things is the requirement for a formalisation of best practice bringing together themes of quality and accountability: clinical governance. Therefore the chapter will look at some aspects of clinical governance.

Much of today's best practice in midwifery centres on normality in childbirth for more women. The words 'normal' and 'normality' engender much discussion. There is no one classification. So the chapter will explore differing definitions of normality in childbirth, and show how having the freedom to offer a woman a normal birth where appropriate, can empower both women and midwives.

# What do we mean by best practice?

Firstly, we need to think about what we mean by 'best practice'. When considering what to write here, I looked up a thesaurus for the word 'best' and was offered words such as top, most excellent, finest, greatest and unsurpassed, among others. The word 'practice' offered meanings such as ritual, procedure and routine as well as the dictionary meaning: 'the process of repeating something such as an exercise many times in order to improve performance', and, 'the performance of a religion, profession, set of customs or established habit' (*Encarta* 1999:1478). Yes, when we are practising midwifery we are performing the customs and rituals of our profession. And, yes, we want to do this in the best way possible. So, best practice is an ideal to which we can aspire. But the aspiration towards best practice in midwifery has surely always been there and in every situation. It is not just a twenty-first century idea. For instance, during the twentieth century midwives practised in hospitals, dunnies under tenement flats in Glasgow, tinkers' tents, one-roomed over-crowded 'single ends', poor 'black houses' on the crofts as well as well-kept homes and opulent mansions with staff for every need. Each of these midwives would be doing her best on an individual level, however difficult the circumstances. Imagine the following scene, described by a midwife practising in 1946.

> I remember [being] called to a case in this [ex-army] camp and you
> went into the room where they lived and everything was happening

in there and there was a mother in labour. In the cot were two little ones and this was her third one. And she was twenty something. She looked like forty something, poor woman. I can see father yet, sitting over the far end, and I remember he was a painter on the Forth Bridge. You know, I was getting so annoyed with him. I felt this – what a situation to be in. Well, she had her baby and they were all right. Then of course she haemorrhaged, this awful thing and I was giving ergometrine and trying to get the uterus [to contract] and she was going into shock and I said to the father, 'Could you get me some heat, hot water bottles?' 'Oh no.' I said, 'Any beer bottles?' 'Oh yes.' I said ,'Well fill them up with hot water, as much as it will stand and bring as many to me.' I can see me packing beer bottles round this woman to give her heat. [I was] there by myself. It was a terrible situation. Yes. Until I could get her stabilised. Again, we were just called at the last minute . . . I'd never seen her before.

*LR 35*

That midwife was practising in very difficult circumstances. But she was practising to the best of her ability and with the equipment she had available. This is the difficulty with trying to define 'best practice'. It has to differ, depending on the place of birth and the kind of care, who is giving the care, how the practice is given, the reason for a particular type of practice and when it is/was being given.

Then there is collective best practice: the best practice which is laid down by protocol, either local or national. An example here is the way we used to handle situations where there was a stillbirth (R Mander, personal communication, 2005). The baby was taken away quickly; the mother did not have a chance to hold or say good-bye. She might have been discharged from the maternity unit as quickly as possible, 'all for the best'. Now our thinking on what is best practice in this situation has changed and we look back on the previous best practice with something akin to shame. Thus, the concept of best practice must change as ideas, fashions, theories, models and personalities come and go.

So best practice is something to strive for, to aspire to. In a way, it is a continual push for betterment both individually and collectively. It also fits within the current concept of lifelong learning. The old childhood rhyme comes to mind:

Good, better, best,
Never let it rest,
Till your good is better,
And your better – best.

*Anon*

# Can we measure best practice?

Best practice, as an aspiration for all, is, because of its intangibility, beyond ordinary assessment and measurement. Nevertheless, as we are all aware, other more accessible and substantial standards can be assessed and considered.

Take, for instance, a newly qualified midwife. When a midwife is first registered she is expected to be 'fit for practice' (Fraser and Cooper 2003:5). The term 'fit for practice' takes us to the holistic knowledge, skills and attitudes of 'competence', its standards and its definition by the United Kingdom Central Council for Nursing, Midwifery and Health Visiting (UKCC): 'the skills and ability to practise safely and effectively without the need for direct supervision' (UKCC 1999, Bower 2002:158). However, to be fit for practice does not imply that the newly registered midwife is able to apply what a midwife with 10 years' experience might call best practice although it has to be remembered that she may be doing the best she can according to her experience. Much of the learning about midwifery focuses on the development of practical interpersonal skills and in most employment situations a system of mentoring is in place to guide the progress of the new midwife. At the same time, to facilitate this development the process of thinking, reflection and development of midwifery theory must also be encouraged and employed on a regular basis. In addition, midwives should be able to articulate their theories and knowledge base. Only then can practice and care be enhanced to a higher level. And then the midwife's 'theory in use' is evident as she makes the most of strategies of care to meet most appropriately the needs of each woman and helps to make sure that the needs are not overlooked (Bryar 1995:6).

Thus, trying to measuring best practice with all its variables of 'who, where, why, what, when and how' is an impossible idea. However levels of practice both collective and individual, can be measured, audited, assessed and improved on. This can be done through systems of clinical governance and supervision (see below). It can also be achieved through:

- Further, more extensive courses. This accords with the concept of lifelong learning and constant work to improve standards (Crichton 2003:997).
- Systems of mentorship which could be extended from mentoring student midwives, the newly registered midwife and those on specific programmes (Thomas and Mayes 1996:61) to a scheme to help all.
- Peer review (Cheyne et al 1999).

- Informal discussion within a safe environment (Hunt and Symonds 1995:61).
- Honest self-examination and assessment.
- Journal keeping. To be used not just to record critical incidents but also to record, reflect and comment on day-to-day happenings.

Thus, while doing our individual and collective best we can assess, measure, reflect and improve on practice and standards whether general or personal.

# The need to be evidence-based

It is generally accepted that to be credible and reliable, current midwifery practice aspiring to be 'best' requires to be evidence-based. Until the late 1970s most midwives did not 'do' research (T Murphy-Black, unpublished paper, 1990). Even as late as 1991 a national survey found that only 8% of midwives had carried out independent research which was not part of course requirements (Alexander 1995:89). Midwives had a tendency to obey the Rules without question as in the following incident:

> In the mid-1980s the Midwifery Professional Officer (MPO) for the National Board for Scotland paid a visit to a group of community midwives. 'And,' the MPO asked, 'Are you still doing routine visits of postnatal mothers and their babies at home twice daily for the first three days and then every day until the tenth day?'
> 'Yes', chorused the midwives.
> 'Why?' asked the MPO.
> 'Because we've always done it', said one. She might as well have said, 'Because it's in the Rules.'
>
> *Anecdotal evidence*

Best practice? Maybe, according to the Rules. But not if you are really thinking about what you are doing, looking at each woman and her situation individually. As the Nursing and Midwifery Council (NMC) Code of Practice (2004:17) says:

> The conditions in which you practise vary widely, whether in the home, in hospital or elsewhere. Your practice should be based on the best available current evidence.

This is much more thoughtful than the old statutory Rules which had to be obeyed without question (Fleming 2002). On the other hand, the new Code puts firmly on the midwife:

- the onus of accountability to each woman
- the necessity to produce the best practice she can
- the requirement to base practice on firm evidence.

Although pre-1970s midwives were still obeying the Rules apparently without question, medical research was well in evidence. However, Mander (2003:64) discusses adverse criticism of medical research occurring in 1972. Commentators remarked on the evidence of current poor medical research along with a lack of scientific rigour identified in medical clinical decision making and emphasised the necessity for strong medical research. An excellent example of a procedure with (at one time) no research base and upheld on a false premise is episiotomy. Medical opinion was that to have an episiotomy would stop perineal tears and would heal more easily than a tear. Routine episiotomy became hospital protocol in many areas. Midwives and women researched the theories and proved them to be wrong. They highlighted the pain and discomfort both short and long term suffered by many women who had had an unnecessary episiotomy because of hospital protocol (Sleep et al 1984). More recent research reinforced the premise that episiotomy would not reduce the incidence of vaginal and perineal tears and, as a direct result, the incidence of long term problems (Logue 1991, Grundy, 1997). What the evidence also showed was that the practice to be of the best, had to centre, not on hospital protocol, but on the woman and her individual needs.

Thus, midwives developed research credibility. This took time. To begin with they were urged to carry out research without first having a full grasp of research principles and methods. Non-researching midwives did not believe the results of their researching colleagues and turned automatically to the work of obstetricians. However, since those early days there has been a considerable increase in research undertaken and subsequently published by midwives (Alexander 1995). The term 'evidence-based practice' came into vogue with evidence elicited from a base of strong research. Evidence-based practice can be defined as:

> the conscientious, explicit and judicious use of current best evidence
> in making decisions about the care of individual patients
> *Sackett et al (1996:71), quoted in Mander (2003:64)*

It forms the foundation of clinical governance which creates a framework within which midwives can strive for continual improvement and excellence in practice.

Thus we see evidence-based practice as 'a new imperative in professional midwifery'. The use of research leading to evidence-based practice has also contributed to the whole concept of woman-centred care and a concerted move in midwifery towards best practice with more autonomy for both women and midwives (Durham 2002:123). Indeed, Calvert (2002:144) states that care that is not evidence based or woman centred is considered to be suboptimal.

Thus, to marry individual and collective best practice together, the practice of evidence-based care means integrating individual clinical experience with the best available external clinical evidence from systematic research (McGuire 2000).

# Clinical governance and the promotion of excellence

Clinical governance is about expanding courses of action that support the continual improvement of standards. In addition, it is about creating an environment that fosters excellence (Proctor 1999) and is a vital component of the effort towards collective and individual best practice.

Clinical governance is

a framework through which NHS [National Health Service] organisations are accountable for continuously improving the quality of their services and safeguarding high standards of care by creating an environment in which excellence in clinical care will flourish

*Pulzer (1999)*

It can be seen, therefore, as a construction on which midwives and others can build a philosophy of continuous improvement in practice through delivering, managing and measuring the quality of the care they give to women and babies (Proctor 1999).

Many principles of clinical governance reflect those of statutory supervision of midwives (Fraser and Cooper 2003:8). Themes linked within the concept of clinical governance include professional self-regulation and lifelong learning. These concepts and themes of clinical governance and supervision are not new to midwifery. They have been included in midwifery rules and codes of practice since the first Midwives Acts in 1902, 1915 and 1918 introduced statutory supervision of midwives (Pulzer 1999). Midwives can further contribute to clinical governance by (Duerden 2003:969, Reid 2005:16):

- auditing and reflecting on personal practice
- identifying issues and participating in reporting critical incidents
- exploring risk management. How do reviews apply to one's own practice?
- use well and wisely the support available from supervisors of midwives.

Supervision of midwives has had a varied history. Early supervisors carried a didactic punitive role. They may still sometimes be seen as a threat when the job of supervision of midwives is approached in a policing manner or, if a midwife is not practising at her optimum but finds this difficult to accept or acknowledge (Duerden 2002). However, supervision of midwives can be seen as a partnership with mutual respect between the two partners as an essential element. The supervisor of midwives and the individual midwife can work in partnership over issues of:

- *Choice.* A midwife may choose her supervisor – an important point but occasionally not known. The midwife–supervisor relationship involves issues of: personality, trust, knowledge of the individual's practice, sympathy, problem solving, the ability to maintain confidentiality and support during change, whether professional or personal.
- *Annual supervisory review.* This is the minimum recommended contact. Ideally, more frequent informal meetings would maintain the partnership but without creating a dependent culture (Duerden 2003:970–971).
- *Accountability.* A midwife is accountable for her practice, also to the NMC and her employer (NMC 2004). This can create a loyalty dilemma demonstrated in a recent example in Peterborough and Stamford NHS Foundation Trust. Peter Beland, midwife, was sacked by the Trust after attending a home birth while the service was suspended. He lost his appeal against his dismissal (Anonymous 2005:8).
- *Advocacy.* Closely linked with accountability is advocacy and midwives are encouraged to be a woman's advocate especially when exercising choice. A dilemma occurs when a midwife sees a choice as inappropriate particularly with regard to maternal or infant safety (Duerden 2003:970, Reid 2005:16).

Thus, if the system of midwifery supervision is well used supervisors of midwifery can give much support and empowerment to midwives. This can be of real benefit to the midwife concerned and the women and infants for whom she cares. Supervision of midwifery fits well within the framework of clinical governance and its aim of excellence in midwifery practice with continuous improvement of standards towards the ultimate 'best practice'.

# Models of childbirth

Best practice or, the best way of doing things, is sometimes called a model. The word 'model' is used frequently to give an example of a specific philosophy of style. Hunt (1997) discusses models of change. We need to acknowledge and activate alteration in practice where necessary. This reflects the idea of models in childbirth on a continuum of practice: if a situation changes the preferred model is flexible enough to vary.

When using the word 'model' to describe best practice a difficulty may arise where differing philosophies collide. This section examines ideas behind two very differing models of childbirth: medical and social. For clarity, the idea of a 'model' requires unpacking. What do we mean by this word? Certainly not someone walking down a catwalk. Interestingly, the definition in the *Encarta Dictionary* (1999:1215) closest to that which we are discussing comes not under 'model' but 'mode': 'Manner or form. A way, manner, or form, e.g. a way of doing something, or the form in which something exists'. Does this mean we should really be saying 'medical and social *modes* of childbirth'? Although this is tempting, for the purpose of this chapter, I shall return to using the accepted word 'model' but agree that the above definition for 'mode' appears to fit. 'Model' is also used quite simply in the context of childbirth as 'describing a working practice' (van Teijlingen 1994:297). The problem in using the word 'model' in this way is that it is sometimes taken to mean a pattern or standard to be used in all situations. It then becomes an ideology, can be used to justify practice and could be seen as a deterrent to moving forwards. The other descriptors used to illustrate thinking behind medical and social models of childbirth are 'working practice' and 'analytical'. Thus we come to three levels of approach of models of childbirth: practice, ideology and analysis. Each model has a different level of approach and these are discussed below under the appropriate heading.

Models are used not only for childbirth, but also in the wider world of healthcare: medical practice, technology, discoveries, advances in surgery, pharmacology, eradication of many diseases, treatment by medical procedures. All these indicate a disease-orientated approach rather than one that looks at the patient as an individual. This fits in with the hospital as opposed to community care being considered the 'best place', the development of medical specialisms and their departments and hospitals, and, the inclusion in the medical model of the care of childbearing women. The latter is characterised by the use of high technology equipment, the use of medical and nursing hierarchical systems and public persuasion to give birth in hospital on the grounds of safety (van Teijlingen 1994:299).

The alternative to the medical model epitomises a holistic approach to healthcare: the social model. This 'covers rehabilitation, prevention of illness and the social management of illness, rather than . . . biological and medical aspects of health care' (van Teijlingen 1994:300). A social model of childbirth parallels this with its emphasis on the fact that the great majority of pregnant women have the potential to have a normal and safe pregnancy without medical intervention. This has also been known as the 'midwifery model' and includes teams, caseload practice, midwife-led care and what became known in the 1990s as woman-centred care (Wrede et al 2001:33). Bryar (1995:119) uses the term 'pregnancy as a normal life event' when discussing a similar model.

## Practice

'Practice' contrasts obstetric and midwifery practice. Practitioners other than obstetricians may operate according to obstetric practice and include not only obstetricians and other doctors working in obstetric units but also others working in obstetric units who follow the directions of the obstetrician, e.g. midwives, obstetric nurses. Similarly, in other settings, e.g. at home, in a community midwifery unit (CMU), or a midwife-led unit, the midwifery/social model will prevail and may include others who practise in the community, e.g. midwives and GPs. So, midwives can be found practising within both medical and social models.

*Obstetric practice/model:*

- regards pregnancy as a medical process and potentially pathological
- regards the pregnant woman as an object
- bases practice on a science orientated perspective
- defines risk as statistical risk
- bases solutions and improvements on measurements of outcome through mortality and morbidity statistics

*Midwifery practice/model:*

- is based on the assumption that pregnancy is a normal event in a woman's life and so emphasises normality
- tends to be a woman's perspective on birth. Women are the main players and women give birth
- encourages psychological well-being to contribute to a best possible labour and birth
- regards each pregnant woman as an individual rather than relying on statistics and risk
- encourages the woman to have a sense of power and active involvement
- sees the experience of childbirth as valuable in its own right
- considers the issue of woman's choice to be very important
- uses working practices which are flexible and forward-moving (van Teijlingen 1994: 306–315).

On examination of the above bullet points, it is fair to say that there could be a coming together of models at some points. As van Teijlingen (1994:314) says, 'It is hard to envisage an extreme example of the obstetrical practice taken to its full extent.' On the other hand, it is possible to imagine full midwifery care of a woman in childbirth being taken to a reasonable conclusion providing all goes well.

## Ideology

Ideologies are to do with beliefs and include a system of values and attitudes with a significant reference group ready to influence the thinking of the ideology (van Teijlingen 1994:316). In the context of models of childbirth, it should be obvious by the model of practice what the practitioner believes. Although this may be true of most obstetricians, some midwives practising within the obstetric model do so, not because they believe specifically in the obstetric model but because of the job situation in the area, local hospital policy or, because of a desire to change and improve practice through gradualism and example. However, some found that they could not give of their best because of the constraints of the model within which they were working. One midwife performed an episiotomy without medical permission in a Scottish maternity unit with a particularly strict obstetric model. On the resultant row, she commented, 'I felt as if my hands were *tied*' (LR 120). Other Scottish research has highlighted the possibility of deterioration in care given by midwives where they had no part or are over-ruled in policy making.

> It is so sad and frustrating to see bad care given by midwives who work in a unit where policy/procedures are dictated by the medical profession ... All illusions or hopes they [mothers] may have are totally squashed by medical intervention and mismanagement
> *Hillan et al (1997:12)*

Those who follow specific ideologies can form strong groups that can be totally opposed to other thinking and intolerant of any alternative. In the biomechanical ideology of the obstetric/medical model, obstetricians argue that the level of risk of a pregnancy can only be seen in retrospect; that it was medical research, technology and assistance which were instrumental in reducing maternal and infant mortality; that the 'normality' of pregnancy is a dangerous fallacy (van Teijlingen 1994:317). However the woman-centred ideology of the social/midwifery model stresses the normality of pregnancy, may use terminology which implies criticism of doctors and hospitals, emphasises the emotional bonding of the mother and the newborn, talks about 'love' and 'life event' in relation to birth.

Woman-centred ideology also speaks about choice and women's active involvement in the process of childbearing (van Teijlingen 1994:319).

## Analysis

At the analytical level, the two models of childbirth are, to their proponents, very nearly ideal. Each claims to know how to achieve the best result. The medical model emphasises the risk of pregnancy but the biomechanical ideology within this model will add that obstetrical practice is best-placed to improve the chances of a good outcome. Women are passive patients, lack knowledge and authority and 'do not know what is good for them'. On the other hand, the social model emphasises the active role of women in childbirth, and woman-centred ideology will add to the importance of midwifery practice in encouraging and stimulating the woman's active involvement. Pregnancy and labour are normal physiological processes. Socially the woman has changed: she has become a mother with all the attendant joys and sorrows that motherhood brings (van Teijlingen 1994:323–327).

So far, the medical and social models of childbirth have shown themselves to be, on the whole, at opposite ends of a spectrum. At one time, a coming together appeared to be, at worst, well-nigh impossible, at best, a long way off. In 1970s Scotland the medically dominated Central Midwives Board for Scotland (CMBS 1971) made it clear that in the labour ward particularly, the midwife should 'carry out measures of treatment as delegated by the medical staff'. Obstetricians were influential in the production of the Peel Report (1970) and the similar Scottish Tennent Report (1973). Both reports, while acknowledging geographical and demographical differences between the two countries, agreed on 100% hospital delivery on the grounds of safety, although there was no supporting evidence for this (Scottish Home and Health Department (SHHD) 1973:2, Campbell and Macfarlane 1994:217–218). Thus, at the time, the medical model was in its ascendancy. However, since then social, midwifery and to an extent, medical, thinking has changed. A movement looking at childbirth as a normal life event has developed along with a trend towards the social/midwifery model of birth. With this movement has come a convergence of attitudes which might mean a more successful partnership between the two models.

## What is normal?

Much of today's best practice in midwifery centres on normality in childbirth for more women. There seems to be no real consensus on the meaning of the words 'normal' and 'normality': ask 10 people what they mean by normal childbirth and you will probably receive 10 different answers. This section explores the concept of 'normal' and 'normality' in childbirth. What do we mean when we say 'normal childbirth'. What is normality? Can you define normality in childbirth or normal birth? Probably anyone, if asked would be able to give some sort of definition but that is the point: there is no one answer. Yet this is what many maternity care practitioners are working towards: normality in childbirth.

At a recent National Childbirth Trust Conference in Belfast in 2004, Naimh McCabe, obstetrician, discussed: 'Normal births in northern Ireland – trends causes and consequences'. She started by asking the question 'What is normal?'. Her possible answers ranged from 'a vaginal delivery' to 'anything that is not a caesarean section'. But these nebulous definitions epitomise the problem: there are many answers to the question. The *Encarta Dictionary* (1999:1290) defines 'normality' as 'the way things are under normal circumstances' with other definitions including:

- usual, conforming to the usual standard, type or custom
- healthy, physically, mentally and emotionally
- occurring naturally, maintained or occurring in a natural state.

These definitions do not explain fully what we want. And they muddy the waters by including 'natural' within the bounds of 'normal'. The next question that has to be asked is: While a natural birth will usually be normal, are all normal births totally natural? Then the word 'usual' comes into the equation in explaining 'normal' and 'normality'. This disadvantages the attempt at a definition even further: as customs change, the meaning of 'usual' changes too. As well as the dictionary with its fundamental but unexciting meanings, Beech and Phipps (2004) discuss varying aspects of what could be included as normal and use women's stories as illustrations of their widely varying birth experiences. These widen the gates towards a meaning but they also demonstrate the size of the task.

A rather unimaginative definition of normal labour/childbirth, is: 'Normal labour occurs at term and is spontaneous in onset with the fetus presenting by the vertex. The process is completed within 18 hours and no complications arise' (Cassidy 1993:149). Where, in this restricted definition, is there evidence of any flexibility, choice or behaviour on the part of either woman or midwife? However, Cassidy enlarges on the theme:

> The physiological transition from pregnancy to motherhood [which] heralds an enormous change in each woman physically and psychologically . . . every system in the body is affected and the experience represents a major rite de passage in a woman's life.

This gives a wider picture to add to Cassidy's previous definition. Here, we are beginning to explore not only the clinically evident features but also some of the broader more abstract characteristics. These are holistic, indicating the importance of the total health and wellbeing of a woman and are of great significance to the achievement or otherwise of a normal birth.

The Royal College of Midwives (RCM) offers a comprehensive description of what normality in childbirth might include and exclude (reproduced in Table 2.1). Box 2.1 adds further components of normal birth including the interaction between mother and fetus (Beech and Phipps 2004:62, Reid 2005:3).

Table 2.1 UK Royal College of Midwives' description of normal birth

| Normality includes | Normality excludes |
|---|---|
| Spontaneous onset of labour | Induced and augmented labour |
| Labour is considered as a continuum | Timing of labour |
| Holistic, alternative methods of pain relief, water, ambulation | Medical methods of pain relief |
| Permit food and fluids | Withholding food and fluid in labour |
| Spontaneous physiological rupture of membranes | Artificial rupture of the membranes |
| Encourage mobility | Restricted mobility |
| Calm, gentle and non-threatening environment, auscultation | Clinical environment – institutionalisation of birth |
| Intermittent fetal monitoring | Continuous fetal monitoring |
| Specific indications only for vaginal examinations, preference for abdominal examinations | Routine vaginal examinations |
| Judicious use of episiotomy | Routine episiotomy |

Box 2.1 UK Royal College of Midwives: components of normal birth

- Birth is a unique, dynamic process
- Fetal and maternal physiologies interact symbiotically
- Birth occurs within 24 hours of commencement of labour
- Minimum trauma occurs to either mother or baby
- Spontaneous onset is between 37 and 42 weeks
- It follows an uncomplicated pregnancy

To add to the RCM's list it is appropriate to include the following state-ment from the RCM *Vision 2000*:

> Maternity services should demonstrate, in their policies and practice, an underpinning philosophy of pregnancy and birth as normal physi-ological processes, with a commitment to positive reduction in unnec-essary medicalisation of normal pregnancy and birth.

In its use of the words 'maternity services' this statement includes, not just midwives but all professionals caring for childbearing women. It highlights for all, the importance of the 'normal' philosophy. It also implies in its inclu-siveness the necessity for those in the maternity services to work together.

So, with a few words and phrases, the whole idea of 'normal' with regard to labour and childbirth has become wider, more thoughtful, caring and kind. Less overtly dramatic perhaps, with fewer professionals around, no urgent beeping, no bells ringing and less chance of watching the cardioto-cograph pushing out yards of paper. But what more drama could one want than a woman going about her labour in her own way with a midwife to support her? And for the midwife, an opportunity and the freedom to provide individual best practice while conforming to the clinical govern-ance philosophy of the pursuit of excellence.

The RCM's Position Statement defines normal childbirth as: 'one where a woman starts, continues and completes labour physiologically at term' (RCM 2004). The RCM is also promoting normality in childbirth through its website and hopes to (Day-Stirk and Palmer 2003):

- generate new understanding and promote a wellbeing approach to childbirth;
- promote normality as a key political agenda item
- lead on what is normal within the whole process of childbearing and expand the awareness and benefits of a normality focus to the childbear-ing process
- provide information
- serve as a global reference resource.

Thus, midwives are committed to challenging the inappropriate use of technology and the promotion of normality (Sinclair 2003). The RCM's website is http://www.rcm.org.uk/

Other definitions, key words, ideas and thoughts enter and add to the 'normality in childbirth' debate. There is evidence that a difficult and/or very medicalised birth impacts adversely on the mother. Our growing understanding of the psycho-neuro-endocrinology (the psyche-brain-hormones) gives us further insights into this. Female bodies are designed to give birth and medicalised disturbance of the important 'hormonal orchestration' of labour and birth will have negative consequences for labour, birth and after. So, more births need to be allowed to be normal life events. Given the right conditions, the female body is genetically encoded to go through the processes of normal birth (Buckley 2004). Indeed, the vast majority of women are capable of giving birth by their own efforts without intervention although this is not widely accepted in this society. This is not a reflection on the physiology of childbirth. It is a reflection of our birthing culture, much of which has been shaped by placing birth within a medical framework (Taylor 2004, Reid 2005:5).

When discussing hormones in this context, we must also take into account the fetal hormones. Soo Downe (2001) reminds us of 'the subtle hormonal dance between mother and infant which is intrinsic and essential to the wellbeing of both in the future'. Here she is discussing 'salutogenic birth' which generates positive short- and long-term wellbeing for the mother, baby, family and caregiver. Salutogenesis or the creation of wellbeing (Day-Stirk and Palmer 2003, Downe and McCourt 2004:19, RCM website) can be summarised by its components:

- *Meaningfulness.* The deep feeling that life makes sense emotionally.
- *Manageability.* The extent to which people feel they have the resources to meet the demands; the knowledge of where/how to get help.
- *Comprehensibility.* The extent to which a person finds or structures their world to be understandable, meaningful, orderly and consistent (Downe and McCourt 2004:19, Reid 2005:5).

Move the ideas of meaningfulness, manageability and comprehensibility into the childbirth arena and there could be a real sense of empowerment for both women and maternity care professionals towards normality in childbirth (Downe 2001).

Downe (2001) acknowledges that the terms 'salutogenesis' and saluto-genic birth are not user-friendly and although she uses them and explains and discusses their use, she suggests that the term 'positive birth' could be used instead. The concept of the creation of wellbeing in the context of birth goes a long way towards empowering women and increasing a feeling of self-worth. The person who copes well with life and has wellbeing is said to have a fundamental 'sense of coherence'. In the birth context the wellbeing maximises a sense of coherence between the woman, baby and family.

Recognition of flexible definitions of normality will help to achieve the promotion of the conditions for physiological birth. To help women with their feeling of wellbeing and to recognise their uniqueness, it is important for midwives to be aware of each woman, consider her needs whether clinical, psychological, emotional or spiritual and be with the woman as appropriate. Given the empowerment of a woman in this situation along with her midwife with freedom to practise, normality in childbirth should be much more in evidence and medical intervention should be minimal (Downe 2001, Downe and McCourt 2004:21).

As noted above, the concept of 'normal' is made less clear by including the word 'natural' within its meaning. Mander (2002:182) points out the theory of Kitzinger and colleagues who said that 'normal' may be used to mean that a phenomenon is a naturally occurring one. In the same way, Righard (2001) also appears to use the words 'normal' and 'natural' as though they were interchangeable. His article's title is *Making childbirth a normal process* but he then goes on to use 'natural' throughout this article. He briefly defines natural childbirth thus, 'My definition of natural childbirth is a birth without medical intervention'. However, 'natural' would also cover such events as breech births and twin births while Kitzinger's theory of 'normal' would not include an episiotomy (Reid 2005:6).

Sandall asks why we are so reluctant to use the word natural. We could therefore also ask: Is 'normal' the right word to use in this context? No one wants to be labelled as 'abnormal'. Sandall suggests that what we are talking about is 'straightforward birth that is as natural as possible, and in which any interventions that are used are evidence-based and do more good than harm' (Sandall 2004, Reid 2005:6).

Thus, this section has demonstrated many variables surrounding the use of the words 'normal' and 'normality' when referring to childbirth: there is no single answer to the question 'What is normal?'. However, most ideas and theories of normality appear to be moving towards a calmer philosophy of childbirth. This includes an attitude and way of working which gives women more informed choice and a greater sense of wellbeing and satisfaction, and gives midwives and other professionals greater opportunities to achieve excellence and the elusive best practice through having the confidence and the freedom to practise normal midwifery.

# Conclusion

In this chapter we have explored the notion of best practice in midwifery and attempted to show the differences between individual and collective best practice. The meaningfulness of individual best practice depends on the midwife herself along with the variables of where, when, how and with whom she is practising. Collective best practice is brought about by local protocol, national guidelines and each country's rules, standards and codes of practice, all based on strong research and evidence.

Measuring best practice, because of the aspirational word 'best', is a difficult, if not impossible task. However, differing levels of midwifery practice are assessed and through varying agents such as mentorship, peer group review, informal discussions, further academic courses, clinical governance and supervision of midwives will move practice and knowledge to a higher level. Thus, the concept of lifelong learning is an ongoing facet of clinical governance and excellence in practice.

Models of childbirth are currently in vogue as a term to describe ideal ways of working. But, in addition, a current hot topic is regarding childbirth as a normal life event together with the social/midwifery model. The phrase, 'models of childbirth' implies striving towards excellence. The problem comes when certain models do not coincide. Models under discussion here are medical and social/midwifery. At their most distant, each appears to be in opposition to the other and reluctant to accept any alternative. But, clinical governance requires that best practice should include collective excellence in clinical practice and both models have their merits. Nevertheless, while there should be recognition of the need for a working together of models where necessary, for midwives to be able to give of their best and for women to have a birth to remember for all the right reasons, the social/midwifery model ought to be the primary aim.

Finally, we have explored some varying definitions and arguments on the issues of 'normal' and 'normality'. Some childbirth practices at variance with each other may affect levels of normality in childbirth and may affect the midwife's ability to be free to practise and to give of her best. The 'normal' philosophy of childbirth epitomises caring and support from all professionals in the maternity services. Thus it demonstrates as far as possible, best practice, individually and collectively.

## Reflective questions

The concept of 'best practice' is abstract and sometimes confusing. Can you think of areas in midwifery practice where your best differs from the 'best' laid down by clinical governance or code of practice? How do you come to terms with this?

Given that professionals in maternity care are expected to work as a team with mutual respect, can you see a coming together of models to the satisfaction of all concerned?

Can you add your thoughts to the normality debate?

Is normal childbirth available for all women who wish it?

If 'yes' how has it been achieved?

If 'no' what has prevented it and what can you do to promote it?

# References

Alexander J 1995 Midwifery graduates in the United Kingdom. In: Murphy-Black T (ed) Issues in Midwifery. Churchill Livingstone, Edinburgh, pp 83–98

Anonymous 2005 News page. The Practising Midwife 8(1):8

Beech BL, Phipps B 2004 Normal births: women's stories. In: Downe S (ed) Normal Childbirth: Evidence and Debate. Elsevier, Edinburgh, pp 59–70

Bower H 2002 Educating the midwife. In: Mander R, Fleming V (eds) Failure to Progress: The Contraction of the Midwifery Profession. Routledge, London, pp 150–169

Bryar R 1995 Theory for Midwifery Practice. Macmillan Press, Basingstoke

Buckley S J 2004 Unlocking the potential for normality. The Practising Midwife 7(6):15–17

Calvert S 2002 Being with women. In: Mander R, Fleming V (eds) Failure to Progress: The Contraction of the Midwifery Profession. Routledge, London, pp 133–149

Campbell R, Macfarlane A 1994 Where to be born? The debate and the evidence. National Perinatal Epidemiology Unit, Oxford

Cassidy P 1993 The first stage of labour: physiology and early care. In: Bennett V, Brown L (eds) Myles' Textbook for Midwives. Churchill Livingstone, Edinburgh, pp 149–167

Cheyne H, Niven C, McGinley M, et al 1999 The PEER Project: evaluating a model of peer review. RCM Scottish Board, Edinburgh

CMBS 1971 Minutes NAS CMBS 1/9 1971 CMBS Minutes. 16 December Appendix IV Comments on the Integration of Maternity Services, pp 1–2

Crichton M 2003 Organisation of the health services in the United Kingdom. In: Fraser D, Cooper M (eds) Myles' Textbook for Midwives. Churchill Livingstone, Edinburgh, pp 989–999

Day-Stirk F, Palmer L 2003 The RCM virtual institute for birth: promoting normality. Midwives 6(2):64–65

Downe S 2001 Defining normal birth. MIDIRS Midwifery Digest 11(3 supp2):S31–S33

Downe S, McCourt C 2004 From being to becoming: reconstructing childbirth knowledge. In: Normal Childbirth: Evidence and Debate. Elsevier, London, pp 3–24

Duerden J 2002 Supervision at the beginning of a new century. In: Mander R, Fleming V (eds) Failure to Progress: The Contraction of the Midwifery Profession. Routledge, London, pp 78–98

Duerden J 2003 Supervision of midwives and clinical governance. In: Fraser D, Cooper M (eds) Myles' Textbook for Midwives. Churchill Livingstone, Edinburgh, p 959–973

Durham R 2002 Autonomy and commitment to life outside midwifery. In: Mander R, Fleming V (eds) Failure to Progress: The Contraction of the Midwifery Profession. Routledge, London, pp 122–132

Encarta World English Dictionary 1999 Bloomsbury, London

Fleming V 2002 Statutory control. In: Mander R, Fleming V (eds) Failure to Progress: The Contraction of the Midwifery Profession. Routledge, London, pp 63–77

Fraser D, Cooper M 2003 The midwife. In: Fraser D, Cooper M (eds) Myles' Textbook for Midwives. Churchill Livingstone, Edinburgh, pp 3–11

Grundy L 1997 The role of the midwife in perineal wound care following childbirth. British Journal of Nursing 6(10):584–588

Hillan E, McGuire M, Reid L 1997 Midwives and woman centred care. University of Glasgow and RCM Scottish Board, Edinburgh

Hunt S, Symonds A 1995 The social meaning of midwifery. Macmillan, Basingstoke

Hunt S 1997 The challenge of change in the organisation of midwifery care. In: Karger I, Hunt S (eds) Challenges in midwifery care. Macmillan, Basingstoke, pp 165–187

Logue M 1991 Putting research into practice: perineal management during delivery. In: Robinson S, Thomson AM (eds) Midwives, research and childbirth II. Chapman and Hall, London, pp 199–251

McCabe N 2004 Normal births in northern Ireland – trends, causes and consequences. National Childbirth Trust Conference, Belfast, 20 October

McGuire M 2000 Identifying gaps in midwifery knowledge and practice. Presentation at RCM Study day, Stornoway, 9 November

Mander R 2002 The midwife and the medical practitioner. In: Mander R, Fleming V, Failure to Progress: The Contraction of the Midwifery Profession. Routledge, London, pp 170–188

Mander R 2003 Evidence-based practice. In: Fraser D, Cooper M (eds) Myles' Textbook for Midwives. Churchill Livingstone, Edinburgh, pp 63–75

NMC(Midwives) Rules 2004. NMC, London

Proctor S 1999 Clinical governance: the new black. RCM Midwives Journal 2(7):204

Pulzer M 1999 Clinical governance and the midwife. RCM Midwives Journal 2 (8):250

RCM 2000 Vision 2000. RCM, London

RCM 2004 Position statement 6 Normal Childbirth. Midwives 7(8):332. Online. Available at: www.rcm.org.uk

Reid L 1997–2002 Archival collection of oral testimonies between these dates. Cited as LR 1–128

Reid L 2005 Scottish normal labour and birth course manual. Scottish Multiprofessional Maternity Development Group, Edinburgh

Righard L 2001 Making childbirth a normal process. Birth 28(1):1–4

Sackett D, Rosenburg W, Gray JA et al 1996 Evidence based medicine: what it is and what it isn't. BMJ 312(7023):71–72

Sandall J 2004 Normal birth: a public health issue. The Practising Midwife 7(1): p 4–5

SHHD1973 Maternity Services: Integration of Maternity Work. Tennent Report. HMSO, Edinburgh

Sinclair M 2003 Editorial. Technology and normality in the 21st century: sharing the power base. Midwives 6:(6) 232

Sleep J, Grant A, Garcia J et al 1984 West Berkshire Perineal Management Trial 1984. BMJ 289:587–590

Standing Maternity and Midwifery Advisory Committee (Chairman, J Peel) 1970. Domiciliary midwifery and maternity bed needs. HMSO, London

Taylor M 2004 Time for an independent voice. The Practising Midwife 7(1):41–42

Thomas M, Mayes G 1996 The ENB perspective: preparation of supervisors of midwives for their role. In: Kirkham M, (ed) Supervision of midwives. Books for Midwives Press, Hale pp 58–70

UKCC 1999 Fitness for practice: the UKCC Commission for Nursing and Midwifery Education (Peach Report). UKCC, London

van Teijlingen E 1994 A social or medical model of childbirth? Comparing the arguments in Grampian (Scotland) and the Netherlands. Unpublished PhD thesis, University of Aberdeen, Aberdeen

Wrede S, Benoit C, Sandall S 2001 The state and birth/the state of birth: Maternal health policy in three countries. In: Devries R, Benoit C, van Teijlingen et al (eds) Birth by design. Routledge, New York, pp 28–50

# CHAPTER THREE

# Midwifery in Australia: emerging from the shadows

JENNY GAMBLE AND BARBARA VERNON

Midwifery in Australia is in transition. For at least the past 50 years, midwifery in Australia has been dominated by medicine and subsumed within nursing. However, in recent years midwives and maternity consumers are asserting that women need access to quality midwifery care. This has resulted in lobbying for alternatives to the medical model, access to continuity of care by a midwife with medical back-up and philosophical approaches that place women and their families at the centre of care. In effect, consumers are actively challenging the barriers to comprehensive midwifery practice.

This chapter will describe the context of midwifery care in Australia, explain the main barriers to midwives assuming their full role, and highlight some of the recent developments that give us hope for the future of the midwifery profession and maternity care in this country.

## Maternity services

Australia is a large continent with a high concentration of people in cities and towns along the coastline. There are approximately 252 000 births each year. Midwives attend the vast majority of these births. The average age of first time mothers has risen to 27.6 years and less than 5% of mothers are younger than 20. Australia has a relatively low perinatal mortality rate (8.0 per 1000 births). However, at 17.5 per 1000 births, the rate more than doubles for babies born to Aboriginal or Torres Strait Islander mothers (Laws and Sullivan 2005:64,67). (Perinatal mortality rate in Australian includes both the fetal and neonatal rates and any baby older than 20 weeks' gestation or weighing at least 400 grams. It is not only live births).

Virtually all maternity services are provided in hospitals (of which there are 540), with only 0.2% of women giving birth at home in 2003 (Laws and Sullivan 2005:10), the latest year for which national statistics are available. More than 97% of births take place in conventional labour wards, with 66% of these occurring in units with greater than 1000 births per annum and only 2.4% occurring in small units with fewer than 100 births per annum (Australian Health Workforce Advisory Committee (AHWAC) 2002:62). Only 2.1% of women have access to a family birth centre staffed by midwives (Laws and Sullivan 2005:10). Such birth centres are located mainly in capital cities and not all birth centres offer one-to-one continuity of midwifery care.

Maternity services in Australia are delivered through complex funding arrangements that are a legacy of federation. We have both a private and a public health system. Both systems receive taxpayer-funded support, however, different levels of Government administer the funding. The private health system is funded by private health funds with significant input from the national Government and the public system has funding managed by state/territory governments.

Around a third of Australia's 250 000 annual births occur in the private system, which is mostly used by mothers with private health insurance. Maternity Coalition Queensland President conservatively estimates around half the cost of births in private care (from Aus$5000 to Aus$19 000 – Medicare Private) is taxpayer funded by the national Government through schemes such as Medicare rebates for doctors' fees, the Medicare SafetyNet, a 30% rebate on Private Health Insurance premiums, and sub-sidised indemnity insurance for doctors (B Teakle, personal communication, 2006).

Public care is provided mainly by public hospitals. Public hospital care is free to women using these services. However, not all public hospitals provide full maternity care. Many, particularly those in rural communities, offer only intrapartum care, and rely on general practitioners (GPs) to provide antenatal care. Postnatal care is generally limited to the post-birth hospital stay, which averages three days or less for most women (Laws and Sullivan 2005:39). It is fair to say, there is little or no public accountability for the outcomes of obstetric care – public or private – despite the high levels of public funding.

The midwifery workforce in Australia reflects the geographical distribution and organisation of maternity services. Of the 12 000 registered midwives currently working, 97% work in a hospital setting and predominantly in either a capital or regional city (86%) (AHWAC 2002:43). Three-quarters of all midwives work in public hospitals. More than 90% of midwives in both public and private hospitals work rostered shiftwork, largely within wards that segregate antenatal, intrapartum and postnatal care of women. Less than 0.4% of midwives work in the community in private practice, either solo or group (AHWAC 2002:44). The average age of midwives is 41 years, and two-thirds of them work fewer than 35 hours per week, with the average being 15–24 hours per week. This reflects that many midwives perform other economic and social roles, such as being primary carers to children or assisting a spouse with running a business.

By far the most alarming statistic about the Australian midwifery workforce is the national shortage and rates of attrition. There is estimated to be a shortfall of more than 1800 midwives in Australia at present. Despite high levels of unmet demand for placements in three-year Bachelor of Midwifery courses (1500 applications for 150 places in 2005 for example), rates of education of midwives are not keeping pace with attrition. Research has confirmed that attrition rates are accelerated through stress and frustration caused mainly by lack of opportunity to practise the full scope of midwifery and to provide non-medicalised primary care to women (Brodie 2002). Resolving the midwifery workforce shortages will take more than educating more midwives.

In this context, it is encouraging that innovative examples of best practice in maternity care are on the increase. A growing number of service providers have a strong commitment to address the needs and expectations of women in a better way and to address the problems facing the sector more creatively. This is increasingly involving reorganisation of the way maternity care is provided, to afford an expanded role for midwives in providing primary care to women, with appropriate medical back-up. Such services, although still in the minority, now exist in every state and territory in Australia and more are in the pipeline. However, there are also significant problems with current maternity services. These problems are briefly explained in this section.

## Problems facing Australia's maternity services

Like many other developed nations, Australia has a problem with rates of medical intervention in childbirth. Currently, about 1 in 4 labours are induced (26%) and more than a quarter of all babies (28.5%) born by caesarean section (Laws and Sullivan 2005:25,29). In some Australian states, such as Queensland, the problem is worse with a caesarean section rate of 32% for 2004, significantly higher than the 21.6% rate for that state a decade earlier. This represents a 50% increase in the number of caesarean sections. Over the same time period the perinatal mortality rate has not changed (Queensland Health Department 2005, 2006) (Figure 3.1).

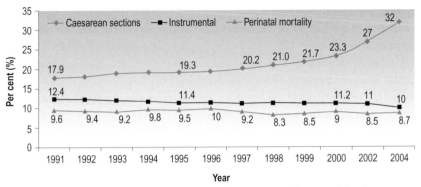

*Figure 3.1* Australian caesarean section and instrumental vaginal birth rates with perinatal mortality expressed as number per thousand. Source: Laws and Sullivan (2005)

An Australian study published in the *BMJ* in 2000 has shown that even healthy, low risk women receive significantly greater numbers of caesarean sections than can be justified on clinical grounds alone, or than is recommended by the World Health Organisation (WHO) as best practice (Roberts et al 2000). Other forms of intervention are also being widely used during the labours and births of healthy, low risk women. The Roberts et al (2000) study of 171 000 births in New South Wales found that of low-risk first-time mothers, labour is induced or augmented with oxytocin for 1 in 3 public patients and a half of all private patients. Epidural anaesthesia is used in between a quarter (public) and a half (private) of labours. Forceps procedures or vacuum extraction are used to deliver 1 in 5 babies born in a public hospital and 1 in 3 born in a private hospital. One in three public women and half of all private women receive an episiotomy. Overall, only a quarter (28%) of public and a fifth (18%) of private first-time mothers give birth without at least one obstetric intervention. The study provides strong evidence that medical interventions in the labours and births of healthy pregnant women are not always clinically indicated or in accordance with evidence-based best practice.

The current medicalised system of maternity care in Australia focuses on early detection and treatment (where possible) of complications. This frequently involves doctors assuming the role of 'team' leaders, and women experiencing many routine medical tests and procedures. Some of these are not supported by the evidence and include among others: routine repeat ultrasound; electronic fetal heart rate monitoring on admission in labour; routine rupture of membranes in labour. Care is usually fragmented involving many healthcare providers. There is typically a limited focus on psychosocial concerns or preventive care, unless it is a medical treatment such as antenatal anti-D or hepatitis B vaccination. Similarly, there is very little emphasis on lifestyle factors that impact on wellbeing and affect outcomes (e.g. obesity, smoking) and inadequate attention to the effective support of disadvantaged women or women with special needs. Indigenous women are particularly poorly servised by our current maternity service, which only exacerbates the comparatively high perinatal mortality rate for their babies.

Within the mainstream services a medical model of care predominates. Women receive fragmented care from multiple midwives and doctors and continue to report that their choices are restricted. Throughout the country it is not uncommon for public and private maternity services alike to actively discourage or restrict women's choices about mobility in labour, choice of birthing positions, the number and type of support people in labour, and use of water immersion in labour or for birth. In one infamous event, a state minister for health took a group of journalists to a local birth centre that had recently been opened and confiscated the plugs to baths that had been installed for the use of women in labour. The effect of such policies and practices is that maternity services often fail to provide the support necessary to promote normal birth. Women frequently report feeling pressured to accept medical interventions they would prefer to avoid, such as induction, augmentation, epidural and even caesarean section.

Another key problem with Australian maternity services is the fragmented way in which care is routinely provided to women, and their lack of access to primary care by a midwife. Women have very little choice in the type of care they access although there is wide variation throughout Australia. In many places, women only have the option of medical model care in the public or private sector despite consumer groups over many years requesting the option of continuity of care by a known midwife and choice of place of birth – home, hospital or birth centre (Maternity Coalition 2002). Demand for continuity of midwifery care is high in every service offering women this option, yet it remains the case that less than 3% of women are able to access birth centre care or home birth services. The majority of women access public hospital antenatal clinics where they typically wait for long periods of time for each antenatal check-up before seeing a midwife or doctor who is a stranger to them. Once in labour they are cared for by another group of midwives whom they have not met before, and by yet a third group of midwives in a postnatal ward.

Women's access to postnatal care has suffered badly under the dominant model of maternity service provision. Postnatal care is largely limited to in-patient care. In the minority of services that offer out-patient care with a midwife visiting a woman in her home, the service typically involves visits from different midwives, each of whom is unknown to the woman. Postnatal wards are frequently very busy with high midwife to mother/baby ratios (e.g. 1 midwife to 8 mothers and their babies). Community based postnatal care is not universally available and services are frequently delivered in an inflexible way. Although approximately 90% of Australian women want to breastfeed, many do not receive the support they need to breastfeed exclusively and rates of breastfeeding drop markedly in the few months after birth (National Health and Medical Research Council (NHMRC) 2003).

A further problem facing maternity services is the shortages of both midwives and doctors. These shortages have increased the pressures on midwives working in hospitals to care for even more women simultaneously than was the case previously, with resulting increases in stress. There is also mounting pressure to substitute midwives with nurses who lack midwifery qualifications. Women in rural communities have been particularly hard hit, with more than 126 rural maternity services being closed in the past 10 years with workforce shortages being blamed. Workforce shortages in both maternity and other areas of healthcare recently prompted a national Government inquiry that has produced recommendations about how more efficient use can be made of the existing workforce (Productivity Commission 2005). Advocates for midwifery are drawing on this report to support arguments that midwifery workforce shortages will only be addressed once the fundamental causes of the shortage are resolved – namely the current barriers to the freedom of midwives to practise.

# Barriers to comprehensive midwifery practice

A range of politico-cultural, legal, regulatory, and industrial impediments currently prevent midwives in Australia from providing the full scope of midwifery care to women in a manner comparable with their colleagues in some other OECD (Organisation for Economic Co-operation and Development) countries. Midwives are actively lobbying for freedom to practise. Seeking autonomy does not mean that midwives want to work in isolation from doctors or other health professionals in providing maternity care. Rather they are seeking the opportunity to work on their own responsibility, in collaboration with doctors and others as indicated by the needs of each woman and her baby. This approach is currently not possible in most maternity services in Australia.

The major changes needed to enable midwives to practise comprehensively relate to:

- developing and expanding midwifery models of maternity care
- legislative and regulatory reforms
- investment in continuing professional development for midwives
- reforming funding mechanisms
- resolving the lack of professional indemnity insurance for self-employed midwives.

In many places there is a shortage of midwives and difficulties recruiting and retaining midwives; a solution to the workforce problem might help to drive some of the much-needed reforms. Changes to midwifery education are slowly being implemented and these will be discussed in this section too.

## Political and cultural issues

The reform process is reliant on strengthening the 'midwifery voice' within the health system. The relative invisibility of the midwifery profession has contributed to the current inappropriate provision of maternity services and the orientation towards technocratic, mechanistic and medical approaches to childbearing (Brodie 2002, Hirst 2005). Recognition of midwifery as distinct from nursing and autonomous in relation to medicine will pave the way for the legislative and regulatory reforms and the full utilisation of midwives.

Although midwifery and nursing were distinct occupations prior to the regulation in the early 1900s, for the past 80 years nursing has subsumed midwifery. This has resulted in disadvantages to both midwifery and the public. Midwifery has not had a strong voice in the corporate health-planning sector. Senior nurses have been required to represent both nursing and midwifery with a natural tendency towards nursing being dominant. This has meant that despite all the evidence linking improved maternal and infant outcomes with strong professional midwifery practice, such practices have not flourished. Successful reorientation of maternity services depends on strengthening and supporting the midwifery profession. For this to happen it is essential that midwifery be recognised as a discrete profession, distinct from nursing, and that midwives routinely have input to policy development, strategic planning, and service evaluation.

Midwives are under-utilised within the current system. Midwives are experts in the care of women experiencing a normal pregnancy, labour and birth and postpartum period. They can recognise deviation from normal, refer appropriately and execute emergency care. However, specialist obstetric staff or visiting medical officers are commonly used in the routine care of normal pregnant and birthing women. This approach is costly, results in unwarranted and avoidable surgery and other medical interventions, and fragments care resulting in dissatisfaction and, at times, distress for women and their families. Midwives provide a better service with less intervention, fewer surgical procedures and are cost effective. Currently many executive managers of maternity services lack the specialty knowledge of the type of service they are managing. It seems that their actions are driven by the need to manage the risk for the health service or themselves rather than the risk to users of the service. Reward for budgetary control, a culture of blame and other external factors work to mitigate the forces for change (Forster 2005:57–67). This does not make for a quality service or appropriate use and care of staff.

Recognition of the need for midwifery leadership to be factored into the public healthcare system (e.g. midwifery consultants, supervisors of mid-wives, midwifery development positions) for the purpose of developing midwifery and midwife-led models of care, is only beginning. In many states and territories there is limited or no co-ordination of midwifery at a corporate health level. Midwifery, as a profession distinct from nursing, is rarely represented through any Government instrumentality at state or national levels of government. In some states, there is even a dearth of basic workforce data on midwifery, with midwives still being registered as nurses, no maternity policy and no public evaluation of the outcomes of the mater-nity service as a whole. Midwifery issues continue to be overlooked or solutions developed to address nursing issues are applied. An example of this is a recent national inquiry into nursing practice and education, com-missioned by national and state health ministers, in which the status of midwifery remained ambiguous (National Review of Nursing Education 2002). The nomenclature throughout the Report is specific to nursing but ministers have assumed that a taskforce established to implement the report has jurisdiction over midwifery as well as nursing.

However, there have been some significant achievements in recent years in terms of securing greater recognition of midwifery as a distinct profes-sion. The federal Government, for example, commissioned a national study of the midwifery workforce, which provided the first comprehensive assess-ment of the workforce for planning purposes (AHWAC 2002). This report has supported the creation of government-funded scholarship schemes tar-geted at midwives, as well as wider public recognition of the extent of, and shortfalls in, the midwifery workforce. There have also been important symbolic changes in the nomenclature of some peak bodies, which are translating into practical projects that focus on the issues facing midwifery. For example, the peak body of Australian regulators renamed itself the Australian Nursing and Midwifery Council in February 2005 to much fanfare in the national parliament house. The peak body of university deans of nursing and midwifery has done likewise, and both university faculties and Government offices in some states are also changing their names to include specific recognition of midwifery.

## Legislative reform

There is a pressing need to align legislative frameworks and maternity policies with evidence-based models of care. Midwives in Australia are granted a licence to practise according to the International Definition of the Midwife, with authority to take full responsibility for the care of women and their babies throughout pregnancy, labour and birth and the early postnatal period (WHO 1992). They need refer to doctors only when there are complications and can execute emergency procedures while help is being summoned.

However, in practice, midwives are unable to assume their full responsibilities as autonomous primary care providers because of out-dated legislation. Specific changes to the legislation regarding prescribing rights within their professional sphere, authority to order a range of diagnostic tests, admitting rights to maternity units and rebates for midwives fees for care provide in the private sector are needed.

## Prescribing rights and ordering pathology tests

Currently, midwives lack the legal authority to prescribe the range of drugs used regularly in the care of normal childbearing women, or to order and interpret the appropriate pathology tests. Regardless, midwives routinely administer drugs such as oxytocin (Syntocinon) and lignocaine in many settings. Maternity units often have medications such as these written up as standing orders and the midwives administer them as part of their normal practice. The midwives complete the documentation on the expectation that the doctor, who may have never seen the woman, will come to sign the order for the medication within 24 hours of administration. In practice, the doctor frequently never signs the order. Besides raising legal issues this can also lead to anxiety, frustration and conflict between the professions.

This issue has been well recognised by various states and national jurisdictions for many years. In 1998, the NHMRC's *Review of Services Offered by Midwives* found that:

> It is clear that in many Australian public maternity hospitals, midwives currently order and interpret routine diagnostic tests during pregnancy, labour, birth and postnatal care. They also administer pharmacological substances that have not yet been prescribed or

signed for by a medical practitioner. Current midwifery practice in many hospitals can be at variance with State/Territory legislation, raising the possibility of difficult legal implications, both for the midwives and the medical staff involved. This situation needs to be clarified by appropriate hospital committees and, if necessary, backed up by legislative amendments.

*NHMRC (1998:13)*

The situation is complicated in Australia because of the federal system of Government. The constitutional power to provide prescribing authority rests with the state/territory governments and, in the absence of a national maternity policy/ framework, it is up to the states/territories to implement reform according to their own agenda and in response to local political pressures.

## Right to admit women to hospital

To fulfil the role of primary care provider, midwives need to be able to admit women to hospitals and birth centres under their own name. This is sometimes referred to as visiting rights. It involves the midwife, rather than the doctor, as the named clinician and therefore responsible for the care of women and babies admitted under their name. The lack of visiting rights for midwives can cause conflict between midwives and doctors because doctors say that they are legally responsible for the outcome of care if they are the named clinician even though the midwife may be providing the care and making clinical judgements on their own responsibility. Many doctors believe that they will be in a legally vulnerable position of being accountable for care provided by clinicians from another discipline (in this case midwifery) without having any control over that midwife's actions.

This problem was also highlighted in the report of the Queensland Review of Maternity Services:

Even if a midwife provides almost all care ... a doctor will still be named in hospital records as the responsible officer for care. Such unclear role delineation sits uncomfortably for both doctor and midwife and needs to be resolved as a matter of priority.

*Hirst (2005:36)*

Midwifery practice has evolved over the past decade in response to the decreasing availability of medical officers particularly in rural areas. For example, Mareeba Midwifery Service, located in a small rural town in north Queensland, is a primary care model of maternity services. All of the care for healthy mothers and babies is provided by midwives at Mareeba Hospital with consultation and referral to the obstetricians at the large regional hospital should problems arise. The service was established as a demonstration site to showcase a model of care that meets the needs of rural communities with small numbers of birthing women. Despite assurances that the appropriate legislation would be changed to support the comprehensive practice in primary care settings such as Mareeba, this has not yet happened.

## Medicare rebates for fees

The Commonwealth Government provides funding of maternity care in the form of payments to doctors and rebates to consumers for relevant services provided under the Medicare Benefits Schedule. Eligibility to claim Medicare funding for antenatal, intrapartum and postnatal care provided to women is limited to doctors including GP, GP-obstetricians and specialist obstetricians. The only way practising midwives can earn an income is to accept an employed position with a public or private hospital, GP or community health service, or to be self-employed and charge women the full cost of their service. Only a minority of health insurance funds currently offer women a rebate when they contract and pay for the services of a midwife.

A recent announcement by the national health minister (January 2006) has indicated that midwives will soon be able to receive Medicare rebates for fees for antenatal 'check-ups' in rural and remote locations, albeit at a lesser fee than the one provided to doctors and only under the direction of a doctor. Yet midwives are able to provide similar services on their own responsibility and with additional benefits to healthy women compared with GPs and obstetricians. Experience overseas (such as in New Zealand, the Netherlands, the UK and parts of the USA and Scandinavia) indicates that granting midwives equitable access to public funding for their professional services results in enhanced maternity services. In particular, there is greater choice and satisfaction for women at reduced cost to taxpayers while safety for mothers and babies is retained.

There have been attempts over the years to have midwives' fees rebated in the same way as doctors' fees are rebated. Changes to funding systems have occurred in other Western countries, such as New Zealand, however the resistance in Australia to recognise and fund midwives as primary care providers is entrenched. The Australian College of Midwives and Maternity Coalition are currently lobbying the federal Government to facilitate full access for women to the Medicare Benefits Schedule for rebates for midwives' fees with the midwife as primary care provider.

# Regulatory reform

If there were politico-cultural recognition for midwifery as a distinct profession from nursing the door would be open to instigate a range of regulatory reforms. These include separate regulatory legislation, national standards of midwifery education, and recency of practice and continuing professional development requirements for annual licensing.

## National regulation of midwifery under a separate Midwives Act

Perhaps the most fundamental change required is the legislation regarding the regulation of midwifery. Currently, each State and Territory has its own regulatory authority. Although some regulatory authorities are beginning to recognise that midwifery is a distinct profession from nursing, tangible evidence of changes to regulate the two professions separately is limited. Several regulatory authorities do not mention midwifery in their name and routinely apply nursing frameworks to midwives and midwifery. Many regulatory authorities do not have a guaranteed place on the board/council for a midwife. Even where individual members of a regulatory board might be a midwife, they typically do not have the authority to represent midwifery as a profession and are only one of a dozen or so (nursing) members.

The key challenge with the regulation of midwifery being undertaken by state/territory regulatory boards whose primary focus is on nursing is that midwifery issues risk being overlooked. Alternatively, it is assumed that nursing frameworks are relevant to midwifery with little evaluation of the impact on the midwifery profession or the quality of care provided to women and their families. There seems limited protection of the roles and scope of practice of a midwife, with boards in some states and territories responding to workforce shortages and associated political pressures by smoothing the way for the use of unqualified or under-skilled staff to assume aspects of midwifery care.

Midwifery needs distinct and visible regulation to maintain and improve standards and protect the public. There is also a recognised need for greater national consistency in the education and practice standards that apply to the midwifery profession. A single national midwifery regulatory authority comprising midwives and consumers would help to strengthen midwifery regulation in Australia. A recent national Government inquiry into the health workforce in general reached the same conclusion recommending single national bodies for both the registration of health professionals and the accreditation of educational curricula (Productivity Commission 2005). It remains to be seen whether the federal and state/territory governments will collaborate to implement these recommendations.

## National standards of midwifery education

As a result of a lack of a national approach to regulation, there is also disparity in relation to the standards of midwifery education. The regulatory authorities in each state and territory accredit midwifery education courses using different yardsticks to determine the adequacy of curricula submitted. As a result, there is currently wide variety in the length, scope and methodology of midwifery education programmes for entry to practise. The predominant education pathway for entry to the profession remains a 12–18 months Graduate Diploma in midwifery, the prerequisite for which is a three-year Bachelor's Degree in Nursing. Regulatory authorities in only three states have thus far paved the way for registration of graduates of three-year Bachelor of Midwifery courses. Mutual recognition arrangements mean that a Bachelor of Midwifery graduate (without nursing qualifications) can still work anywhere in Australia (if they can find an employer), but universities in four of the eight states are still being prevented from offering the Bachelor of Midwifery degrees despite high demand for places in such courses from would-be midwives.

In 2001 the peak professional body for midwives, the Australian College of Midwives, developed national midwifery education standards. These initially applied only to the three-year Bachelor of Midwifery programmes introduced in Australia at that time. However these standards are currently being reviewed with the objective of achieving an agreed national standard for all education programmes leading to entry to practise as a midwife. The revision is taking place in consultation with students, educators, regulators, employers, and the profession, with a view to maximising the acceptance and use of the standards once they are finalised.

## Recency of practice and continuing professional development

At least two of the eight regulatory boards that authorise midwives to practise, do not currently have the power to require a midwife seeking re-registration to have recent midwifery practice in order to gain an annual practising certificate. For example, a registered nurse who also has gained a midwifery qualification and registration as a midwife but never practised as a midwife is able to renew her annual licence to practise midwifery simply by declaring recency of practice as a nurse (not a midwife).

There are currently no requirements to demonstrate continuing professional development (CPD), although at least one regulatory board has moved recently to address this and others are considering it. Midwives in Australia currently lack any national guidelines for their CPD. In the absence of a national, professionally endorsed framework, many midwives depend on their employers to determine their professional development needs and provide them with access to suitable opportunities to address those needs. Midwives in rural areas report particular difficulties in accessing CPD, not just because of their relative lack of access to courses but also because of the inability to find someone to backfill their shift to free them to travel and attend training. The Australian College of Midwives has recently commenced a project to address this gap, possibly with funding support from the national Government, which will create the first national CPD framework for midwives by early 2007.

## Industrial reform

While there are small pockets of innovation in the provision of maternity services, which have sometimes been accompanied by the development of specific industrial agreements for midwives in that facility, this is not the norm. Concerns remain about the ability of the healthcare system to re-orientate from a mechanistic view of childbirth that has resulted in maternity services being designed as an acute surgical service.

Most Australian women still experience maternity care as a series of outpatient appointments for the purpose of investigation and diagnosis, an acute hospital stay for the extraction of the baby and short hospital recovery period (average 2.4 days) (Laws and Sullivan 2005). The focus on acute care services using a medical model has resulted in industrial arrangements that mimic the needs of an acute surgical unit. Midwives predominantly work shifts to cover 24 hours, and the associated industrial arrangements focus on staff/patient ratios, skill mix, adherence to policy, and budgets. The autonomous practice of midwifery and the role of midwives as primary carers are lost in this bureaucratic system. There has been only limited recognition that midwives interested in providing continuity of care to women require separate industrial arrangements from those designed for nursing.

The role of the midwife in applying the principles of primary health care and participating in health promotion, illness prevention, community development, and providing holistic care of the woman and her family has yet to be widely accepted and is rarely implemented. Midwives dedicated to providing midwifery models of care often struggle under industrial arrangements that do not recognise their knowledge and skills or the new ways of working. This contributes to burnout and feeling undervalued (Hirst 2005:38).

New industrial arrangements are just beginning to emerge for midwifery. As demand from women for greater access to continuity of midwifery care grows, employers, unions and the midwifery profession are slowly rising to the challenge of finding new ways to remunerate and structure this way of working. However, industrial agreements that support midwives in using their full skills and reward clinical judgement, autonomous practice and the level of responsibility and accountability inherent in the role of primary care provider, continue to be the exception rather than the norm.

## Professional indemnity

A final key barrier to autonomous midwifery practice in Australia is a lack of professional indemnity insurance for self-employed midwives. Most midwives in Australia are employed by either public or private hospitals and can access professional indemnity through the union. However, for the small minority of midwives who are self-employed, it has not been possible to purchase professional indemnity insurance since July 2001. Union membership does not confer access to the union sponsored professional indemnity for midwives who are self-employed.

The market for professional indemnity for private midwifery care has been tenuous for a long time. Insurers tend to be wary of midwives providing home birth in the light of claims by obstetricians and their professional bodies that home birth is dangerous and, the occasional successful claim against the insurer of a home birth midwife. Other issues have combined to make it difficult to encourage insurers to reconsider their assessment of self-employed midwives. These include: inadequate regulation of the midwifery profession; inconsistent education standards for midwives; lack of compulsory requirements for CPD; and, lack of nationally endorsed standards for practice and codes of ethics. Also, the relatively small number of midwives in private practice, and their limited earning capacity have been key factors that make it uninviting for an insurer to carry a book for midwives when the potential maximum payout for an obstetric case in Australia recently reached a landmark Aus$12 million in a court ruling against an obstetrician (B Vernon, EO Australian College of Midwives, personal communication from discussion with insurers, 2005–2006).

The inability to purchase professional indemnity insurance has made private midwifery even more challenging than it already was in the absence of rights to order tests, prescribe relevant drugs and admit women to hospital if needed. It also has significant legal implications. In a move to provide greater protection to consumers of all private healthcare services, the state and territory governments have all legislated over the past five years to require all health professionals providing private services to hold their own professional indemnity insurance. This policy is intended to ensure that in the absence of any Government schemes to provide such compensation, any consumer who successfully sues a negligent health care professional, is able to access adequate compensation.

This policy, while commendable from a consumer protection viewpoint, has created an additional barrier to midwifery practice in Australia. In the face of market failure in this area of insurance, self-employed midwives are unable to comply with this legal requirement. In most states and territories the regulatory authority responsible for each of the different health professions has been charged with ensuring that this requirement is met. The response of the nurses' boards has varied, with most not actively enforcing the requirement when processing re-registrations for self-employed midwives. However, in one territory in 2005, the Board was required by the Government to enforce this requirement, and refused to re-register self-employed midwives living and working in that jurisdiction. The resulting consumer driven political campaign resulted in the government's providing professional indemnity cover to a handful of midwives to enable them to continue to offer women the choice of continuity of care and birth at home. However, the outcome of the campaign was by no means guaranteed and considerable financial hardship was borne by the affected midwives.

There are signs that professional indemnity policies may be available to midwives once again in coming years. However, an ongoing barrier is the small number of midwives interested in taking out such policies, which makes providing insurance products uneconomic for underwriters. Until the political and legal barriers to midwives being able to work as fully autonomous and responsible health professionals are removed, it seems unlikely that many more midwives will choose to be self-employed. Thus, a lack of professional indemnity will continue to be yet another barrier to midwives' freedom to practise.

# Opportunities and positive developments

Maternity services and the midwifery profession in Australia are at a critical juncture. With growing shortages of both midwives and doctors (especially in rural areas), escalating rates of medical intervention in childbirth, and rising costs, the way maternity services are currently organised is not sustainable. Nor are they producing the best possible health outcomes for women and babies. These circumstances pose threats for the midwifery profession but also open up opportunities for reform. In particular, some developments within the past five years provide hope for the future.

## Consumer group action

For the first time, Australian women and their families have a national consumer advocacy group: Maternity Coalition. This group is a non-profit, non-political and non-sectarian national umbrella organisation committed to the advancement of best-practice maternity care. It acts as a peak body for the plethora of small local maternity groups, as well as having membership from individual women, midwives and other interested individuals.

Maternity Coalition brings together activists with a wide range of skills and extensive experience as advocates, educators and researchers in the area of childbirth and women's health for effective lobbying, information sharing, networking and support in maternity services. The organisation actively supports consumer participation at all levels of health policy planning, decision making and service delivery and has been highly effective in putting maternity services on the political and media agendas and promoting women's access to midwifery models of care.

In 2002, Maternity Coalition launched a blueprint for reform of Australia's maternity services called the National Maternity Action Plan (NMAP) (Maternity Coalition 2002). It was widely circulated and endorsed by many organisations, individual consumers and professionals. NMAP was written by pregnant women and mothers committed to seeing that women have the choice of a known midwife to care for them throughout pregnancy, birth and the first few weeks after the birth, with medical backup if needed.

Maternity Coalition has formed strategic partnerships with other organisations and successfully lobbied for an independent review of maternity services to be conducted and implemented in at least four states and territories. Its advocacy has also served as a catalyst to the creation of several new birth centres and the re-opening of several threatened rural maternity services. Nationally, Maternity Coalition has launched a campaign to have private practice midwives receive rebates for fees using the same mechanism that rebates doctors' fees: Medicare. One of the strategic partnerships formed by Maternity Coalition is the Australian College of Midwives. They have signed a Memorandum of Understanding and work in partnership to achieve shared goals.

## Midwifery leadership

Ten years ago, Australian midwives Professor Lesley Barclay and Linda Jones wrote,

> Midwives frequently identify themselves as victims . . . and see obstetricians or nursing organisations as opponents. It is time we as midwives looked hard at ourselves and considered that we may be deficient in political acuity and strength. . . . Midwives have not led

improvements in services for women. Except for the courageous few, midwives remain hidden within the system. While many complain about the status quo few actually are effective in changing it. Those midwives that do speak out are often not supported by their colleagues.

*Barclay and Jones (1996:129)*

While these words still ring true, it is also true that things have changed. On the one hand services for women have deteriorated. Increasing intervention rates, and an intense 'preoccupation with technological intervention, medical dominance and hospital routines' (Barclay and Jones 1996:127) have resulted in fragmented and depersonalised care being the norm. The transition to motherhood is made even more difficult with the inadequate provision of information to women and a dearth of postpartum and child health services. However, the midwifery profession in Australia is coming of age and reaching a critical mass of reform oriented midwives in clinical practice, research, education, and management/policy. A growing number of midwives with a reform orientation have research and higher degree education and apply midwifery models/principles of care to research and policy development.

The professional association for midwives, the Australian College of Midwives, has also grown as an organisation. The strategic vision of the College is to be the leading organisation shaping Australian maternity care by 2015. This is the first time that midwives, as a professional body, have publicly acknowledged their key role in the provision of maternity care rather than just their role in strengthening the midwifery profession.

With clearer goals and direction and a better understanding of political processes, the College is becoming much more active in setting professional practice and education standards. In recent years the College has produced standards for midwifery education and led the way in the development of new Bachelor of Midwifery Education programmes, which are now offered by six universities in three states. The changes to midwifery education with the introduction of Bachelor of Midwifery programmes will facilitate change in practice and will help to broaden the role of midwives within the healthcare system. Importantly, these new midwifery programmes are comparable with midwifery education in other OECD countries.

The College has also developed National Consultation and Referral Guidelines for Midwives that delineate the scope of autonomous midwifery practice and specify the circumstances in which referral to a suitably qualified medical practitioner is warranted (Australian College of

Midwives 2004). Further, the College is now collaborating closely with regulators, promoting the kinds of reforms that are needed to produce greater consistency in the quality of midwifery practice across Australia. Projects to support midwives with continuing professional development and reflection on their own practice are also being developed in 2006.

The College is also playing a key role in providing the means for midwives to network with one another, and in raising public awareness of midwifery issues and the need for reforms to maternity services. The cumulative effect of these initiatives is that there is stronger collective midwifery leadership in Australia than ever before.

## Conclusion

Freedom to practise midwifery according to the International Confederation of Midwives definition has been, and continues to be, highly constrained in Australia. Medical and nursing influences on the organisation and delivery of maternity care for many decades has obliged midwives to settle for a role that is restricted, controlled and largely disconnected from the women for whom they care. Lack of insurance, visiting rights and access to appropriate drugs and equipment has limited the option of self-employment to all but the most determined midwives. Education programmes for midwives have, until recently, been predicated on becoming a nurse, and regulation has deprived midwives of the authority to undertake normal midwifery practices, like ordering and interpreting tests, on their own responsibility. As a result, the midwifery profession in Australia has generally suffered low self-confidence, high levels of stress, and problems with retention.

Yet despite these significant barriers to the freedom of midwives' practice, the future looks bright. There is growing recognition of the role and significance of midwifery by governments, regulators, educators and the community. Midwives themselves are coming to see their roles differently and to agitate for greater freedom to practise. Consumer advocacy, combined with existing pressures for reform arising from workforce shortages and spiralling costs, are resulting in the slow but steady creation of innovative services that provide midwives with much greater professional freedom and responsibility. Regulatory reforms and moves towards greater national consistency in education and practice standards are helping to lay the groundwork for midwifery to have a strong, capable and well-respected role in Australian maternity services.

> ## Reflective questions
>
> Change is difficult to effect. What ideas could you offer to help to change a maternity unit from an 'acute surgical service' using only a medical model to something that is more woman-friendly?
>
> 'The midwifery profession in Australia is coming of age and reaching a critical mass of reform oriented midwives in clinical practice, research, education, and management/policy.' Midwifery everywhere needs leaders and potential leaders. Could you become one of these? What skills would you require to become a leader?

The views expressed in this chapter are those of Jenny Gamble and Barbara Vernon and not necessarily the views of the Australian College of Midwives.

## References

Australian College of Midwives 2004 National consultation and referral guidelines for midwives. Online. Available at: http://www.acmi.org.au/text/publications/publications.html (accessed 10 February 2006)

Australian Health Workforce Advisory Committee 2002 The midwifery workforce in Australia 2002–2012. Australian Health Workforce Advisory Committee, Sydney, pp 43–44

Barclay L, Jones L 1996. Where to now? Priorities and problems for midwives in the future. In: Barclay L, Jones L (eds) Midwifery: Trends and Practice in Australia. Churchill Livingstone, Melbourne, pp 127–135

Brodie P 2002 Addressing the barriers to midwifery – Australian midwives speaking out. Australian Journal of Midwifery 15(3):5–14

Forster P 2005 Queensland Health Systems Review. Independent Review of Queensland Health's Systems, Brisbane, pp 56–67

Hirst C 2005 Re-birthing: Report of the review of maternity services in Queensland. Independent Review of Queensland Health's Systems, Brisbane, p 16

Laws PJ, Sullivan EA 2005 Australia's Mothers and Babies 2003. AIHW Cat. No. Per 29 Sydney Australian Institute of Health and Welfare National Perinatal Statistics Unit. Online. Available at: http://www.npsu.unsw.edu.au/ps16high.htm

Maternity Coalition 2002 National Maternity Action Plan (NMAP). Online. Available at: http://www.maternitycoalition.org.au/ (accessed 9 February 2006)

NHMRC 1998 Review of services offered by midwives. Online. Available at: http://www.nhmrc.gov.au/publications/_files/wh26.pdf (accessed 9 February 2006)

NHMRC 2003 Dietary guidelines for children and adolescents in Australia incorporating the infant feeding guidelines for health workers. Online. Available at: http://www.health.gov.au/nhmrc/publications/synopses/dietsyn.htm (accessed 9 February 2006)

National Review of Nursing Education 2002 Our Duty of Care 2002. Canberra, National Review of Nursing Education

Productivity Commission 2005 Australia's Health Workforce, Research Report. Online. Available at: http://www.pc.gov.au (accessed 9 February 2006)

Queensland Health Department 2005 Perinatal Statistics, Queensland 2004. Queensland Health Department, Brisbane

Queensland Health Department 2006 Perinatal Summary Statistics 1987–2004

Queensland. Health Information Centre Publications Online. Available at: http://www.health.qld.gov.au/hic (accessed 9 February 2006)

Roberts CL, Tracy S, Peat B 2000 Rates for obstetric intervention among private and public patients in Australia: population based descriptive study. British Medical Journal 321:137–141

WHO 1992 Global action for skilled attendants for pregnant women. Appendix 4The international definition of the midwife. Online. Available at: http://www.who.int/reproductive-health/publications/global_action_for_ skilled_attendants/rhr_02_17_11.html (accessed 9 February 2006)

## Additional resources

Australian College of Midwives website: http://www.acmi.org.au

Access this site for:

- The College's strategic plan
- Standards for Midwifery Education
- National Guidelines for Referral and Consultation for Midwives

Maternity Coalition website: http://www.maternitycoalition.org.au
Access this site for:

- The National Maternity Action Plan (NMAP)
- Further information about the maternity consumer movement in Australia
- Links to an online discussion list called *ozbirthing Community*

Australian Nursing and Midwifery Council (ANMC) website: http://www. anmc.org.au

Access this site for:

- National Competency Standards for the Midwife

# CHAPTER FOUR

# Embracing change: maintaining standards

## ELAINE MADDEN

The *Changing Childbirth* (1993) initiative aimed to ensure that maternity services focused on the individual woman, and sought to develop maternity care that was accessible, responsive and effective. *Delivering Choice* (1994) the Northern Ireland response to this document reiterated these recommendations for women to have continuity, choice and control during their childbirth experience. Midwives in Northern Ireland embraced these recommendations and hoped to redress the established medical model of care and develop innovative midwifery practices at the point of care.

In Northern Ireland there are examples of midwifery developments and initiatives in each trust. Skilled midwives committed to normal/natural childbirth are pushing back the boundaries. The Craigavon midwifery-led unit has achieved many milestones. Since its opening in 2000 until October 2005 midwives in Craigavon have undertaken 950 water births and lead the way in providing water births in Ireland. In Down and Lisburn Trust Midwifery Services Manager Rosemary Hood and her team led the establishment of team midwifery, and worked hard to initiate the first midwifery-led unit. Sadly, this has not been accomplished before Rosemary's retirement in 2006. The Royal/Jubilee Maternity Services developed both caseload and team midwifery and have build-up 10–15% of women receiving total midwifery-led care.

However we must acknowledge that the same restrictions and constraints that influenced midwifery practice elsewhere in the UK also have an impact on Northern Ireland and affect freedom to practise autonomously. Lack of midwifery autonomy usually means that women are cared for using the medical model. As a rule, this includes a high level of intervention for women in labour. Yet, almost 500 midwives in Northern Ireland responded to a survey stating clearly that they preferred non-technological birth (Sinclair and Gardner 2001).

Statistics show that in Northern Ireland intervention levels are indeed high. More than 21 500 babies are born annually in the Province. Of these, over 25% are born by caesarean section, another 12% by instrumental delivery and more than 33% of the labours will have been induced (Birthchoice 2006). A high level of intervention by itself is not unique. Downe et al (2001) found that the majority of childbearing women experienced some type of intervention in labour. But these figures will have a subsequent effect on, for instance, home birth figures, as intervention in childbirth is less when the birth takes place at home. Figures for home births in the UK vary widely from 5.8% in Devon with those for Northern Ireland coming in at an average of 0.24% (Birthchoice UK 2006).

While Northern Ireland is not unique with its high intervention rates for women in labour, the trend of movement of care of the majority of childbearing women from the medical to the midwifery/social model is perceived to be slower. Women's choice, possibly made without knowledge of the benefits of the midwifery model of care, is a major factor in this. The midwives of the four countries of the UK have worked together within, first, the Nursing and Midwifery Council (NMC) and, previously, since 1983, the United Kingdom Central Council (UKCC). Since the 1990s midwives have worked towards changing practice from the medical model to the midwifery/social model of care (Department of Health (DoH) 1993, Scottish Home and Health Department (SHHD) 1993, Department of Health and Social Services (DHSS) 1994, Welsh Office 1996). Progress has included:

- the establishment of midwife led units; birth centres
- some independent midwifery practice
- several consultant midwifery posts
- the offer of woman-centred care, along with a willingness to return normality to birth in larger units where appropriate.

Through these measures, midwives have greater freedom to practise.

In Northern Ireland these developments have not yet been fully exploited: there are currently no consultant midwives, no independent midwives and no standalone midwifery birthing centres. The first direct entry group of student midwives to undertake a BSc (Hons) Midwifery Sciences (three years) in Northern Ireland is still currently in training, while, for instance, in Scotland the first group of similar students started their midwifery education in 1992. However, we have not seen the recruitment and retention problems that have affected other areas of the UK. In addition, dedicated one-to-one midwifery care is provided for all labouring women throughout the Province. Also, there have been local Government policy changes and approvals that support the establishment of birthing centres and consultant midwife posts although to date no trust has committed to establishing these options.

This chapter will attempt to identify factors which have influenced midwifery practice in Northern Ireland and explore issues which may have restricted the development of freedom to practise. The chapter will first give an overview of what has happened in the past 30 years in the field of maternity care in Northern Ireland. It will explore what progress is being made towards freedom to practise midwifery and the ambition for midwives to be with woman. It will examine changing strategies and take a look at concerns and hopes for Northern Ireland as this region of the UK moves towards more peaceful times. It offers a hopeful pointer with a summary of a case study of a recent beautiful birth before trying to pull the threads together in the conclusion.

# How did we get here?

It seems appropriate at this point to pause and briefly look back. In 1963, 32% of babies were born at home; six years later this had declined to 17%. By 1970 the number of home confinements was so low that few pupil midwives were able to witness a single home delivery. In 1970 the Peel Report (DoH 1970) advocated 100% hospital delivery. The Central Midwives Board expressed concern about ensuring that pupil midwives attended and witnessed sufficient home confinements to give them experience of that environment (Towler and Butler-Manuel 1975) Most contemporary practising midwives have had all their intranatal training in hospital under the hierarchical lead of consultant obstetricians and have had little opportunity to observe and care for a woman in normal labour at home. Kitzinger (2005:105) suggests that the real problem now is not resistance from obstetricians but from midwives themselves who have not been used to practising autonomously and 'have no confidence in or understanding of homebirths'. From the woman's point of view, research revealed that many women asking for a home birth did not choose an easy option: to get what they wanted was like 'climbing a mountain' (Ng and Sinclair 2002).

Thirty years ago in Northern Ireland, like the rest of the UK, the senior medical staff within each maternity unit had the traditional role at the top of the hierarchical establishment. Within my own unit it was routine practice for a midwife to 'scrub' for the senior consultant undertaking a perineal repair to hand him what he needed. It was not the midwife's role to perform artificial rupture of membranes (ARM), obtain intravenous access or undertake repair of a tear or an episiotomy even if they had personally performed the episiotomy.

Antenatal care had similar protocols. The medical team provided antenatal care in hospital. The midwife could assist by testing urine and taking blood pressures; however, only the medical person in attendance wrote (minimally) in the maternal notes, which remained within the hospital filing system to await the next visit. Medical and midwifery records remained separate.

When a woman was in labour, any problems were referred according to protocol: senior house officer (SHO), registrar and then consultant. Local guidelines and policies in many units governed practice with clear limitations for all midwives. This policy was intensified during the latter decades of the twentieth century when the 'war zone' of Northern Ireland affected the development and use of technological control offered through induction of labour and other medical interventions. For women especially in the 1970s, anecdotal evidence from midwives practising during those years suggests attending for elective induction meant less worry about driving through a troublespot. Therefore higher induction rates were situation driven to protect women's exposure to difficult situations in labour.

Medical staff had to approve many aspects of care. An SHO with six months or less experience was the first contact for midwives; this included SHOs' responsibility for signing reassuring cardiotocographs (CTG) even though they could still be receiving instruction from senior midwives on assessing CTGs: it was still their responsibility to sign the reading. It could be that some midwives have become institutionalised into a hospital hierarchical system through their previous nurse training and acquiesce with medical staff in perpetuating this culture (O'Connor 2000). Autonomy as a concept was not encouraged.

# Making progress

There has been progress throughout the UK: like their counterparts elsewhere, Northern Ireland midwives now undertake a number of procedures which used to be medical prerogatives for instance: performing ARM where appropriate; suturing; assessing and acting on CTG readings; inserting cannulae and giving intravenous medication; topping up epidurals; undertaking total antenatal care; undertaking scanning and checking Doppler flow. The introduction of multi-professional courses such as the Advanced Life Support in Obstetrics (ALSO) course and Neonatal Life Support (NLS) has encouraged midwives and obstetricians to work and learn together in a collaborative and co-operative manner. Midwives are embracing the remit of an autonomous midwifery role accepting decision making and responsibility for their practice and can be identified as independent practitioners (Northern Ireland Practice and Education Council for Nursing and Midwifery (NIPEC) 2005).

It is necessary to remember that rules and standards require midwives to refer to medical staff when necessary. However, some midwives persist in working within the model of medicalised care. This is the model to which they have been used and frequent referral to medical colleagues may be perceived as due to lack of confidence. Obstetricians report that their attempts to work in partnership are met with resistance from some mid-wives who do not wish to take responsibility or participate in the decision making process (M McMechan, personal communication, 2006).

Progress will continue with continuous professional development. Con-temporary midwives undertake examination of the newborn courses, fetal assessment courses and multi-professional courses on obstetric and neona-tal emergencies. They are becoming more competent and skilled, adapting and changing their practice and role to meet the needs of contemporary women in a technological society. As this happens and midwives also acquire new interventional skills, once only the remit of obstetricians, are they more autonomous than the midwives of previous decades? Do they have freedom to practise and the opportunity to offer best practice and care appropriate to individual users of the service?

The Royal College of Midwives (RCM) has recognised this important question. The College has launched a campaign, recognising challenges but hoping to refocus midwives on normality of childbirth (RCM 2005). The aim is to inspire and support normal birth practices and seeks to redress the balance between over-medicalisation of birth and the normal physio-logical birthing process. As noted by the RCM (2005), interventions, which may be inappropriate, must not be the first choice; to undertake a collabo-rative approach to intervention may mean a loss of traditional midwifery skills. This is highlighted in a comparison of Northern Ireland statistics with those of birth units in Great Britain (Dr Foster 2005). This work demonstrates that we have work to do to promote a normal birth culture and develop midwifery expertise and autonomy.

The RCM is right to acknowledge the challenges of the campaign. To practise within the constraints highlighted above makes it difficult for midwives to develop the confidence to be free to make decisions, practise autonomously and give of their best. Fleming (1998) explored the main issues affecting and influencing true autonomy and, refuting the notion of midwifery autonomy, declared that medicalisation of birth was a major factor in the decline of midwifery status. Also, although midwives claim to be autonomous practitioners, investigation revealed an inability to artic-ulate what makes them autonomous (Fleming 1998). In addition, midwives responding to a qualitative study (Pollard 2003) did not feel that their midwifery education had equipped them for professional autonomy. However, the same study noted that midwives educated by the direct-entry route appeared to be more capable of exercising autonomy than were their nurse-trained midwifery counterparts. And, there was doubt whether genuine midwifery autonomy was possible within the present system. Some respondents also suggested that many midwives do not support their own or other midwives' professional autonomy.

As noted in Chapter 2, midwives now need to consider the notion of best practice and how it can be achieved. To do this, it may be useful to take an observational approach:

- use a reflective approach in daily practice; take time to examine the day that is past and what you achieved, or what went wrong.
- observe contemporary midwives; possibly use a peer review situation to talk about practice.
- seek to define autonomous practices.
- ask questions.

Questioning peer as well as personal practice may be awkward but is necessary in the pursuit of best practice. For instance: are midwives, highly skilled in working with technology and equipment in the labour ward setting, providing true autonomous midwifery care or still working at the behest of an established system? Are they with woman or with machine and technological aspects of birth? A problem of distinction arises: machines and technological aspects of birth are necessary – for those women who require them. Thus to use high-tech aspects of care will be best practice for these women. But the midwife who has freedom to practise and who is trying to apply best practice will be able to decide or participate in the decision to use the technology. And she will also be able to recognise the normal labour and not comply with inappropriate intervention. In addition, she will gain important recognition for the uniqueness of midwifery knowledge and practice.

Results of a survey of midwives' attitudes to CTG indicated that midwives reject the notion of being dependent on machines. However, the survey also suggests that midwives who trust machines are more disposed to their use and the more competent midwives are in using machines, the more they trust them (Sinclair 2001). Instinctive midwifery behaviour used to be developed through observing interactions between midwives and women in natural labour in their own environment. It is possible that using and trusting machines and being institutionalised into medicalised labour ward cultures has eroded the development of this behaviour. Midwives must now reflect on changes that have affected their practice and think about their future direction. Northern Ireland midwives are in a position to examine, explore and learn from the experiences of colleagues in the other countries of the UK and elsewhere who have already established many midwifery-led initiatives. If we are to be free to practise we must be able to speak and act in this way. Medical staff do not have to state they are autonomous practitioners: they demonstrate it through their manner and approach.

# With woman

Evidence suggests that midwives and midwifery are the cornerstone of good maternity care (Wagner 1994). Tew (1998) supported this belief and stated that midwives practising their skills without technological aids are the most effective guardians of childbirth. Yet the current climate does not appear to support this. In Northern Ireland, as in the rest of the UK, the general practitioner (GP) usually is the first contact for all pregnant women to access maternity services. In Northern Ireland, further referral is in most instances to an obstetric consultant. This is not only a Northern Ireland issue: Davis (2003) highlighted that in order to strengthen normality in childbirth, midwives should be the first point of contact for pregnant women (RCM 2004).

As the main focus of care for childbearing women in Northern Ireland has moved from the community to the hospital there has been a change in the perception of what a midwife does. This has resulted in an erosion and undervaluing of the experience and skills of midwives by a public who seem genuinely confused about the midwife's role and frequently refer to midwives as nurses (Hunt 1995). Perhaps this is not surprising: much midwifery practice is considered to be 'high tech' and midwives are perceived as intensive care nurses (Hunt 1995). This point can be reinforced by personal experience:

- With over 20 years' midwifery practice and, at the time, a labour ward sister, I was asked by a close family relative if I ever saw babies being born.
- A pregnant woman attending a booking interview with a colleague, asked if midwives actually delivered babies.

There is an idea within Northern Ireland that only obstetric doctors are in attendance at birth. How widespread this is and what the public perception of the midwives' role is, requires further investigation. However, mistaken public perception of the role of the midwife can be seen as another hindrance to midwives in their quest for freedom to practise. When childbearing women from England come to attend our units we are often surprised that they insist on having midwifery care. At the same time, we are heartened that this is the culture that is growing within Great Britain. In Northern Ireland too, we need to promote the role and raise the profile of the midwife. If women know what their choices are and what a midwife's remit is, then hopefully more will ask for a normal birth with midwifery care whether this takes place at home or in hospital. But the undervaluing of midwifery skills and the imposition of change in maternity care have occurred not only in hospitals. In primary health care O'Connor (2000) claimed that maternity care is the only sector where the primary healthcare provider has all but been obliterated. Based on current home birth statistics, and equally negligible DOMINO figures, some community midwives are in danger of losing skills and confidence in dealing with intrapartum care. They are increasingly seen as predominantly concerned with postnatal care and confused with health visitors (Symonds and Hunt 1996). Therefore, both hospital and community midwives need to acknowledge the constraints in their current freedom to practise in order to address the issues and redefine their role and work towards greater autonomy.

Another factor, which contributes to less time 'with woman', is administration. Recent reports (Department of Health, Social Services and Public Safety (DHSSPS) 2005) demonstrate that the erosion of administration on our working day takes up to 30% of time away from hands-on care. Whilst recognizing the requirements to keep accurate and contemporaneous records the pressures of paperwork are frustrating to many healthcare professionals. Current policies, protocols and guidelines influence practice in hospital and community. A surge in clinical governance and quality issues has meant that trusts strive to produce documents covering best practice advice. All concerned are advised to document all care provided, fully and explicitly; the focus appears to have shifted to completion of paperwork rather than providing hands-on care.

Some administrative paperwork is necessary; it is also essential in, for instance, education and research. Improved education and access and contributing to evidence-based knowledge have supported the midwife to increase her knowledge and skills. Today's midwives have the benefit of years of research and evidence-based guidelines from resources such as the National Institute for Health and Clinical Excellence (NICE) and the Clinical Resource Efficiency Support Team (CREST). Most hospitals have local protocols and guidelines for any childbearing event during pregnancy, labour and the postnatal period. These documents are necessary as a contribution towards the aim of best practice and yet thinking about, discussing and writing them takes up a great deal of multi-professional time. And, if midwives are to be involved in true partnership with other healthcare professionals then they must play their part in developing and contributing to the writing of local documents. Similarly, the role of the midwife needs to be identified as equally important within the team providing up-to-date maternity care.

It could be argued that concentrating on developing education, equality of status and technical skills and the writing of documents has had a detrimental effect on intuitive midwifery. Yet, take the situation of the lone midwife in 1946 attempting to cope with a postpartum haemorrhage in very poor circumstances (see Chapter 2). We admire her ability, her independence and her ingenuity. But we have moved on from the use of beer bottles as we have progressed from routine perineal shaving and enemas as best practice examples. Today, a similar haemorrhage would bring support from a wide range of professionals; even at home a midwife, along with her skills, would have more equipment, a phone to hand and possibly a second midwife present, even before additional help comes. In each case the midwife will use 'best practice'. Surely the added research, status and technological skill could be made to work alongside intuitive aspects rather than to their detriment. Therefore, all these attributes should work together to improve care for the childbearing woman – if the system, and midwives, will allow them to.

In Northern Ireland, as elsewhere, we are struggling to define the midwifery role and seek to develop patterns of multi-professional working relationships. We are attempting to fit into a Department of Health system (DoH 2000) to streamline healthcare according to targets and overriding challenges such as waiting lists and trolley waits. Maternity care is not a high priority. So, if maternity care is not an issue at higher levels, midwifery is not seen as an issue either. The majority of midwives are vastly limited in their practice by the nature of where they work (Kirkham 1989). This affects both midwives and women.

In 2005 the RCM launched its major new UK-wide initiative: the Campaign for Normal Birth (see above). Midwives in Northern Ireland must find the motivation to get involved in the debate and take up the challenge of revisiting normality. We must address the issues of normality. Also, we need to establish our roles and define the autonomous role for the midwives of the future. Being autonomous does not mean working in isolation: we need to build and develop a collaborative approach within an equal partnership with other members of the multi-professional team; we need to comment and have our opinions counted and considered; we need to participate in multi-professional teaching sessions, joint audits and developing local guidelines. However, there still remains the bigger challenge of raising the midwifery profile and getting recognition for the significant role recognised at higher levels.

# Changing strategies

Raising the profile of, and acquiring recognition for the role of the midwife requires individual and collective application. Change is not a new concept for midwives: through the centuries midwives have competed with doctors and the developing specialism of obstetrics for their place with woman (Donnison 1988, Loudon 1992). In the twentieth century each of the countries of the UK as well as elsewhere has seen change as birthing customs and fashions come and go.

When the Peel Report of 1970 accelerated the change for childbearing women from birth at home with a midwife, to birth in hospital with varying numbers of staff, this also accelerated the decline in midwifery status (Tew 1998). Change in place of birth brought change in care. The majority of women who could give birth normally entered a medicalised environment, which has evolved into a climate of interventions and increased scientific and technical management. This has grown to the extent that more than 25% of babies in Northern Ireland are delivered by operative methods. The report, *Changing Childbirth* (1993) challenged maternity services to offer 'continuity, choice and control' to its users. The equivalent Northern Ireland document, *Delivering Choice* (1994) reiterated the recommendations and challenged midwives to fulfil their roles as autonomous practitioners and improve care by implementing and advocating midwifery managed schemes. At this time funding was made available to 'pump prime' midwifery projects and facilitated their initiation in each trust. Senior midwives in each trust worked towards implementing the midwifery care most applicable to their setting.

However, in 1979, Northern Ireland had 17 consultant units and 19 GP units. Currently (2006), there are 11 consultant units and no GP units. Plans continue in Northern Ireland to centralise maternity services. The ethos within Northern Ireland appears to value medicalisation and technology and place the midwifery/social model of woman-centred care at the bottom of a list (DHSPSS 2003).

On the other hand, Mander and Fleming (2002) reveal a contemplative perspective, outlining a changing attitude in current practice. They encourage midwives to examine seriously whether or not they have changed practice for the better through the years. We need to reflect upon the challenge that Mander and Fleming present:

- Do our current working practices reflect progress?
- From a personal perspective, are we really autonomous or do we just think we are?
- Is our best practice best for the users of our service?

- What can the individual midwife do to demonstrate and fulfil autonomous practice?

It is necessary also to think about what we are doing as a group. Women in Northern Ireland book into a system of care, provided by a variety of professionals. A recent audit of the woman's childbearing journey in one Northern Ireland setting highlighted the number of professionals even low-risk women met from booking to discharge. The range of contacts was from 15 to 50: antenatal care meant contact with 8–10 healthcare professionals including six midwives. Care during labour and childbirth could lead to meeting another 10–15 different professionals (J Rodgers, unpublished work, 2006). We aspire to a 'best' of one-to-one midwifery care and continuity of care. Whilst some have attained this through the caseload midwifery approach and that is to be commended, the reality is that many women continue to be cared for by a range of professionals. Therefore, we must actively address these findings and with this aspiration in mind ensure that we are working together at all levels to promote a midwifery agenda to facilitate and implement change.

Other work has had more positive results. In one maternity unit in Northern Ireland a practice development co-ordinator undertook to explore the notion of change in order to develop a shared vision for the future. Workshops engaged midwives of differing age and experience in Values Clarification Exercises and in Practice Development Processes (McCormack et al 2004). Using the medium of the workshops and with the help of an objective facilitator, midwives were able to identify and articulate their current situation and a possible future direction to make their vision a reality. They identified five key areas that they want to focus on for the future.

- Developing woman-centred care
- Defining normality/promoting normality
- The midwives' role
- Improving practice through challenge and support
- Organising care to make the best use of existing resources

The midwives involved also used the facilitator to help them identify action plans for each of these themes and are responsible for implementing them. Empowering midwives to take responsibility for their future should allow them actively to engage in the transition process.

As the midwives progressed through the Practice Development workshops, their comments demonstrated the frustration and feeling of constraint which they have experienced within the unit. It is likely that their dissatisfaction epitomises opinions held elsewhere. However, participating in the workshops also helped midwives to:

- accept the need for change to a firmly established culture
- realise that to effect change, they also need to appreciate the extent to which current attitudes and practices within the profession maintain the existing collective culture and thus influence junior and student midwives.

Individual scrutiny of practice has helped those midwives who have gone through the process of values clarification and reflection to agree the necessity of revisiting the idea of woman at the centre of care and the need to re-establish the role of the midwife.

Much of today's struggle for best practice in maternity care centres on normality in childbirth for more women (Chapter 2 p 10). The argument for promoting situations and practice where normal childbirth can be encouraged would therefore seem to be clear. After all, choice, continuity and control as issues only appeared when birthing women were removed from home to hospital with little control over their care. Once the problems were identified, maternity services in the UK began to change, not all at once and not all at the same speed. Nevertheless, midwife-led quality initiatives sprang up:

- birth centres appeared
- midwife-led projects progressed
- consultant midwife posts were advertised and applied for
- independent midwifery took on a higher profile
- in some areas midwives welcomed increasing home births
- elsewhere, midwives' confidence grew as some became the autonomous lead practitioner in childbirth.

In Northern Ireland the fight to establish a stand-alone birth centre continues. Although there are pockets where midwives demonstrate their freedom to practise, the move towards midwifery autonomy appears to have not reached the same scale as in some other areas of the UK. Yet, Northern Ireland midwifery has undergone significant changes in the past decade as various initiatives to bring about peace have improved the quality of life for its various communities (Barrowman and Clarke 2003). Devolution and setting up of the Northern Ireland Assembly had a positive impact on service delivery with members of the Legislative Assembly demonstrating a keen interest in developing the health services, including maternity services. However, the Legislative Assembly is currently under suspension (2006) and delivery of change is slow.

Yet the confidence of midwives in Northern Ireland is growing. The development of a midwifery-led unit at Craigavon established a precedent within the Province. This has been a big step: however the midwifery-led ward is situated within a maternity unit and the midwifery team involved have required strength and commitment to establish and maintain their remit. These midwives are just one example of the move towards midwifery-led care in Northern Ireland. There are a number of other midwives who continue to make a difference. In other units (Dr Foster 2005) women are offered complete midwifery care. These initiatives have been established against opposition from some GPs, some medical consultants and sadly with sometimes little support from midwifery colleagues. The midwives involved repeatedly reported opposition to their efforts to move forwards (Madden et al 2003).

Thus, the seeds of the strategies for change in midwifery in Northern Ireland are sown and nurtured. Whether or not they take root remains to be seen.

# Northern Ireland: concerns and hopes

In Northern Ireland in 2006 the fight to establish a stand-alone birth centre continues. There are no independent midwives, no consultant midwives and it may appear therefore that we are slower to take up these innovative midwifery practices demonstrated elsewhere. Is Northern Ireland really lagging behind the rest of the UK? This section will briefly explore the issues and highlight hope for the future.

## Demography

Different factors affect the need of a population for health and social care. These include population size, age and gender balance. Other key factors are associated with the socioeconomic profile of the population and level of deprivation. The population of Northern Ireland is around 1.7 million people and 21 600 births are expected per annum (DoH 2005). Compared with Great Britain, Northern Ireland has a higher proportion of its population in younger age groups: 22% of Northern Ireland's population is under 15 compared with 19% in Great Britain. Currently, the Northern Ireland population is smaller than in Wales. However, Northern Ireland has the fastest growing population in the UK: the birth rate per 1000 population in 2000 was 12.7 in Northern Ireland, 11.4 in England, 10.3 in Wales and 10.5 in Scotland (McWhirter 2002).

## Health and social factors

In Northern Ireland, management of health and social services are integrated and this raises a number of unique organizational issues. There are additional issues regarding socioeconomic deprivation, the impact of the 'Troubles', the extent of rurality, and the provision of regional services. Northern Ireland has a relatively high level of deprivation associated with a long history of socioeconomic problems. This particularly occurs in pockets of the population affected during the periods of civil disturbance. Conflict and political unrest for over 30 years within Northern Ireland with associated problems leave a legacy that will not be resolved quickly. The long-term impact of deprivation will continue to have a major impact on health and well being in Northern Ireland (DoH 2005).

A number of indicators testify to relatively high levels of material disadvantage in Northern Ireland. Family Expenditure Survey data show that household income and expenditure in Northern Ireland are markedly lower than in the UK as a whole. The proportion of people on most social security benefits is also much higher than in the UK (DoH 2005). Another factor is the infant mortality rate (IMR). The IMR for Northern Ireland has declined over the past 40 years, but it has done so more slowly than in most comparator countries. At 6.4 deaths per 1000 live births in 1999, the Northern Ireland IMR is above the European Union (EU) (population-weighted) average of 4.9. Over the past 30 years the IMR has dropped considerably across the UK. However, compared with the other UK countries, Northern Ireland still has the highest IMR (DoH 2005). Similarly, Northern Ireland rates for congenital malformations at birth are very much higher than the rates for England and Wales.

## Practice roles

Thus, there are situations in Northern Ireland affecting midwifery practice which are not relevant in the other UK countries. Given the problems, progress so far on so many motivated and innovative roles and initiatives is to be commended. Midwifery opportunities continue to be developed in Northern Ireland: a particular example centres round a role for midwives with specific interests in ethnic minority issues. These include addressing language barriers and developing and providing suitable and appropriate parenting skills (I Campbell, unpublished work, 2005). Other midwifery roles are also evolving and under recommendation including: antenatal screening; diabetic in pregnancy care; bereavement support and breastfeeding support; and roles in quality and effectiveness, risk management, complementary therapies and practice development.

Another example of progress highlights breastfeeding: Northern Ireland has one of the lowest breastfeeding rates in the world. Midwives aim to reverse this trend by striving towards gaining UNICEF UK Baby Friendly Status. Currently three trusts have full accreditation and six have certificates of commitment. Change therefore is in the air. Like other professions, midwifery in the UK has coped with great change over the past decade (Davis 2003). Most of these changes relate to: access to university education, including higher degrees; diversifying the arena of practice to include public health; strengthening normality in childbirth; and, the growth of midwifery research. Although progress in Northern Ireland may have been slower than in Great Britain, the changes that have occurred in our units over the past decade can also be attributed to the same factors.

## Education

To prepare the midwife of the future it is essential to offer her an education that provides her with the knowledge and skills necessary to practise safely and effectively. Midwifery practice and education are inextricably intertwined (Pairman 2000). Two universities in Northern Ireland provide midwifery education, one with pre- and post-registration and one with post-registration courses. Over the past decade midwives have made use of the post-registration programmes of study available at both locations; however, there were few midwives at doctorate level in the universities to support and encourage more midwives to progress in academia. Midwives wishing to do this had to seek supervision from universities in the other countries in the UK. The difficulties are shown in research figures obtained in 1999. A sample 500 midwives out of the 1086 practising midwives in Northern Ireland were questioned. Of these, only 53 had a degree, 2 had a Master's and none had a PhD (Sinclair et al 1999).

However the situation is changing. In recent years a number of visionary midwives have embarked on pathways and courses in university which should lead to higher degrees. Within the next two years this first group of midwives will complete their studies at doctorate level and, within clinical and academic settings will lead and encourage more midwives to pursue higher standards of learning and support best practice. From an organisational point of view, education to Master's level and beyond enhances credibility and increases influence (Currie 2004). The ability to undertake research and debate, discuss and challenge current systems from a higher academic level will bring midwifery professionals to a position where they can shape change within the healthcare systems.

NIPEC is also vital in ensuring a high midwifery profile on the universities' education agenda. NIPEC undertakes to promote high standards of midwifery and nursing education, training and development in a variety of ways at strategic, operational and advisory levels. It has a pivotal role in the quality assurance of all DHSSPS commissioned midwifery and nursing programmes in Northern Ireland including those that lead to all recordable qualifications with the NMC (NIPEC 2005). NIPEC has ensured the involvement of an expert practising clinical midwife at all consultations.

## Leadership

Raising the midwifery profile through higher education increases credibility and acknowledgement of 'the midwifery voice' at strategic levels. The subsequent effect of this is the opportunity for natural evolution of midwifery leadership. Breedagh Hughes, RCM Northern Ireland Board Secretary, suggests that lack of representation at department (DHSSPS) levels was a factor influencing the midwifery situation over the past decade (B Hughes, personal communication 2006). It was 2001 before Ruth Clarke was appointed as the first dedicated midwife to represent midwifery at the DoH. The World Health Organization (WHO) recently described midwives' lack of influence on national health care policies as an 'anomaly' to be corrected (WHO 2000).

Lack of influence equates with invisibility. One way to give visibility to midwives is through leadership programmes. A midwifery leadership programme has been available elsewhere in the UK since 2002. This aims to provide midwifery managers with support to enable them to develop critical midwifery leadership competencies. It could be argued that the pool of midwifery managers in Northern Ireland is not big enough to make this a feasible option here; there is also a problem regarding funding for Northern Ireland midwives to access the course. There is an established midwifery managers' network in Northern Ireland but there is a need to: widen the group to include lead midwives and support midwives in senior roles but without management remit; develop a strong succession planning approach to the profession; and, use strong leaders to encourage midwives to make changes.

The RCM (2006) recently launched a three-day executive and development coaching programme to enhance the leadership skills of midwifery managers. This is a vital opportunity for Northern Ireland midwives to meet their peers throughout the UK. There are 1273 midwives in Northern Ireland compared with 26000 midwives in England, 3300 in Scotland and nearly 1600 in Wales. The current midwifery leaders in Northern Ireland need to use the RCM's learning opportunity to share knowledge by sending potential future midwifery leaders to network with those who have already met and overcome challenges to progress midwifery initiatives and women-centred care. Thus, collaboration and learning from others' experiences can occur, and the results brought back to Northern Ireland.

As well as taking in knowledge from elsewhere, however, midwives in Northern Ireland are also able to disseminate what is happening here. For instance, the International Confederation of Midwives in Brisbane 2005 accepted nine research papers from Northern Ireland midwives. This is a remarkable achievement for this small region. We acknowledge a continuing strong medicalised culture in much of maternity care in Northern Ireland. Nevertheless, there is a desire among midwives to bring about change, and foundations for change have been laid.

## Women's choices

The range of choice available for women is enshrined within the concepts of woman-centred care and freedom to practise midwifery. However choice has led some women in Northern Ireland down another route: that of consultant obstetrician antenatal care. This is particularly unique to Northern Ireland as private maternity facilities are not available; others' perceptions of private care would be entirely different from that which is offered here. When private care is provided to a woman in Northern Ireland, an obstetric consultant undertakes total private antenatal care. However, on admission to hospital, the woman enters the National Health Service (NHS) system; NHS midwives provide the midwifery care within the NHS irrespective of the type of antenatal care.

Due to constraints and quirks of data collection it is difficult to obtain exact numbers of women choosing private care; the National Sentinel audit assessed the rate as 8% at least, but could account for 20% (Royal College of Obstetricians and Gynaecologists (RCOG) 2001). And when we ask the women 'Why?' the usual reply is 'For continuity of care'. On further investigation this is often because they are seen by different medical staff at each antenatal clinic visit. Centralisation of the maternity services has led to fragmentation of care and women could meet up to 10 different healthcare professionals during the antenatal period (J Rodgers, unpublished work, 2006; see also p 62). We can appreciate why women choose to pay for a consultant obstetrician to try to ensure continuity of care.

Conversely, women report that they lack enough information about the risks and benefits of medical procedures and therefore their choice, not truly informed, is dubious (Johanson et al 2002). The National Childbirth Trust has also suggested that women are constrained by the culture of existing maternity services (Newburn 2002). An additional problem with private maternity care is its possible contribution to caesarean section levels. At over 25% (Birthchoice 2006), the caesarean section level in Northern Ireland is the highest in the UK. One of the reasons given for this is private practice (N McCabe, unpublished work, 2004, Reid 2005). In 2001 the overall rate of caesarean sections for Northern Ireland was 24% but women who opted for private obstetric care had a 40% caesarean section rate (RCOG 2001).

Maternity care practitioners need to listen to what women want, offer them choices in care, and include the continuity of carer that they are looking for. They should not have to go down the private route for this.

## Case study

Women's choice and freedom to practise for midwives can work together. To illustrate this, this section presents briefly the circumstances surrounding a home birth I had the privilege of attending recently. The story demonstrates how the mother, Laura, exercised her right to choose and, how the midwives involved used their ability from differing aspects, to be free to practise (Madden 2005).

Laura, 37 years and married to Gregg and mother of Ben, was expecting her second child. She stated her desire for a home birth early in her pregnancy, first to her GP and then to a community midwife. That midwife responded negatively. However plans went ahead: Laura had a named midwife; she preferred not to have any scans; she wanted a water birth at home; it was important that she and Gregg should be in control of the experience; and, they wanted Ben to be involved.

When Laura was 38 weeks pregnant, her named midwife went on holiday. This was pre-arranged and Laura met the community team covering for the named midwife beforehand. However, when they arrived for a home visit they made it clear that they were not comfortable with the plans and not happy to 'allow' the birth in water. It took strength for Laura to carry on with her plan. She and Gregg felt awkward and uncomfortable as they felt they were not conforming and under considerable pressure from professionals.

Laura took the problem to the Association for Improvements in Maternity Services (AIMS). The AIMS representative advised her to see the consumer representative for the Eastern Health and Social Services Board (EHSSB). Via the EHSSB, Laura and Gregg reached the assistant directorate manager of the unit concerned. From that point, Laura received encouragement and enthusiasm from those she met and felt able to share her vision and hopes for the birth. She agreed that the hospital team would provide back-up for the community on-call team. In addition, any midwife who was not happy with the plans would not be put on either rota.

Laura went into labour nine days after her due date. Around her were: her birth partners (carrying out acupuncture, reflexology, reiki and spiritual healing), her family (Ben too), and the midwives (one community and two from the hospital). The burning oils aided an atmosphere, which was calm, candle-lit, quiet and focussed on Laura. 'Baby Lucy floated into a world of gentleness and an atmosphere of calm and music'.

This was my first experience of a home birth in 25 years as a midwife. It was quite memorable. All the midwives involved at the birth have commented on how privileged we felt to have been present at and included in Lucy's birth (Madden 2005).

## Discussion

Here we had a situation where Laura demonstrated from the beginning of her pregnancy what her choice was to be: birth at home. It was after she became comfortable enough with sympathetic midwives that she felt able to articulate her further vision of what she wanted the birth to be like. In the end Laura gave birth in the way she visualised, but she had to be steadfast in the face of some opposition – not from the medical profession but from some midwives.

However, we can argue that each of the midwives involved was given the opportunity to be free to practise. Firstly, the midwives who did not want to participate in the birth were able to decide not to. It is true that the first community midwife Laura encountered, rather than opting out immediately, tried to obstruct Laura from having a home birth. However this midwife was able to choose to opt out. Similarly, the other midwives who chose not to participate when they voiced their unhappiness were free make decisions about their practice.

There could be a problem here. When we say midwives want autonomy or to be free to practise we expect them to want to opt for woman centred care and the midwife/social model. But autonomy may also give midwives the freedom to opt out of giving this kind of care. So, as noted in Chapter 6 (p 116) 'should we give midwives the freedom to choose not to use [the clinical pathway for normal labour] and whom does that freedom best serve?'. In Northern Ireland we are giving the opting out midwives the opportunity to update their future practice to meet their needs. However, the fact remains that some midwives are reluctant to embrace the midwifery/social model.

On the other hand, the midwives who attended Lucy's birth demonstrated their commitment to freedom to practise by helping Laura and Gregg to achieve the birth of their choice. Not only that, they were able to do this: nobody stopped them. What is that but a demonstration of autonomy?

# Conclusion

Many midwives in Northern Ireland aspire to autonomy, freedom to practise, not in isolation but in a multi-professional partnership, to a best practice, which would enable them to be with women and offer normal birth to more women. This chapter has explored and acknowledged problems in maternity care in Northern Ireland. Here there are high rates of intervention in labour along with a largely medicalised model of care in labour. Midwives, linked with the other midwives of the UK, officially through the NMC and in other ways through peer group meetings, still appear to lag behind the rest in initiating new schemes. Yet many examples of good practice are in place. For instance, our established one-to-one care during labour is a standard that must not be brought down.

I have tried to identify and discuss factors which have led to the current situation and highlight where progress has and is being made. Exploration from a midwifery perspective, through Northern Ireland's recent past revealed a progress of strategies for change, both negative and positive. We examined Northern Ireland's concerns and hopes through demography, health and social factors, practice roles, education of midwives, leadership in midwifery and women's choices, all with a part to play in the development of midwifery practice. Slowly emerging, and highlighted in the story of a home birth in Northern Ireland, is the fact that progress towards freedom to practise midwifery is happening.

Johanson et al (2002) identified the factors that impacted on changing a culture as the right attitude, leadership, teamwork, support and commitment to best practice. This chapter notes the requirement for leadership at Government level but also the need for midwives to work in partnership not only within the midwifery profession but also with the women who use the maternity services. Many midwives within Northern Ireland have a commitment to provide best care but within current settings are struggling for true autonomy.

However, there is a strong desire to establish and promote the role of the midwife and redress the imbalance of power between the medical and midwifery models. There is evidence of innovative practice within every trust and attempts to raise the midwifery profile throughout the Province. The challenge is now for Northern Ireland midwives to embrace the need for change, and build on the groundwork already begun, to establish their true identity. Northern Ireland to date may have no consultant midwives, no independent midwives and no stand-alone midwifery-led birthing centres, but a growing number of midwives is working to redress these issues. The status quo is not an option.

## Reflective questions

Some midwives do not feel that their midwifery education equips them for professional autonomy. Do you think that your midwifery education is taking/has taken you in the right direction for you to be able to be free to practise midwifery? If 'no' what can you do about it? If 'yes' how can you maintain this for your own practice and to help the practice of your colleagues?

# References

Barrowman L, Clarke R 2003 Northern Ireland in changing midwifery environments. British Journal of Midwifery 11(10):s12

Birthchoice. Maternity statistics. Online. Available at: http://www.birthchoiceuk.com (accessed 6 May 2006)

Campbell I 2005 Making a difference for non-English speaking women. Poster Display, International Congress for Midwives, 25–28 July, Brisbane, Australia

Council Directive of 21 January, 1980, (80/155/EEC). Official Journal of the European Communities, No L 33/8, 11280

Currie C 2004 Master's degree why bother? British Journal of Nursing 13(19):1123

Davis K 2003 We must be the first point of contact for pregnant women. British Journal of Midwifery 11(10):S6

DoH 1970 Peel Report Standing Maternity and Midwifery Advisory Committee. Domiciliary midwifery and maternity bed needs: report of a sub-committee. HMSO, London

DoH 1993 Report of the Expert Maternity Group, Changing Childbirth. Part 1. HMSO, London

DoH 2000 Millennium Executive Team Report on Winter 1999/2000. Online. Available at: http://www.dh.gov.uk/assetRoot/04/01/46/90 (accessed 6 May 2006)

DHSS 1994 Report of the Northern Ireland Maternity Unit Study Group, Delivering Choice. HMSO, Belfast

DHSSPS 2003 The Centralisation of Belfast Maternity Services Analysis of Responses to the Consultation Document March 2003. Online. Available at: http://www.dhsspsni.gov.uk/index/health_and_social services review (accessed 8 March 2006)

DHSSPS 2005 Centralisation of Belfast Maternity Services Announcement of Ministerial Decision. Online. Available at: http://www.dhsspsni.gov.uk/hss/maternity (accessed)

Donnison J 1988 Midwives and Medical Men: a History of the Struggle for the Control of Childbirth, 2nd edn. Historical Publications Ltd, London

Downe S, McCormick C, Beech B 2001 Labour interventions associated with normal birth. British Journal of Midwifery 9(10):602–606

Dr Foster. Welcome to the Dr Foster Good Birth Guide. Online. Available at: http://www.drfoster.co.uk/localservices/birthGuide.asp (accessed 4 April 2006)

Expert Maternity Group 1993 Changing Childbirth Part 1. HMSO, London

Fleming V 1998 Autonomous or automatons? An exploration through history of the concept of autonomy in midwifery in Scotland and New Zealand. Nursing Ethics 5(1):43–51

Hunt S 1995 15th Dame Rosalind Paget Memorial Lecture, The social meaning of midwifery. Midwives Chronicle 108(1292):283–8

Johanson R, Newburn M, Macfarlane A 2002 Has medicalisation of child-birth gone too far? British Medical Journal 324(7342):892–895

Kirkham M 1989 Midwives and information giving during labour. In: Robinson S, Thompson A M (eds) Midwives Research And Childbirth, Volume 1. Chapman and Hall, London, 117–138

Kitzinger S 2005 The Politics of Birth. Elsevier, Edinburgh

Loudon I 1992 Death in Childbirth. Clarendon Press, Oxford

Madden E 2005 A birth vision. Midwives 8(2):68–71

Madden KE, McDaid K, Donaghy H et al 2003 Midwife-led care. Royal College of Midwives Professional Development Forum Development Seminar Auditorium, 5 November, Lagan Valley, Lisburn

McCormack B, Manley K, Garbett R (eds) 2004 Practice Development in Nursing. Blackwell Publishing, Oxford

McWhirter L 2002 Health and Social Care in Northern Ireland: a Statistical Profile, 2002 edition. Online. Available at: www.dhsspsni.gov.uk/publications (accessed 6 March 2006)

Mander R, Fleming V (eds) 2002 Failure to Progress: the Contraction of the Midwifery Profession. Routledge, London

National Childbirth Trust, media centre. http://press.nct.org.uk/pressrelease?prid (accessed)

Newburn M 2002 A birth policy for the National Childbirth Trust. MIDIRS Midwifery Digest, 12:122–126

Ng M, Sinclair M 2002 Women's experience of planned home birth: a phenomenological study RCM Midwives Journal 5(2):56–59

NIPEC 2005 An exploration of nursing and midwifery roles in Northern Ireland. Online. Available at: http://www.nipec.n-i.nhs.uk

Northern Ireland Maternity Unit Study Group 1994 Delivering Choice. Department of Health and Social Security, Belfast

NIPEC 2005 Northern Ireland Practice and Education Council for Nursing and Midwifery An exploration of nursing and midwifery roles in Northern Ireland. Online. Available at: http://www.nipec.n-i.nhs.uk (6 March 2006)

O'Connor M 2000 Midwifery for all or midwifery for none? Midwifery Matters, Issue 87:14–18. Online. Available at: Association of Radical Midwives website: http://www.midwifery.org.uk (accessed 6 March 2006)

Pairman S 2000 International trends and partnerships in midwifery education. Adapted from a paper presented at the International Confederation of Midwives Asia-Pacific Region Conference, October, Bali. Online. Available at: http://www.midwife.org.nz (accessed 6 April 2006)

Pollard K 2003 Searching for autonomy. Midwifery June 19(2):113–124

RCM 2004 Home birth 'as safe as hospital'. Online. Available at: http://www.midirs.org/midirs

RCM 2005 Campaign for Normal Birth. Online. Available at: http://www.rcmnormalbirth.org.uk/

RCM 2006 Campaign for normal birth. RCM professional page-leadership courses. Online. Available at: http://www.rcm.org.uk (accessed 6 May 2006)

Reid L 2005 Making normal birth a reality: sharing good practice and strategies that work. Report of NCT Conference, Belfast, 30 September 2004. The Practising Midwife, 8(1):44–45

RCOG 2001 National Sentinel Audit. Online. Available at: http://www.nice.org.uk (accessed )

SHHD 1993 The Provision of Maternity Services in Scotland: A Policy Review. HMSO, Edinburgh

Sinclair M 2001 Midwives' attitudes to the use of the cardiotocograph machine. Journal of Advanced Nursing 35(4):599–606

Sinclair M, Brown G, Jones A 1999 Project-based learning in midwifery education. The Practising Midwife 2(2):19–22

Sinclair M, Gardner J 2001 Midwives' perceptions of the use of technology in assisting childbirth in Northern Ireland. Journal of Advanced Nursing October 36(2):229

Symonds A, Hunt S C 1996 The Midwife And Society: Perspectives, Policies and Practice. Macmillan Press, London

Tew M 1998 Safer Childbirth? A Critical History of Maternity Care, 3rd edn. Free Association Books, London

Towler J, Butler-Manuel R 1975 Modern Obstetrics for Student Midwives. Lloyd-Luke Medical Books, London

Wagner M 1994 Pursuing the Birth Machine. The Search for Appropriate Birth Technology. ACE Graphics, Australia

Welsh Office 1996 Welsh Maternity Services Review. HMSO, Cardiff

WHO 2000 Conference Scope and Purpose. Second WHO Ministerial Conference on Nursing and Midwifery Munich, Germany, June EUR/00/5019309/2

World Health Organisation Online Available at: http://www.who.int./ health-services-delivery/nursing/index.htm

## Additional resources

Babyworld. How to arrange a home birth. Online. Available at: http:// www.babyworld.co.uk/information/birth/homebirth/how_arrange.htm (accessed 4 April 2005)

Birthing the Future. All About Birth. Holland's lesson. Online. Available at: http://www.birthingthefuture.com/AllAboutBirth/hollandslesson. php (accessed 4 April 2005)

National Childbirth Trust, media centre. http://press.nct.org.uk/ pressrelease?prid (accessed 4 April 2005)

Northern Ireland Maternity Unit Study Group (1994) Delivering Choice. Department of Health and Social Security, Belfast

Office for National Statistics website: http://www.statistics.gov.uk/

# CHAPTER FIVE

# Midwifery practice in Ghana and Malawi: influences of the health system

JULIA HUSSEIN, ANN MATEKWE-PHOYA, JANET
ANSONG TORNUI AND TAMUNOSA OKIWELU

Few midwives trained as health professionals today practise entirely in isolation from some sort of formal support or institutional structure. Their training is usually organised and regulated by educational governing bodies linked to the health sector. Midwives may go on to practise as community or facility providers of care and those practising in the public sector will usually take up employment by a health authority. Similar arrangements would generally exist in the private sector. Even for the minority of midwives who practise independently or in very remote locations, most will have reason to utilise essential equipment, drugs or referral systems provided by a health system. The term health system is thus used in this chapter to describe the wider context or environment within which midwives practise, including the systems which train, govern and regulate midwifery practice, provide essential supplies and equipment, set up referral mechanisms and organise private and public care provision. These are all factors which determine the environment in which midwifery care takes place, and therefore how midwives practise.

The health system's influence on midwifery practice is the reason why we see this chapter on midwifery and the health system as an essential part of how midwives define their role and practice. A midwife's 'freedom to practise' is often a function of the health system, as the environment within which they practise. This very situation can be seen in a positive light, with the health system providing the 'enabling environment' necessary optimally to manage a pregnancy or delivery (Graham et al 2001, Bell et al 2003a). This may be in normal birth or when complications occur and if additional resources are required. Instead of functioning as a support mechanism,

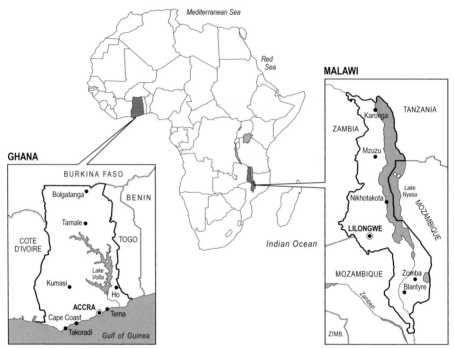

*Figure 5.1* Political map of Africa, with inserts detailing Malawi and Ghana
Sources: Malawi map, https://www.cia.gov/cia/publications/factbook/geos/gh.
html; Ghana map, http://www.cia.gov/cia/publications/factbook/geos/gh.html;
Outline map of Africa, http://www.cdli.ca/CITE/maps.htm

factors in the health system can however also act as barriers and hindrances
to the practice of a midwife. In this chapter, we explore the realities of how
the health system can affect the practice of midwives in two sub-Saharan
African countries, Ghana and Malawi (see Figure 5.1).

# The global maternal health context

Why have we chosen to highlight the situation of midwives in these two
countries? To answer this question, we need firstly to consider the role of
midwifery in the global maternal health context. Every year, more than
half a million women around the world die due to reasons related to childbirth and pregnancy (World Health Organization (WHO) 2005). More
than 97% of these deaths occur today in the less developed countries. In
terms of numbers of maternal deaths, the burden is suffered almost equally
between Africa (47.5%) and Asia (47.8%), as shown in Figure 5.2 (UNICEF/
UNFPA/WHO 2004).

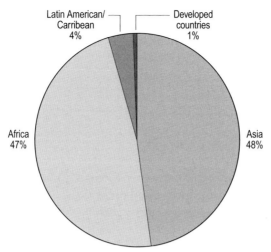

*Figure 5.2* Proportion of maternal deaths by world regions. Source: UNICEF/ UNFPA/WHO 2004

However, in terms of the risk experienced by a mother with each delivery, the countries with the greatest burden are predominantly those in sub-Saharan Africa with countries such as Sierra Leone and Malawi having the highest maternal mortality ratios of over 1000 deaths per 100 000 live births (AbouZahr 2003). These are over 100 times greater than the maternal mortality experienced in countries such as the UK (13 deaths per 100 000 live births) and Sweden (2 deaths per 100 000 live births) (UNICEF/ UNFPA/WHO 2004).

The full scale of the daily tragedy of deaths in many developing countries is not captured by these numbers of death alone. Many more women survive long, difficult and dangerous labours, only to be left physically and psychologically scarred by socially embarrassing and debilitating conditions. It is estimated that 15–20 million women will develop serious long-term disabilities including chronic pain, urinary incontinence and infertility (Ashford 2002) as a result of pregnancy or childbirth. For the same reasons that pregnant women suffer, millions of babies die – and many of those who survive bear the burden of disability throughout their lives.

It is perhaps useful to reflect that in many developed countries, this same situation was taking place not so long ago. One of the most influential texts written on the historical patterns of maternal deaths was Irvine Loudon's

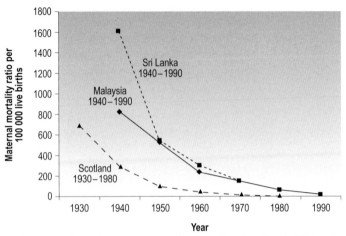

*Figure 5.3* Historical declines in maternal mortality: Scotland, Malaysia and Sri Lanka. Sources: Loudon 1992, Pathmanathan et al 2003

treatise in 1992. Loudon examined records from several countries in Europe and North America to as far back as the 1800s, investigating trends in maternal deaths in the context of social, political, economic, demographic and medical advances of the time. For example, only 70 years ago, more than a thousand women in Scotland died every year in childbirth. Bleeding, prolonged labour, 'toxaemia' or high blood pressure, abortion and puerperal fever were the main causes of death. The year 1935 marked the beginning of a period of dramatic change. In the space of the 15 years between 1935 and 1950, Scotland experienced a drop in maternal deaths by a remarkable 83%. Historical evidence available from countries such as Sweden and the UK, and more recently from other developing countries like Sri Lanka and Malaysia, suggest that the same pattern of declines in maternal mortality have repeatedly been achieved (Figure 5.3).

These carefully documented events across the world are not simply a matter of historical interest. Estimated numbers of maternal deaths today in some of the poorest countries in the world are comparable to what was happening in Sri Lanka and Malaysia as recently as the 1940s, and in Scotland and the UK in the 1920s and 1930s. The causes of death remain the same, although the world has changed in many ways. Antibiotics, blood transfusion, new drugs to prevent and treat bleeding in labour; better anaesthesia, better training in midwifery and obstetric skills are all thought to have led to the observed improvements in the countries where maternal mortality has reduced (Loudon 1992, Pathmanathan et al 2003). Even though these modern day technologies are available in most developing countries, the question remains as to why we still struggle to reduce the number of maternal deaths in many parts of the world.

The reasons for this are complex. Some will say that reducing these deaths must await economic development, despite examples such as Sri Lanka where the decline in maternal deaths occurred despite relatively poor indicators of economic development. Others continue to seek 'magic bullets' in the form of new clinical technologies: a suppository to prevent and treat haemorrhage, a pill to swallow which will induce abortion in unwanted pregnancies or a once off jab to increase uptake and compliance for family planning. But none of these technologies can be the sole answer, as they need to take into account women's perspectives and needs, and be delivered through well functioning health systems and by competent providers of care.

Making better maternity care services available and accessible is therefore important. There are many diverse and confusing strategies proposed to improve services for maternity care (Berer and Sundari Ravindran 1999, Bullough et al 2005, Hussein and Clapham 2005), although these are all united in their common goal of reducing maternal mortality and improving maternal health. In 1994, the Programme of Action of the International Conference on Population and Development (ICPD) at Cairo gained consensus and recognition from 179 countries that the reduction of maternal mortality is a key priority for development. In September 2000, 191 nations adopted the United Nations Millennium Declaration, further acknowledging the burden that pregnancy-related deaths and disability place on poor populations. One key strategy is now being recommended by the WHO – to reduce the number of maternal deaths by providing skilled attendance at delivery (Box 5.1). To underscore the importance placed on this strategy, the percentage of deliveries with health professionals is included as an indicator to measure progress against the Millennium Development Goal, along with the target of reducing maternal mortality by 75% by 2015. This strategy thus places the skilled attendant – in most cases, a professional midwife – centre stage in global efforts to reduce maternal mortality.

Most midwives who practise in the rich, developed Western world will, thankfully, never see a maternal death throughout their careers. But for the vast majority of women in the rest of the world, pregnancy and childbirth is still a dangerous journey from which there may be no return. We cannot allow this scandal to be repeated over and again in this twenty-first century

Box 5.1 International statement on the importance of midwifery skills

Having a health worker with midwifery skills present at childbirth, backed-up by transport in case emergency referral is required, is perhaps the most critical intervention for making motherhood safer.

*Safe Motherhood Technical Consultation, Colombo (1997)*

(Graham 1998). It is for this reason we have chosen to focus on the practice of midwives in Ghana and Malawi – countries which have been successful in placing high political priority on reducing maternal mortality and where midwives have had a long established tradition of professionalism and high standards of training. We explore the challenges placed on midwifery practice in relation to the health system and illustrate how midwives in these countries have been constrained or enabled in their 'freedom to practise'.

## The historical development of midwifery in Ghana: foundations of a health system

On the western coast of Africa, north of the equator (Figure 5.1), Ghana is a country rich in natural resources such as gold, timber and diamonds. The country has made considerable social, economic and political progress, with a gross national income (GNI) of over US$380 per capita (Table 5.1). Populated by 21 million people, literacy rates in Ghana are reported to be 55% in women (Ghana Statistical Service 2004). A number of health indicators in infant mortality and overall life expectancy have shown consistent improvements since the 1960s (Ghana Statistical Service 2004, WHO 2005) despite the HIV epidemic, which was first identified in Ghana in 1986, but has not reached the proportions seen in other parts of Africa. The 2002 adult HIV prevalence was reported to be 2% in 2003 (Ghana Statistical Service 2004).

Concerns of poverty and the health of the population are important issues in Ghana – more than a quarter of the population in Ghana are thought to live below the extreme poverty line (Gayn-Baffour 2005). Maternal health has featured as a crucial need in recent reviews of sectoral readjustment efforts in Ghana, with data indicating persistent and unacceptably high maternal mortality ratios, estimated to be as high as 540 per 100 000 live births (UNICEF/UNFPA/WHO 2004). Indicators of antenatal care and delivery care with health professionals show continued but slow improvements (Bell et al 2003b) over the past decade.

Table 5.1 Malawi and Ghana: key indicators at a glance

| Indicator | Malawi | Ghana |
|---|---|---|
| Total population (people) | 12 million[1] | 21 million[6] |
| Gross national income per capita, US$ | 170[2] | 380[2] |
| Female literacy | 49%[3] | 55%[3] |
| Life expectancy at birth (years) | 42[3] | 58[3] |
| Infant mortality rate per 1000 live births | 76[3] | 64[3] |
| Under five mortality rate per 1000 live births | 133[3] | 111[3] |
| Total fertility rate | 6.1[3] | 4.1[3] |
| Maternal mortality per 100000 live births | 1120[1] | 540[7] |
| Antenatal care coverage | 93%[4] | 92%[6] |
| Proportion deliveries with health professionals | 57%[4] | 47%[6] |
| Physicians, density per 100000 population | 1[5] | 9[5] |
| Midwives, density per 100000 population | 26[5] | 84[5] |

Sources of data:
[1] National Statistical Office Malawi 2001
[2] World Bank 2005
[3] World Health Organization 2005
[4] National Statistical Office Malawi 2005
[5] World Health Organization 2004
[6] Ghana Statistical Service 2004
[7] UNICEF/UNFPA/WHO 2004

# History of midwifery in Ghana

The role of the midwife in the healthcare delivery system in Ghana was founded as far back as 1917 over concerns of infant wellbeing (Ofosu-Amaah 1981). Concerned about the high mortality among infants, the Government at the time set up a committee to investigate the causes. The committee's report revealed that poor midwifery practice and particularly inadequate postnatal care to both mother and infant were the main causes of the high infant mortality rate. The committee recommended that the Government should open maternity hospitals and train midwives to attend to mothers and their babies.

Consequently, in 1927 the Government selected two districts in the capital city of Accra to start domiciliary midwifery in Ghana. Two African midwives trained in England were employed to work there. These midwives were encouraged to work with and give practical demonstration to traditional midwives to improve their skills. A year later, the Korle Bu Maternity Hospital was opened in Accra to provide professional midwifery care and training. This hospital remains the main teaching hospital and reference centre in Ghana to this day. In 1930, the first batch of the locally trained midwives graduated. In 1931, legislation for the training, examination, registration and practice of midwifery was promulgated. In 1932, the first midwives' ordinance was passed and the Central Midwives Board constituted. All midwives who graduated from 1930 were thus formally issued their certificates of registration.

As the years went by, other maternity hospitals and midwifery training schools were opened in the various regions of Ghana. There are also many private maternity homes and hospitals scattered throughout the country which participate as training sites, leading to a wide network of midwifery training facilities.

## Training and regulation

Initially, there were two categories of nurses who were trained as midwives – the Qualified Registered Nurse (QRN) and the State Registered Nurse (SRN). The period of midwifery training for both was 18 months. Later, the period of training for the SRN was reduced to 12 months. This was when 3 months of midwifery training was introduced into the SRN curriculum. The QRN continued to train in midwifery for 18 months but this training was phased out in 1970.

There are presently three categories of midwifery training programmes in Ghana. The one-year post basic SRN programme is described above. A two-year post basic Enrolled/Community Health Nursing Programme selects candidates after an entrance examination. Training takes two years after which they are awarded certificates to practise as midwives. The direct midwifery (Diploma) programme is a three-year programme designed for senior secondary school graduates. Students are required to submit one client care study and a group research project during the programme which forms part of the requirement for the final licensure examination. Both public and private sector maternity units are used for the students' clinical experience where there are preceptors or experienced midwives to supervise them. In 1999, a thesis-based graduate programme at the University of Ghana was implemented, thus furthering the status and recognition of nursing and midwifery as professions, with a PhD programme planned for the future (Ogilvie et al 2005).

Apart from the district, regional and national health authorities that control the activities of the midwives, the Nurses and Midwives Council for Ghana is mandated to: maintain professional standards; inspect and supervise the midwife both in public and private institutions to make sure that standards are maintained. The Ghana Registered Midwives Association is an association of private practitioners, and also supervises its members and ensures maintenance of standards. The association organises workshops and courses for its members to upgrade their knowledge and skills in practice. Every midwife is required to have an update of not fewer than five days in every three years before the renewal of their professional identification number by the Council.

# The Ghanaian health system and practice of midwifery

Public health services in Ghana are organised in five tiers – national, regional, district, sub-district and community. The sub-district facilities comprise health centres, health posts and clinics. About two-thirds of the 100 districts have a district hospital. In each district, the district Director of health services heads the district health management team and oversees all health services. Each of the ten regions has a regional health director, and eight of the ten regions have regional hospitals. These regional hospitals act as referral hospitals for the district level. At national level, there are three psychiatric hospitals and two university teaching hospitals. Other providers in the health system include the police and military health facilities.

Ghana has a large private health sector. It is estimated that between 50% and 70% of health care services are provided outside the public sector. These private providers include religious organisations, employers, private practitioners and charitable organisations, along with an informal private sector such as dispensers and traditional practitioners of all kinds. There is some evidence to suggest that the quality of maternity care provided may not be as high in the private for profit sector as in the Government or mission facilities (Hussein et al 2004).

In Ghana a professional midwife is a person who, having been admitted into a midwifery school which is duly recognised by the state, has successfully completed the prescribed course of studies in midwifery and has acquired the requisite qualification to be registered and or legally licensed to practise midwifery. She must be able to give the necessary supervision, care and advice to women during pregnancy, labour and the postpartum period, to conduct normal deliveries on her own and to care for the newborn and the infant. This care includes preventive measures, the detection of abnormal conditions in mother and child, the procurement of medical assistance and the execution of emergency measures in the absence of medical help. She is also a health counsellor and educator for her clients, family and community at large. Her work should involve antenatal education and preparation for parenthood and extend to certain areas of gynaecology, family planning and child care. She may also have expanded responsibilities to deal with complications, performing procedures according to her training, for example to conduct deliveries by vacuum extraction. She may practise in hospitals, maternity homes and health centres in both the public and private sectors.

Ghana health policy has well laid out guidelines and protocols for staffing of the different health services (Ministry of Health, Republic of Ghana 2000a, b). Maternity units are staffed by at least one professional midwife who should have access to a range of essential emergency obstetric care drugs and supplies. Instrumental vaginal deliveries can also be conducted at this level. The maternity units in district hospitals are staffed by a team of midwives, along with at least one doctor. Drugs and equipment are limited at district hospital level, but most will be capable of providing anaesthesia and conducting operative deliveries 24 hours a day. However, the interest and experience of the doctor in obstetric care will differ, and quite often the main responsibility for emergency obstetric care will fall upon a senior midwife. At regional and national level, a team of midwives, with a fully qualified obstetrician or experienced surgeon, as well as anaesthesiologist will be available.

Despite these clearly defined roles, women in Ghana are utilising maternity services only selectively. Surveys of women's utilisation for professional delivery suggest only slow changes (Bell et al 2003b, Ghana Statistical Service 2004). The barriers experienced are similar to those seen in many developing countries. Geographical and financial barriers have been identified. In Ghana, user fees were payable for delivery care services for several years even in public facilities, but increasing realisation of the effects of financial hardship barrier faced by the poorest, especially for maternity services, led to the introduction of universal fee exemption for delivery care in 2003. This policy is meant to increase the utilisation of skilled care at delivery and thus contribute to reducing maternal mortality. Other factors leading to the relatively low utilisation of services include a lack of confidence in the services (Opoku et al 1997), poor attitudes of health personnel and mistrust of health professionals (D'Ambruoso et al 2005).

Ghana's well-structured system with a long history of placing emphasis on the value of professional midwives has resulted in organised midwifery practices and regulation in Ghana. Despite the advantage of this strong foundation, the leadership in nursing and midwifery is thought to be relatively weak and indeed deteriorating, with few opportunities for nurses and midwives to participate in decision-making processes (Odoi 2003). Ghana has also recently faced a disturbing exodus of health professionals to other countries (Martineau et al 2004, Mensah et al 2005). The documented poor attitudes of midwives (D'Ambruoso et al 2005) are other symptoms of dissatisfaction and insecurities within midwives which are not well addressed within the Ghanaian health system.

# Midwives in Malawi: a critical resource for healthcare systems

Malawi is a small land-locked country south of the equator in sub-Saharan Africa. Densely populated with 12 million people, Malawi is among the poorest countries in the world with a GNI per capita of US$170 (World Bank 2005). There is a large inequality in the distribution of income with 63% of the population living below the absolute poverty line. More than 80% of the population engages in subsistence farming and food insecurity is prevalent due to the high cost of agricultural inputs and dependency on unpredictable rainfall. Literacy in Malawi is low: 51% of women are not literate (National Statistical Office Malawi 2001).

Health indicators for the country are among the worst in the world (Table 5.1). Infant and under-five mortality in the past five years has shown some improvements. Currently, infant mortality is 76 per 1000 live births – a drop from 104 in 2000. Similarly, under-five mortality has dropped from 189 per 1000 live births in 2000 to 133 in 2004 (National Statistical Office Malawi 2005). However, life expectancy at birth stands at only 42 years, partly due to the HIV epidemic. The estimated human immunodeficiency virus (HIV)/acquired immune deficiency syndrome (AIDS) prevalence in adults aged between 15 and 49 years of age is one of the highest in the world at 14.4%. Levels of HIV infection in the adult population have remained constant for the past seven years; among adults in urban areas it is over 20%. Heterosexual transmission accounts for 90% of HIV infection in the country. Vertical transmission of HIV from mother to child contributes about 9% of infections and unsafe blood products contribute to about 1% (Malawi National AIDS Commission 2004).

A Malawian woman today will have, on average, six children in her lifetime. Antenatal care uptake is high, with 93% of women seeking these services. Only 57% of deliveries occur with a health professional present (National Statistical Office Malawi 2005) with slow improvement from 53% in 1992 (Bell et al 2003b). In contrast to the improvements in child mortality, maternal mortality has remained consistently high in the past decade with an estimated 1120 deaths per 100 000 live births (National Statistical Office Malawi 2001). The major determinants of this high ratio include the high fertility rate, poor access to quality obstetric care and the effects of HIV/AIDS.

## The health system

Nearly all formal healthcare services in Malawi are provided by three main agencies. The Ministry of Health provides 60% of services; the Christian Health Association of Malawi 37%; and the Ministry of Local Government provides 1%. Private practitioners, commercial companies, the armed forces and non-government organisations provide the rest, with a very small private for profit sector. Health facilities managed by the providers cited above form an extensive and comprehensive infrastructure comprising dispensaries, health centres, community hospitals, district hospitals and central hospitals. Dispensaries and health centres offer primary health care as the first point of entry into the formal healthcare system. The district and central hospitals provide secondary and tertiary care. These health facilities enable at least 54% of the rural population to access formal health services within a 5 km radius. This proportion increases to 84% in urban areas.

Despite this orderly and comprehensive health infrastructure, barriers to access of health services exist, and include geographical and financial factors for many communities. Financial barriers are experienced by those communities served by health facilities operated by organisations or private clinics which charge user fees. Government facilities do not charge user fees although the quality of care in government facilities can be adversely affected by critical staff shortages, inadequate supplies or essential equipment. Lack of electricity and running water is an additional problem for rural health facilities. Difficulties of geographical access particularly in rural communities are compounded by poor transport and communication systems, especially for timely referral.

The health work force in the different types of health facilities includes a number of health professions. Medical doctors are in general and specialised practice although their numbers for the size of population in Malawi are relatively low with only 1 physician per 100 000 population (WHO 2004). Their role is supplemented by clinical officers and medical assistants. Dentists, pharmacists, nurse-midwives, laboratory and radiography technicians and physiotherapists are the other types of health professionals represented in the health system. Nurse-midwives form the majority of health workers, acting as the backbone of the healthcare system as they manage nearly 95% of health centres. There are two categories of nurse-midwives in the country, the professional nurse-midwife, also known as the registered nurse-midwife; and the enrolled nurse-midwife or nurse-midwifery technician.

# Educational preparation of the professional midwife

Professional midwives in Malawi are required to train firstly as a registered nurse; consequently a registered nurse-midwife in the Malawian context is a graduate nurse who has completed four years of university education (Bachelor of Science in Nursing) and an extra year of midwifery. Before starting the fifth year of midwifery training, the prospective student midwife is expected to pass a licensing examination as a general nurse. Prior to 1993, registered nurse-midwives were trained at diploma/certificate level for four years (three years as a general nurse and one year as a midwife). Between 1975 and 1995 training in midwifery was compulsory for every nurse. The midwifery compulsory training policy was part and parcel of the second national health plan of the country (1973–1985) which placed emphasis on the delivery of maternal and child health services. Nurse-midwives are therefore viewed by Government as a comprehensively trained health worker who could provide a package of maternal and child health services with minimum support or back-up from medical doctors.

Compulsory midwifery training was suspended in 1995 as experience showed that not all nurse-midwives practised midwifery and it was felt that the costs of the extra year of training were not well utilised. With the high maternal mortality in Malawi, and current constraints experienced in providing skilled care to all births, the Malawian Government is considering reintroducing compulsory midwifery training.

The second category of nurse-midwives in the country includes the enrolled nurse-midwives who are trained at nursing colleges or schools. The training is either for three disjointed years (two year general nursing and one year midwifery), or a continuous three-year integrated nursing/midwifery curriculum.

# Regulatory structures

The training and practice of nurse-midwives in the country is regulated by the Nurses and Midwives Council of Malawi, established under the Nurses and Midwives Act of Malawi in 1965 and 1995. Regulation is implemented through the setting of the syllabus to be followed by all nurse training institutions including the university and the administration of licensing examinations to graduates who have successfully completed their training. This examination assesses acquisition of prescribed competencies as well as safety to practise independently. The Council also prescribes the scope of practice for each category of nurse-midwife. In addition to general nursing and midwifery procedures, the Registered Nurse Midwife (RNM) in Malawi is licensed to carry out a number of specific procedures related to complications of pregnancy and childbirth. These are to provide antenatal care including external cephalic version, conduct normal deliveries including twin deliveries, deliver malpresentations, perform vacuum (ventouse) extraction and manual removal of placenta, resuscitate an asphyxiated baby through intubation, suture first and second degree tears, give parenteral fluids including antibiotics and blood, insert intra-uterine devices for family planning and carry out manual vacuum aspiration for incomplete abortion (Ministry of Health and Population 2004).

The Enrolled Nurse Midwife (ENM) has the same scope of practice except for delivery of malpresentations, vacuum extraction, manual vacuum aspiration and intubation. The syllabus for this category has now been revised to include these skills as these nurse-midwives practise alone in health centres where most rural women deliver. Nurse-midwives working in the Government and church related facilities perform these tasks without any interference from medical doctors. Nearly 98% of all births assisted by health workers are attended by midwives (National Statistical Office Malawi 2005). Despite the introduction of a medical school in Malawi, with increasing availability of medical doctors and clinical officers in district hospitals, these changes have not brought in any limitation to the scope of practice for the midwife. One challenge is, however, the availability of cases for training purposes – at the teaching hospitals, both medical and midwifery students have to compete against each other to gain sufficient experience.

## Status and practice of midwives in Malawi

Nurse-midwives in Malawi enjoy a high level of status and prestige as independent practitioners. There is recognition that the nurse-midwife is properly trained to provide a wide range of maternal and child health services. Due to the shortage of medical doctors, clinical officers and medical assistants, the Government has created an enabling policy environment in the regulation of the nursing and midwifery professions. The high standards of training enable the nurse-midwife to function in a wide range of settings. For example, at health centres, enrolled nurse midwives function as managers of the facility, but also as a clinician and midwife, conducting general outpatient clinics for adult patients, under-five clinics for both well and sick babies, family planning, antenatal and postnatal clinics as well as caring for women during labour and delivery.

At district hospitals, the nurse-midwives undertake the functions outlined according to the scope of practice established by the Nurses and Midwives Council, as described earlier. In most cases, it is the midwife who undertakes the care of all women in labour, managing obstetric complications such as eclampsia and puerperal sepsis using standing order treatment protocols and making clinical judgements on the need for specific procedures. In the case of operative deliveries, it is often the senior nurse midwife who makes the decision while the clinical officer or medical doctor merely confirms the diagnosis and performs the procedure.

Although the healthcare system has conferred a high professional status and responsibility on the nurse-midwife there are few appropriate mechanisms for reward or provision of a conducive work environment for nurse-midwives. The salary remunerations are poor and not commensurate with the role and high degree of responsibility of the midwives. Career mobility is limited as there are few senior grades in the system. It is not uncommon to find a nurse-midwife who has served on post for years without promotion. Workloads are heavy, and the short supply of nurse-midwives has meant that many working in rural areas and smaller health centres are expected to provide 24 hour care singly. The remoteness of some rural health centres, the road infrastructure and poor communication systems make many postings undesirable. Female health staff especially can feel unsafe and far from relatives, while also having to face challenges of caring for their families and providing a good education for their children. Given these conditions, it is perhaps unsurprising that Malawi is losing a critical resource – with an exodus of the most capable nurse-midwives from the public to the private sector, from rural to urban locations and from Malawi to other countries.

# Health systems and the freedom to practise: key issues

Both Ghana and Malawi have legacies of a well-organised and regulated health system with potential to provide an enabling environment for the practice of midwifery. However, given the context of poverty, a continent wide epidemic of HIV, and in the case of Malawi, these problems compounded by acute food shortages in recent years, the challenges of maintaining the health system are clearly resulting in dissatisfaction and low performance of many midwives, who form the backbone of health care service delivery.

Some of the factors commonly identified as unsatisfactory by nurses and midwives in a wide range of developing countries include: risky work environments; understaffing; high workloads; poor working conditions; and scarce material resources and salaries (Buchan and Calman 2004). Our descriptions of midwifery practice in Malawi and Ghana reflect these issues well. Most of them are clearly related to how the health system functions.

To synthesise these country specific experiences, we identify three key issues pertinent to the health system that have arisen out of our two country situations:

- Support and regulatory mechanisms and their effect on morale and motivation.
- The added stress on the practice of midwives from the HIV/AIDS epidemic in sub-Saharan Africa.
- Human resource challenges and the freedom to practise in the context of the global workforce.

## Support, regulation and motivation

Standards of professional education and training are high in Malawi and Ghana, equivalent to the training levels achieved by midwives in more developed countries. These high training standards are matched by the high levels of competency required – levels which are perhaps higher even than those expected of most midwives in the UK today. The model of childbirth followed in Malawi and Ghana is a composite of obstetric and midwifery practices (see Chapter 2, p 18), with midwives particularly in Malawi having extremely high levels of responsibility and independence from obstetricians for the management of complications in childbirth. There are fewer than 1–2 doctors for every 100 000 Malawians (the comparative WHO average is 1 in 10 000) (African Development Fund 2005, WHO 2005), and only three full time obstetricians practising in Malawi during the last human resource development survey (Ministry of Health and Population Malawi 1999a). Thus, the brunt of responsibility for care of women experiencing both normal and complicated pregnancies has fallen to midwives.

To what extent does the situation above address issues of freedom to practise? On the one hand, the situation described is enabling in nature, in that the regulatory bodies in Ghana and Malawi have been sufficiently flexible and responsive to local needs by licensing midwives to undertake responsibility for dealing with obstetric complications. The range of roles described for the two countries are to some degree matched to the needs identified within each. In Ghana, with slightly higher physician to population ratios than Malawi (Table 5.1, WHO 2005), their midwives can focus more on preventive and caring aspects of midwifery, whereas in Malawi, the needs for midwives to take on a leading clinical role are more acute. Indeed, this type of responsive approach to regulation can facilitate the availability of suitably trained staff, especially in rural locations where doctors and obstetricians are often unavailable (Bergstrom 2005). On the other hand, a number of disadvantages are apparent. The additional burden on midwives to provide care for complications undermines the important role they play in addressing 'social' and 'normality' needs. Given that we accept that bio-medical and woman-centred care are both required to contribute to a comprehensive view of maternity care, expanded scopes of responsibility expected of the midwife are likely to have consequences on the quality of care provided to women during pregnancy and childbirth, whether they experience complications or not. This will manifest itself in the form of maternity services that are not 'women-friendly' and contribute to the reluctance of women to utilise services, seeing them as places where they are treated in a rude and unfriendly manner.

There are other effects of this expanded scope of work which raise issues of quality. In both Malawi and Ghana, the pressures on human resource availability have led to the establishment of intermediate grades such as the enrolled nurse and shortened midwifery training. The danger is that with the limited training provided to these cadres of staff, it is uncertain as to whether supervision and continuing in-service education provided within the health system is sufficient to give the necessary support to these cadres. Furthermore, as happens in both our focus countries, as well as in many other developing countries, these are the individuals that tend to practise in the more remote and inaccessible areas with minimal support. Thus, a paradox of shorter training but limited continuing supervisory in-service support can become the reality of too many health service systems.

On balance, the systems of regulation and legislation in Ghana and Malawi are positive examples of how the health system has enabled an 'expanded' level of responsibility among midwives according to need. There is, however, also opportunity here to demonstrate how health systems can fail to support midwives' practice. The resource stretched health system in Malawi is well documented and acknowledged (Ministry of Health and Population Malawi 1999b), with profound shortages of essential drugs, supplies and equipment. Shortfalls in the number of health personnel and problems of maldistribution have also been highlighted. Too many facilities cannot provide simple infrastructure such as curtains, screens or a separate room to provide basic privacy to a woman in labour, simply because there are too many other priority needs. Some facilities also lack beds to accommodate all mothers, and the floor or sharing beds can become the order of the day. There are delivery units without running water due to the lack of resources to maintain old and outdated water supply systems. These 'failures' of the health system cannot but restrict 'best practice' and fail to see through the high expectations of the health system on midwives working in extraordinarily difficult conditions. The crucial consequence of this lack of support is demotivation and disillusionment.

# Practising midwifery in the context of high HIV prevalence

Throughout sub-Saharan Africa in particular, HIV/AIDS is increasing the demand on health services, as well as affecting the supply of services through availability and performance of health workers (Buchan and Calman 2004). The negative effect of HIV/AIDS on the health system is most pronounced in sub-Saharan Africa where 'near collapse' of health systems has been attributed to increasing workloads and effects on health workers (WHO and World Bank 2003).

Of the two countries described in this chapter, the high prevalence of HIV in Malawi cannot be ignored. Its effect on rising levels of maternal mortality since 1992 has been documented (National Statistical Office and ORC Macro 2001, Phoya and Bicego 2001) and remains a cause for much concern. A limited but growing body of knowledge on HIV and pregnancy exists (Berer 1999, Bullough 2003, McIntyre 2005). In addition to the effects of HIV/AIDS in pregnancy, this burden of disease has effects on the health system through the availability, quality and uptake of care (Graham and Newell 1999).

The HIV epidemic can be postulated to work through a range of means within the health system through its effects on health workers – midwives in particular and those working in countries where maternal mortality is highest (Graham and Hussein 2003). We have already explored the consequences of working in a health system where physical resources such as supplies and drugs are limited. HIV compounds this effect and diverts attention, funds and supplies away from essential services such as maternity care, in an effort to deal with the acute epidemic of HIV. In addition, it places additional resource needs on services such as blood transfusion and infection control.

Another consequence of the HIV epidemic works directly through the health workers themselves. The effects are complex and relate to new recruitment, retention of existing staff, and to the attitude of providers. In terms of recruitment, midwifery and some surgical specialities especially may be seen as 'high-risk' areas, discouraging potential applicants to enter training. This is a serious concern, especially when other factors such as arduous training, unsociable working hours, poor remuneration and low status already contribute to difficulties recruiting in midwifery schools. The retention of existing staff is also a key area which HIV has affected. Increasing death rates among health workers due to HIV is one obvious consequence – a situation well supported by evidence. As many as 50% of deaths in Government employees in Africa are estimated to be caused by HIV/AIDS (Tawfik and Kinot 2001). In Malawi, death is the most significant cause of losses in terms of numbers (Ministry of Health and Population Malawi 1999a) with death rates overall highest in the nursing/midwifery cadres. Of all deaths, 9% occur before the age of 40, and deaths of nurse-midwives are thought to account for over 40% of losses of this cadre to the health system. Apart from death, ill health and attendance at funerals also contribute to unavailability of staff for up to 50% of their working days (USAID/AED/SARA 2003, Buchan and Calman 2004).

The stigma of HIV also has real consequences on how health providers practise. Health workers may be reluctant to provide adequate care to those whom they think are infected due to real or perceived risks to themselves. The actual risk of HIV/AIDS transmission from patient to provider is small (Ippolito et al 1999) but taboos and insufficient knowledge levels among nurses and midwives need to be rectified. For example, it has been shown in several African settings that fear of contagion is common but less so if knowledge levels were high. Nevertheless, most health workers believed that their access to information on HIV/AIDS is inadequate (Mill et al 2004, Walusimbi and Okonsky 2004). The beliefs and attitudes of the health workers in high HIV prevalence settings is likely to affect their attitude to women and their motivation, with consequent effects on quality of care and utilisation of services.

The consequences of HIV on human resource availability within the health system already illustrate how the existing shortages of trained and experienced midwives in developing countries have been, and can continue to be, exacerbated.

## The brain drain: freedom to practise in the global workforce

Current levels of nursing and midwifery personnel in both Ghana and Malawi are poor. Ghana has 84 nurse-midwives per 100 000 population, while Malawi has 26 nurse-midwives per 100 000 population (WHO 2005). In comparison, the UK has more than 500 nurses and midwives per 100 000 population. Apart from deaths, resignation and retirement are the other main reasons associated with depletion of health workers in our two focus countries. Recruitment is usually constrained by funding and administrative decisions not meeting needs, while the capacity of training institutions to produce the numbers required to build up human resource capacity is limited (African Development Fund 2005). This low availability of nurses and/or midwives is exacerbated by a particular lack in remote and rural areas (Buchan and Calman 2004).

Over the period of five years from 1998 to 2003, the annual outflow of registered nurses to the UK from Ghana has increased six times. In Ghana, the Nurses and Midwives Council Register recorded 915 nurses requesting verification of their professional certification in 2002, giving an indication of the number of nurses intending to leave the country. In Malawi, recorded migration only to the UK increased from 1 nurse in 1998 to 47 in 2003 (Buchan and Calman 2004) – small numbers, but numbers which a small country with few numbers of trained professionals can ill afford. This marked migration, which is also seen in a number of other Sub-Saharan countries such as Nigeria, South Africa and Zimbabwe, is related to the factors discussed earlier – low pay, poor career prospects and lack of recognition. These motivational issues are compounded by the stresses on the health system and on the individual resulting from the HIV crises. Developed countries offer better prospects and also the opportunity to enhance education (Buchan and Calman 2005). From a health systems perspective, the negative implications of these migrations are clear. However, the resulting international inequities in healthcare have also been put forward from a rights perspective. Current Government policy responses are felt to be inadequate and misrepresentative of the ethical dilemmas, with under estimation of the pressures faced by health professionals (Mensah et al 2005). At an individual level, it is indeed difficult to be critical of a midwife, whose freedom to practise in environments conducive to self-advancement and better prospects for themselves and their families cannot and should not, be denied.

# The way forward

Having addressed the issues highlighted above as those arising from our case studies, what strategies can be suggested to pave the way forward for the future?

Continued improvements in the status and recognition of midwives as key members of any health workforce must be placed as a fundamental priority. Current expectations on the performance and role of midwives as health service providers should be matched by robust representation at policy level. Midwives can have a stronger voice in countries by investing in the development of active societies and organisations which can represent them. Profound health policy changes are required. Addressing the needs and motivational factors of midwives must reap long term benefits in the retention of midwifery care which will be of high quality, and accountable.

In sub-Saharan Africa especially, the added stress of dealing with HIV situations has to be dealt with. The recognition of risk must be prioritised. Provider perspectives of the effect of HIV on their practice cannot be ignored – information needs, safety aspects and dangers posed to health workers must be understood and acknowledged. Actions to address them are necessary, requiring changes in the way health systems work. Resources to combat HIV need to be channelled not only from a disease perspective, but also from the provider side.

As for the global workforce, the freedom to practise as a midwife must be respected. It should not be the policy of well resourced, attractive to live in, developed countries actively to recruit health professionals from poorer countries simply for their own needs. Neither should immigration laws be passed to prevent those seeking professional development and experience.

The midwifery profession has a heritage and a history of being part of the global movement to reduce maternal and infant mortality and morbidity. We have seen how the foundation of the professionalisation of midwives in Ghana and Malawi has provided a strong basis for the health systems of these countries. Midwives will nevertheless depend on the health system to provide a functional environment which supports the provision of high quality care. The community concerned with supporting the practice of midwifery care faces a number of key challenges today, and few of these problems can be solved without taking on a wider outlook. This outlook needs to reach beyond the perspective of a midwife as an individual practitioner to include the complex influences of the health system as a whole, and further to that, extend outside the boundaries of single nation states to consider also the effects and consequences of key global issues.

## Reflective questions

Midwives play an important part in every country's health system. Taking Malawi as an example, please reflect upon how 'failures' of a health system can restrict 'best practice' in midwifery.

How does the health system in your country influence midwifery practice?

Can you think of other ways which demonstrate a need for improvement with regard to midwifery and the influence of the health system?

## References

AbouZahr C 2003 Global burden of maternal death and disability. British Medical Bulletin. 67:1–11

African Development Fund 2005 Appraisal Report. Support to the health sector programme. Republic of Malawi Health Development Division,

Social Development Department, North-East-South Region, African Development Fund

Ashford L 2002 Hidden Suffering: disabilities from pregnancy and childbirth in less developed countries. Population Reference Bureau, Washington

Bell J, Hussein J, Jentsch B et al 2003a Improving skilled attendance at delivery: a preliminary report of the SAFE strategy development tool. Birth 30(4):227–234

Bell J, Curtis S L, Alayón S 2003b Trends in delivery care in six countries. DHS Analytical Studies No 7. ORC Macro and International Research Partnership for Skilled Attendance for Everyone (SAFE), Calverton, Maryland

Berer M 1999 HIV/AIDS, pregnancy and maternal mortality and morbidity: implications for care. In: Berer M, Sundari Ravindran TK (eds) Reproductive Health Matters Safe Motherhood Initiatives: Critical Issues. Blackwell Science, Oxford, pp 198–210

Berer M, Sundari Ravindran TK 1999 Preventing maternal mortality: evidence, resources, leadership, action. In: Berer M, Sundari Ravindran TK (eds) Reproductive Health Matters Safe Motherhood Initiatives: Critical Issues. Blackwell Science, Oxford, pp 3–9

Bergstrom S 2005 Who will do the caesareans when there is no doctor? Finding creative solutions to the human resource crisis. British Journal of Obstetrics and Gynaecology 112:1168–1169

Buchan J, Calman L 2004 The global shortage of registered nurses: An overview of issues and actions. International Council of Nurses, Geneva

Bullough C 2003 HIV infection, AIDS and maternal deaths. Tropical Doctor 33(4):194–196

Bullough C, Meda N, Makowiecka K et al 2005 Current strategies for the reduction of maternal mortality. British Journal of Obstetrics and Gynaecology 112:1180–1188

D'Ambruoso L, Abbey M, Hussein J 2005 Please understand when I cry out in pain: women's accounts of maternity services during labour and delivery in Ghana. BMC Public Health 5:140

Gayn-Baffour G 2005 The Ghana Poverty Reduction Strategy: Poverty diagnostics and components of the strategy. Online. Available at: http:// www.casmsite.org/ (accessed 28 December 2005)

Ghana Statistical Service (GSS), Noguchi Memorial Institute for Medical Research (NMIMR) and ORC Macro 2004 Ghana Demographic and Health Survey 2003. GSS, NMIMR and ORC Macro, Calverton, Maryland

Graham W 1998 The scandal of the century. British Journal of Obstetrics and Gynaecology 105:375–376

Graham W, Newell ML 1999 Seizing the opportunity: collaborative initiatives to reduce HIV and maternal mortality. The Lancet 353:836–839

Graham W, Hussein J 2003 Measuring and estimating maternal mortality in the era of HIV/AIDS. Workshop on HIV/AIDS and adult mortality in developing countries, Population Division Department of Economic and Social Affairs, United Nations Secretariat, New York 8–13 September UN/POP/MORT/2003/8. Online. Available at: http://www.un.org/esa/population/publications/adultmort/GRAHAM_Paper8.pdf (accessed 5 December 2005)

Graham WJ, Bell JS, Bullough CHW 2001 Can skilled attendance at delivery reduce maternal mortality in developing countries? Studies in Health Services Organisation and Policy 17:97–130

Hussein J, Clapham S 2005 Message in a bottle: sinking in a sea of safe motherhood concepts. Health Policy 73:294–302

Hussein J, Bell J, Nazzar A et al 2004 The Skilled Attendance Index (SAI): Proposal for a new measure of skilled attendance at delivery. Reproductive Health Matters 12(24):160–170

Ippolito G, Puro V, Heptonstall J et al 1999 Occupational human immunodeficiency virus infection in health care workers: Worldwide cases through September 1997 Clinical Infectious Diseases 28(2):365–383

Loudon I 1992 Death in childbirth. Clarendon Press, Oxford

Malawi National AIDS Commission 2004 Malawi National HIV/AIDS estimates 2003. Government of Malawi, Lilongwe, Malawi

Martineau T, Decker K, Bundred P 2004 'Brain drain' of health professionals: From rhetoric to responsible action. Health Policy 70(1):1–10

McIntyre J 2005 Maternal health and HIV. Reproductive Health Matters 13(25):129–135

Mensah K, Mackintosh M, Henry L 2005 The skills drain of health professionals from the developing world: A framework for policy formulation. AfricaFocus Bulletin March 29 2005

Mill JE, Opare M, Fleming DS 2004 Ghanaian nursing students' knowledge and attitudes about HIV illness. Africa Journal of Nursing and Midwifery 6(2):5–12

Ministry of Health and Population Malawi 1999a Malawi National Health Plan Vol 3: health sector human resource plan. Ministry of Health and Population, Lilongwe

Ministry of Health and Population Malawi 1999b Malawi National Health Plan 1999–2004. Ministry of Health and Population, Lilongwe

Ministry of Health and Population Malawi 2004 Program of Work. Ministry of Health and Population, Lilongwe

Ministry of Health, Republic of Ghana 2000a Vision 2020. Government of the Republic of Ghana, Accra

Ministry of Health, Republic of Ghana 2000b National Reproductive Health Service Policy and Standards. Government of the Republic of Ghana, Accra

National Statistical Office Malawi and ORC Macro 2001 Malawi Demographic and Health Survey 2000. National Statistical Office and ORC Macro, Zomba, Malawi and Calverton Maryland

National Statistical Office Malawi and ORC Macro 2005 Malawi Demographic and Health Survey 2004 Preliminary Report. National Statistical Office and ORC Macro, Zomba, Malawi and Calverton Maryland. Online. Available at: http://www.nso.malawi.net/ (accessed 28 December 2005)

Nurses and Midwives Act 1995 Government of Malawi. Lilongwe, Malawi

Odoi MH 2003 The present leadership crises in the Ghana nursing service: 'A critical problem and a big challenge to Ghanaian nurses'. West African Journal of Nursing 14(2):142–4

Ofosu-Amaah S 1981 The maternal and child health services in Ghana (their origins and future). Journal of Tropical Medicine and Hygiene 84(6):265–9

Ogilvie L, Opare M, Allen A et al 2005 Laying the foundation for nursing research in Ghana. Online. Available at: http://www.aucc.ca/_pdf/english/programs/colloquium/3b-Opare-Ogilvie.pdf (accessed 13 December 2005)

Opoku SA, Kyei-Faried D, Twum S et al 1997 Community education to improve utilisation of emergency obstetric services in Ghana. International Journal of Obstetrics and Gynaecology 59(suppl 2) S201–207

Pathmanathan I, Liljestrand J, Martins JM et al 2003 Investing in Maternal Health Learning from Malaysia and Sri Lanka. The World Bank, Washington DC

Phoya A, Bicego G 2001 Malawi Demographic and Health Survey 2000. Chapter 12. National Statistical Office and ORC Macro, Zomba, Malawi and Calverton Maryland

Tawfik L, Kinot S 2001 The impact of HIV/AIDS on the health sector in Sub Saharan Africa: the Issue of Human Relations, the SARA Project. Washington DC

UNICEF/UNFPA/WHO 2004 Maternal Mortality in 2000: Estimates developed by WHO, UNICEF and UNFPA. Department of Reproductive Health Research, WHO Geneva

USAID/AED/SARA 2003 The health sector human resource crises in Africa. An issues paper. United States Agency for International Development Bureau for Africa Office of Sustainable Development, Washington DC

Walusimbi M, Okonsky JG 2004 Knowledge and attitude of nurses caring for patients with HIV/AIDS in Uganda. Applied Nursing Research 17(2):92–99

World Bank 2005 World Development Indicators Gross National Income per capita 2004 for Ghana and Malawi. Online. Available at: http://devdata.worldbank.org/data-query/ (accessed 28 December 2005)

WHO and World Bank 2003 High Level Forum on the Health Millennium Development Goals Improving Health Workforce Performance Issues for Discussion session 4. Online. Available at: http://www.eldis.org/health-systems/dossiers/hr/documents/IssuePaper4.doc (accessed 8 December 2005)

WHO 2004 Global Atlas of the Health Workforce. Online. Available at: http://www.who.int/globalatlas (accessed 7 December 2005)

WHO 2005 The World Health Report 2005 Make every mother and child count. WHO, Geneva

# CHAPTER SIX

# Does being a principality with an assembly government help midwives in Wales to be free to practise?

SANDY KIRKMAN AND POLLY FERGUSON

Wales is a small country with a long history, an ancient language and a big heart. Rather like the New Zealand of the recent past, it has more sheep than people 9.8 million sheep, 2.92 million people (Welsh Assembly Government 2004) and it neighbours a bigger country sharing a not-always-friendly spirit of rivalry. In the same way that Kiwis hate to be mistaken for Aussies, Welsh people do not like to be thought English. Even more controversially, New Zealand midwives have recently stormed ahead of their Aussie sisters in terms of offering diverse patterns of normal midwifery care. When the National Maternity Action Plan was launched in Australia in September 2002, the authors had drawn heavily on the experiences of their New Zealand, Canadian and UK colleagues for innovative ways in which midwife-led community midwifery care could be funded and provided (Maternity Coalition Australia, Association for the Improvement of Maternity Services (AIMS) 2002). Welsh midwives too feel that they can teach their larger neighbouring countries a thing or two. However, it was not always so and this chapter aims to examine the progress of midwifery in Wales beginning in the 1970s and ending in the noughties.

Wales shares some problems with other small, mountainous countries such as Scotland and parts of Ireland. The population is not evenly distributed over the country, but is concentrated in small areas. In the south-east there are the cities of Newport, Cardiff and Swansea, and in the north the centres of Aberystwyth, Bangor and Wrexham. In the west there are the towns of Carmarthen and Haverfordwest. The mountains and lakes in the central and north of the country present a hazard of road and rail navigation. It is a long (four to five hours), tricky journey from the north to the south whether by road or by rail. This has led, quite understandably, the units in the north to identify with centres of excellence in Liverpool and in Cheshire as they are simply more accessible. Wales has an overall annual birth rate of around 37 000 in the past decade (Confidential Enquiry into Stillbirths and Deaths in Infancy (CESDI) 2001). These births take place mainly in 16 larger maternity units with annual delivery rates between 700 and 3500 a year. There are also 12 small units with delivery rates of between 200 and 15 per year (Welsh Office 1996) (Figure 6.1). These absolute numbers of units and of deliveries therein or thereby, vary from one re-organisation of care delivery to the next. They are set to change again with the implementation of the latest Welsh Assembly Government paper *Designed for Life* (2005) which includes radical proposals for the number and size of district general hospitals.

I am reminded of a great orchestra playing a well-known work and the intermittent arrival of new themes that will be heard later on. The main work, in Wales, in the 1970s and 1980s was probably hospital-based, consultant-led, little-choice maternity care but, small sounds from new themes broke through here and there. Even in 2005 (at the time of writing) we are concerned that midwives working in Wales who read this chapter will think that we believe that all was dark up to a certain point, and then all was light. Life is just not that simple: good work has been done through-out the span of the chapter, as has bad, thoughtless work. Even more puzzling to the reductionists, is the fact that there are selfish and rude midwives who, even today exist alongside kind and woman-centred obstetricians. This chapter seeks to trace the influences on midwives in Wales and their freedom to practise. Some influences are exclusively Welsh, for example the Welsh Health Planning Forum's *Protocol for Investment in Health Gain* (Welsh Office 1991) and the *All Wales Normal Labour Pathway* (National Assembly for Wales 2004). Other influences have been felt from further away, for example UNICEF's 1991 Baby Friendly Hospital Initiative. The various documents will be proposed and their impact on care assessed. In particular the chapter will examine the work and influence on maternity care in Wales of the Normal Labour Pathway (NLP). Thus, through these explorations, the question posed at the beginning of the chapter may be answered at the end of it.

# Midwifery in Wales post-Peel

In line with England, the Peel Report (1970) exerted a massive influence on maternity care in Wales. The home birth rate began a decline which

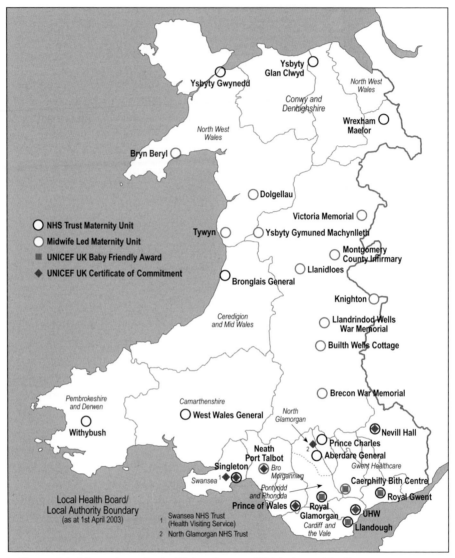

*Figure 6.1* Maternity units in Wales. Source: Welsh Assembly Government (http://www.wales.gov.uk/subihealth/content/keypubs/breast/maternity-units-map-e.pdf)

saw it reach less than 1% of all births by the late 1980s. Some units were closed and large regional units began to specialise in obstetric-led maternity care. This emphasis on technicality led, for example in South Wales, to the proliferation of appliances with the name 'Cardiff' in them. These include the Cardiff inhaler (Jones et al 1971) and the Cardiff pump (Francis et al 1970) which carefully controlled the dose of intravenous oxytocin in response to the cardiotocograph (CTG) recording. Cynics would say that the pump made everyone but the paediatrician redundant once it was set up and running well. Fortunately, my memory of it was that it hardly ever ran well and often had to be disconnected. Midwives in labour wards were becoming skilled technicians and, pre-Sleep et al (1984) the episiotomy rate was often over 50%, yet midwives were not allowed to suture the perineum. Pre-Drayton and Rees (1984, 1989) most women received a shave, enema and bath on admission in labour, and induction of labour was the norm.

Of course, this is not to assert that all midwifery in Wales was like this, nor indeed every labour conducted in the major units. There have always been talented and skilled midwives who could offer normal midwifery care even in the midst of a high-tech unit. In the rural units in North Wales, Powys and West Wales, midwives will not recognise this high-tech pattern of care as, in the main, they never adopted it in the first place. Then, as now, statistics from the rural units show that, for example, Carmarthen has a home birth rate three times that of the rate for the whole of Wales.

The realisation that moving childbirth into hospital was a major legislative and procedural error with far-reaching consequences in re-casting birth as a pathological problem needing expert intervention dawned slowly. However, there are always the few early change agents who have vision and drive, and it is to these seemingly disparate publications and groups that we now turn in an attempt to see how we got from where we were, to where we are today.

# Drivers for change

In collecting information for this chapter we have had some interesting conversations with friends and colleagues, asking them 'What do you think made us re-think our policies during the 1980s?' or 'What reports/publications do you think made us begin to change towards woman-centred, midwife-led practice?'. The following section represents the main drivers which colleagues stated had made them think, or to which they were referred as young midwives as templates on which to build their practice.

## The *Short Report* and *Maternity Care in Action*

The first national impact for midwifery managers in Wales came in the *Short Report* (House of Commons Social Services Committee 1980). The perinatal mortality rate for infants born in Wales was seen to be higher than in England and higher even than in some of the poorer English regions. Furthermore, the report made dismal reading as, time and again, the brief evidences printed showed that midwives had failed to heed the most blatant signs that things were not well. They had failed to recognise deviations from the norm and had not sent for medical aid in time, or at all. This was a sobering moment and heads of midwifery began to debate how they could lead an improvement in midwifery care in Wales. In London, the Maternity Services Advisory Committee (MSAC) was set up in answer to the findings of the Short Report, and it produced three reports under the title *Maternity Care in Action*. Part one was published in 1982 concerning antenatal care, part two in 1984 concerning intrapartum care and part three in 1985 concerning postnatal and neonatal care (Department of Health and Social Security (DHSS) 1982, 1984, 1984).

London may seem far away today but, pre-devolution 'England and Wales' was an entity and what concerned England automatically concerned Wales at the time. In addition, the committee included lay members, obstetricians and senior midwives. Of the latter the Chief Area Nursing Officer for South Glamorgan (then a county containing three big maternity units) and a consultant obstetrician from the unit in Cardiff, were on the committee. The three little booklets contained checklists to see if services were measuring up to 'best practice' as extrapolated by the committee from the *Short Report*. These booklets were used in Wales and began the changes in maternity care which were to see the perinatal mortality rates level out with, and then become from time to time, better than the rates in the rest of the UK. These little booklets were radical in their own way. In booklet one are the words:

> continuity of personal care that every woman should receive
>
> *DHSS (1982:1)*

> Taking full account of her wishes
> treated as a responsible partner . . .
>
> *DHSS (1982:8)*

On the other hand, they show their age by asserting that the general practitioner (GP) is the best person to *lead* the mother's maternity care. They stated that women who do not attend for antenatal care are in some way flawed, and that (in booklet two) hospital confinement has been *shown* to improve maternal and neonatal health. Both the *Short Report* and the subsequent MSAC guidance have been criticised by Marjorie Tew (1992) for their naïve acceptance of flawed statistical evidence regarding the safety of hospital birth. However, looking back to what happened in the 1980s, the people involved tried to do the best that they could on the evidence that they had and believed at the time.

Notwithstanding their flawed basis, the booklets were a start. They gave experiential and empirical (rather than evidence-based) checklists which aimed to improve maternity care.

## The next steps – Association of Radical Midwives, Royal College of Midwives, *Know Your Midwife*

In 1986 the Association of Radical Midwives (ARM) published its document *Vision for the Future of Maternity Services* which proposed midwife-led, woman-centred, one-to-one care. This paper was the result of two years of research by a group who later became Midwives Information and Resource Service (MIDIRS), now a well respected journal and resource for evidence-based practice. Members of the ARM gave evidence to the Winterton Committee in the early 1990s and were glad to see their precepts embedded in the resultant report (House of Commons Health Committee 1992). In 1988 the Royal College of Midwives published *Towards a Healthy Nation* which made many of the same points as *The Vision*, moving the desire for midwife-led, woman-centred, holistic midwifery care further to the front of midwives' thinking. Both the ARM and the RCM are rightly pleased that their visionary publications were out before Winterton and the subsequent *Changing Childbirth* (Department of Health 1993). However, that too can be said for Caroline Flint and colleagues (1989) and their Know Your Midwife work which was followed up very quickly in South Wales.

## Know your midwife in the Rhondda valley 1987–1989

Some major changes in the delivery of care in Wales can be shown to have three parents. Primarily there is the desire to give the woman a better service, secondly a political driver, and the third, less respectable parent is often expediency. All were true in this case. Local managers were impressed by early reports of Know Your Midwife work in London and began to adapt it to a group of midwives attached to a GP practice in Tonypandy. The political driver was that the local unit (Llwynypia) in which women had previously delivered their babies had its maternity beds closed and offered antenatal care (ANC) only. Thus the women had to travel 40 km (25 miles) of narrow and congested valley roads to have their babies in a unit with midwives whom they had never met. So, expediently, during the time that the local women were campaigning to keep Llwynypia open, the Know Your Midwife scheme was started to at least give them continuity of carer. It was formally assessed (Lester and Farrow 1989) and was seen to offer major benefits to women, babies and midwives. It shared some of the findings of Ann Oakley's later work (1992) where the women who received the extra care seemed to report more ill-health than the 'controls'. It may just be that the women who grew to know their carers better, felt more valued and would both report more ill-health and feel more empowered to go and to do something about it.

The same three-parent mechanism went on to give us the first stand-alone midwifery led unit in Wales and one of the first such units in Britain. In 1995 the women of Aberdare were told that they must go 16 km (10 miles) across the mountain to their nearest district general hospital – in another valley – for their births. This was because the anaesthetists and paediatricians would not cover the local hospital. The ensuing midwife-led unit celebrated its tenth birthday this year. It stands in one of the valley areas with a high social deprivation score, yet has consistently achieved outcomes comparable with those in the least deprived areas. The withdrawal of medical care has been priceless to the midwives in South Wales allowing the commencement of three stand-alone and two attached midwife-led units in the past decade. It is to be hoped that the medical staff never realise how valuable their fits of pique are to us.

## *Protocol for investment in health gain: maternal and early child health* (Welsh Office 1991)

Midwives in Wales were rightly very pleased with this document from the Welsh Office as a driver for change. It pre-dated both Winterton (House of Commons Health Committee 1992) and Cumberlege (Department of Health 1993) and was radical in the best Welsh tradition. It explicitly set both 'choice' and 'control' as measurable targets alongside harder parameters such as improvements in infant mortality and morbidity. The publication also targeted 'continuity of carer' as a desirable aim, along with

- clinical audit
- reduction in cigarette smoking in mothers
- prevention of handicap
- increases in breastfeeding rates
- reductions in the rates of dental caries in under fives.

With the benefit of hindsight, some of the projected dates were unrealistic, but they gave managers something to aim for and a target on which to set their sights.

## UNICEF Baby Friendly Hospital Initiative (1991)

The seemingly bland initiative, the Baby Friendly Hospital Initiative, has been responsible for major changes in the look and feel of maternity units in Wales. As midwives strive to achieve baby friendly status for their unit, the free advertising, bottles, milks, diary covers and pens have all disappeared from view. The initial breastfeeding rates have been quite easy to track. However, the rates of mothers still breastfeeding at six weeks postnatal have varied as they depend on the method of recording via links with the health visitors in different areas.

## Winterton, Tew and Cumberlege (1992/1993)

Having seen what went before it was with a sense of anticlimax that Welsh midwives greeted the findings of the Winterton Committee (House of Commons Health Committee 1992) and the subsequent *Changing Childbirth* (Department of Health 1993) report. Though both addressed the situation in England, Welsh midwives were pleased to see just how far the reports went in, for example, naming the midwife as lead carer. The cynical response was that they made wonderful rhetorical reading but, as no changes were funded, they were perceived as a method of offering something unachievable. Marjorie Tew gave evidence to the Winterton committee and published the first edition of her *Safer Childbirth?* in 1992. Careful reading of the text shows how data can be manipulated or even distorted to meet the ends of those who strive to maintain the status quo. As with other documents we have considered, it is not possible for us to say with any precision what individual practitioners have used to give them freedom to practise normal midwifery. It is entirely possible however, that a midwife finding herself in conflict with a received view (hospital is safer; birth is only normal in retrospect) could ably forward an opposite view if she used data from Tew.

## Health Evidence Bulletins Wales (Maternal and Early Child Health) 1998

The Health Service Bulletins (Welsh Office 1998) were part of a series of 12 Cochrane-like reviews which were compiled in Wales for the use and benefit of professionals in a number of fields. Practitioners could look up the healthcare intervention that they were interested in, and find the evidence listed on a continuum from 'likely to be beneficial' down to 'likely to be ineffective or harmful'. To make it more user-friendly each statement was shaded between white and dark grey showing to what extent any benefit had been shown. This was a great help to clinicians: for example, to a colleague who wished to keep a woman with a twin pregnancy on bed-rest which was quite common 20 years ago. If she looked up 'bed-rest in pregnancy' she would find a mid-grey box and the assertion that randomised controlled trials had not yet suggested any benefits.

## MIDIRS first series of informed choice leaflets/internet in general

MIDIRS first series of informed choice leaflets has become so familiar that it tends to be invisible. It is only when researching a chapter such as this that one is reminded of the power of those leaflets. Prior to the informed choice leaflets the practising midwife was thrown onto a range of disparate resources when trying to answer the questions of her client both honestly and with up-to-date evidence-based material. With the leaflets information was all gathered into one place and the whole series won a 'plain English' award for readability and openness for women.

Centres varied in their willingness to buy full sets of the leaflets for all women. However, in Wales, that was set to change. Between 1998 and 2002 the maternity units in Wales were the setting for a large DOH-funded project about informed choice jointly carried out by the Universities of Sheffield and Glamorgan (Stapleton et al 2002). This led to half of the maternity units in Wales receiving the leaflets gratis, and half acting as controls. No clear advantage to using the leaflets could be demonstrated statistically, but the exercise brought many midwives and women into contact with the detailed information for the first time. More recently, MIDIRS has updated and expanded the whole series and made them available online.

The woman who uses today's maternity services has the capacity to be more fully informed than at any time in the past. As the growth of the internet and personal computers in homes has taken place, women are free to look for statistics about their choices, place of delivery, mode of delivery and much other material. The impact of a well-informed client on the behaviour of the professionals is hard to quantify, but it must make an impact.

## Junior hospital doctors and the European Working Time Directive/advanced midwifery (specialist) practitioners/consultant midwives

The European working time directives (93/104/EC) which became law in the UK in October 1998 at first excluded doctors. However, from 2004 the directives have applied to doctors and will be phased in over a five-year period. The 58 hours per week doctors were allowed to work in 2004 will be reduced to 48 by 2009. In light of this it became expedient to create jobs in midwifery where the midwife could act as an advanced or specialist practitioner. There is a lively network of some 30 such midwives in Wales and their jobs have certain common features although each trust has interpreted the role somewhat differently. Advanced midwife practitioners (AMPs) take on the role of the junior hospital doctor in relation to 'clerking' gynaecology patients, assisting at gynaecology operations and acting as first point of contact by night. In relation to midwifery they act as first point of referral in the labour ward and some have taken on such operative tasks as ventouse delivery, low forceps, and suturing of the perineum. Some have a remit for in-house staff development and carry out training such as advanced life support (obstetrics) (ALSO). It is hard to see how the work of the AMP in relation to acting for the 'gynae houseman' can further or enhance the role of the midwife. However, in practice, the AMPs that we know assert that they enjoy this extension of the role and that it brings dividends in enhancing relationships with medical colleagues. Time alone will tell.

The consultant midwife role arose in a different way and does not show the same expediency as the AMP role. The consultant midwife role arose from the National Nursing leadership project and was announced in 1999 with the first appointments being in 2000. By January 2001 the RCM had a consultant midwives group of 36 in the UK. We have consultant midwives in Wales but have sought to widen the remit of the posts so that, for example, one post has a main agenda of 'vulnerable women', one of 'teenage mothers' one of 'normality' and one of 'sexual health'. Two of the four posts are currently occupied by practising midwives but the job descriptions are written (in conjunction with the local higher education institution) to be wider and thus allow non-midwives to occupy some posts. In these cases midwives would, of course, prefer it if a midwife were to be successful at interview but, when the posts are not labelled as exclusively for midwives, then little can be done except for midwives to field the very best candidates.

These two developments have opened up opportunities for midwives who want to stay with women rather than gaining a higher salary (or grade) by going into teaching or management. If the consultant grade becomes commensurate with the consultant grade in obstetrics then midwives will begin to have much more to say at a strategic level.

# Realising the potential: delivering the future in Wales (Welsh Assembly Government 2002)

*Realising the Potential: Delivering the Future in Wales* made radical suggestions on tight time-lines. For example it stated that, by 2003, midwives would have a recognisable base in the community. This would give women easy access to them and thus, midwives would become the first point of contact for pregnant women. In addition, the document stated that the All Wales Clinical Pathway for normal labour would be implemented by 2003 (see below). The document also aims for a 10% home birth rate by 2007. The current home birth rate is 2.7% for all of Wales with small pockets of over 6%.

The heads of midwifery were rightly proud of their document and it is no bad thing to be ambitious in terms of time-scale and reach. It may be worth noting that few, if any of the 18 key principles in the document are on track to be accomplished in time.

## The clinical pathway for normal labour

The idea of developing a clinical pathway grew slowly and was influenced by many factors. The one that first focused midwives' thoughts was the *National Sentinel Caesarean Section Audit Report* (Thomas and Paranjothy 2001), which identified Wales as having the highest caesarean section rate in the UK. This galvanised us into action and began the informal discussions amongst heads of midwifery, senior midwives, the Royal College of Midwives and the midwifery officer at the Welsh Assembly Government. These preliminary 'chats' were to demonstrate the strength of working in a small country where midwives know each other and are keen to work collaboratively and collectively. This strength gave a base for listening to each other and developing new ideas. The aim was to produce results that have a positive impact on the care that women receive. Ultimately this should have some effect on reducing caesarean section rates. However, this was not the sole intention: the primary objective was to examine what midwives could do to reduce unnecessary intervention in labour and birth.

A groundswell of midwives recognised that we had lost our confidence, skills and enthusiasm for normal birth. We had become resigned to the interventionist way of birth as an inevitable consequence of 'progress'. Nevertheless, this did not sit comfortably with most midwives. Although new technologies have certainly benefited women with high-risk pregnancies, the blanket use of many of these interventions may have been a consequence of our complacency. Slowly we had become used to relying on a CTG machine to inform us of when a labouring woman was having a contraction. The use of epidurals certainly relieved the midwife of having to support and encourage a woman through the relentlessly frequent contractions of the late first stage of labour. Instead of being that ever present support, encouraging a woman through each contraction, we had become observers, witnessing and meticulously documenting the process of labour and birth.

At the same time the Welsh Assembly Government was keen to encourage National Health Service (NHS) trusts to use clinical pathways. The Welsh Assembly Government had previously produced guidance on how to formulate and use clinical pathways (National Assembly for Wales 1999) and some NHS trusts had developed very successful pathways for specific medical conditions. The Welsh Assembly Government (1999) defined a pathway as:

> a template or blueprint for a plan of care. It is a guide to usual treatment patterns, but does not compromise the need for clinical judgement. It is not intended to prevent clinicians from using their professional judgement in the way that they care for individual patients.

Pathways are ideal for use in specific conditions where there is multiprofessional/agency input into the care a person receives. They offer evidence based guidelines to which each professional group signs up, so that everyone receives the best co-ordinated care from the least number of healthcare workers.

The Welsh Assembly Government was keen to support the development of a clinical pathway for normal labour as an exercise in collaboration. To do this, it used an all-Wales reference group of midwives who would be able to consider its value and appropriateness. It agreed to fund the cost of a midwife who would be seconded to work with the midwifery officer on this project. The initial intention at this stage was that the Pathway would be available to all maternity units in Wales that wished to adopt it. The initial secondment was for two days a week over a three-month period. However, as the work and interest grew, the secondment was extended to a total of 18 months. This enabled the Pathway to be developed, for training to be carried out in all NHS trusts and the Pathway to be piloted in two maternity units.

## Setting up an all-Wales steering group for the Pathway

The steering group for the Pathway was multi-professional. However, each maternity unit in Wales was represented by one of its midwives and thus clinical midwives formed a large proportion of the group. The midwives were nominated by their heads of midwifery; the only requirement was that they have a passion for normal birth. As well as clinical midwives, the group had representation from the Royal College of Obstetricians and Gynaecologists (RCOG), the Royal College of Midwives and the Royal College of Paediatrics and Child Health. Also on the group were: a user representative who is an active member of AIMS, and of the National Childbirth Trust (NCT), and chair of a south Wales Maternity Service Liaison Committee. The group also contained a head of midwifery education.

From the start of this project steering group members were engaged and excited by being a part of the process. This was a vibrant, challenging and supportive group that showed enormous commitment from the first meeting onwards. At times, the group's enthusiasm almost led its members into 'throwing the baby out with the bath water'; however, the obstetrician representing the RCOG contributed greatly here as he helped the group to steer away from such extremes. Respect for each other within the group showed: all members were able to challenge each other without offence being taken. If this approach could be adopted elsewhere in the maternity services we could effect change much more quickly.

The steering group established certain principles. The first principle that was agreed, and adhered to from start to finish was that anything could be debated. However, once a majority decision had been made, we would all accept that decision, work with it and support it. At this early stage it was agreed that the Pathway would be reviewed annually and anyone could raise any concern for discussion. If new evidence emerged, amendments to the Pathway would be made on an annual basis.

## Defining normality

The first task of the steering group was to define normality. The group appreciated that this is not a simple exercise with an absolute and right answer. However, there had to be agreement on a working definition to support the development of this Pathway. Pragmatism was key to this work. Whilst it is interesting and valuable to philosophise on the concept of normality, in day to day clinical practice we needed a straightforward practical definition as a place to start.

We started with labouring woman in mind. Normality for her, we thought, would be an environment where she could relax in privacy, a spontaneous onset of labour, minimal intervention, the opportunity to mobilise, eat and drink, with minimal use of pharmacological pain relief. Normality would not include artificial rupture of membranes, continuous monitoring and the use of epidurals.

# Idealism versus pragmatism

The next task was to sift through research based evidence and relevant National Institute for Health and Clinical Excellence (NICE) guidance on caring for and supporting women through normal birth. It was necessary for us to identify where robust evidence existed and where it was missing. Where research evidence did not exist, the task would be to debate and discuss best practice and to achieve consensus on a way forward.

The greatest challenge was to consider the balance between two extremes. The first is the idealistic concept of labour as a continuum that does not need timing and where the plan for each woman's labour is almost seen as a blank sheet of paper. The second is the rigid adherence to a set way of managing birth, with little or no variation for each woman. Here there was fascinating, honest and informative debate. If we are honest, most births are 'managed' using guidelines based on local policies. There was fairly rigid adherence to the rule that an acceptable rate of progress in cervical dilatation was 1 cm an hour. Local polices might state that progress in labour should be assessed by vaginal examination four hourly. In practice, we found from initial benchmarking, that most women were examined two to three hourly, and that those were the recorded examinations. We all know that some are not recorded.

The steering group reviewed the evidence related to progress in labour. Thornton and Lilford (1994) considered that there has been little scientific evidence for the present consensus on 'managing' labour. Active management of labour, with an expected rate of cervical dilatation of 1 cm an hour (O'Driscoll et al 1988) was used in many maternity units in Wales. The steering group agreed that this rate of cervical dilatation was inappropriate as it is part of a package of interventions that, in normal births were considered invasive and unnecessary.

The steering group considered whether or not we needed to define an acceptable rate of cervical dilatation at all. To do this causes intervention if slow progress is 'diagnosed'. Progress in labour, we all agreed, is not just about cervical dilatation. It is the presence of regular painful contractions that increase in length, strength and duration, descent of the fetal head and cervical dilatation, all assessed alongside the labouring woman's emotional and physical wellbeing. However, whether we like it or not, we all have a notion of what is agreed as acceptable progress and to ignore this would be dishonest. The steering group focused on Albers' (1999) observational multi-centre studies of 4000 women in normal labour. These studies, from the USA, suggested that a rate of cervical dilatation of 0.5 cm in an hour did not adversely affect outcomes of labour. The steering group agreed to this as the definition of progress as it offered some boundaries but gave women more time, without compromising safety. We were also clear that deviation from this rate of progress is not necessarily an indication for intervention. Rather, it is an indication for evaluating the situation, bearing in mind other factors such as the force and frequency of contractions and the position and condition of the fetus.

## Defining unnecessary intervention

Philosophical debate on what constitutes an intervention is necessary but invariably leads to the response that everything we do is an intervention. Being a midwife is an intervention because we are offering our knowledge, skills and experience to women to guide them through their pregnancy and birth. By so doing we are altering the course of events. If we accept that our very presence is an intervention then from there we can begin to debate what is necessary and what is not. This is what was debated. Every action from taking a blood pressure and pulse to offering food and drink, encouraging mobility and giving telephone advice was considered. Sometimes we found little evidence to support the current practice of, for instance, admission CTG traces on all women. Sometimes we found confusing evidence, for example, on the level of body mass index above which there is an increased risk to women in labour.

When there were differing practices across Wales with no clear research-based evidence we took a majority decision. One example of this is the definition of active labour. There is no standard definition – no right or wrong. But, we know that hospital is not the best place for women who are not in established labour: this encourages and increases the use of analgesics and oxytocics (McNiven et al 1998). The group wanted to encourage women to stay at home in early labour and encourage midwives to support women in doing so. The Pathway defines active labour as established when the cervix is fully effaced and more than 3 cm dilated in the presence of regular, painful contractions. Ideally, women would not need one-to-one care from a midwife, at home or hospital until active labour commences. This is what we aim for. It relies on women being well informed and confident and on midwives being encouraging and supportive. The representatives from the NCT and the AIMS assisted the group in developing a leaflet for women, explaining the concept of the Pathway. This has been invaluable for working in partnership with women to support them in achieving a normal birth.

## Documenting care

The Pathway provides the documentation format for normal labour. Documentation is by exception: this means that if everything is normal as defined by the guidance throughout the pathway, the partogram is considered to be acceptable documentation of care. If there are any deviations to care then freehand thorough recording of events is essential.

This way of recording the care and progress takes a little getting used to. After years of training in writing everything down, many midwives understandably felt wary and vulnerable. The ticking of a box to say that refreshments had been given felt somehow insulting for some midwives. But what is the difference in ticking a box or writing long hand that you have given tea and toast? The difference is that it has significantly reduced the time taken up in record keeping. Gone is the awkward moment when a midwife has to decide, in millilitres, how much blood was lost during the third stage of labour. Now she has to sign to say that blood loss was within normal limits. Now that we spend less time record keeping we have more time to support women in labour and that has to be celebrated. On the other hand, it is such a novelty that perhaps some midwives will have to re-learn how to be with women.

## Freedom or shackled?

The intention of the Pathway was to reduce unnecessary intervention in labour and to give midwives the freedom to practise based on evidence and partnership. It is obvious to me that for many midwives, the Pathway has achieved this aim; for some it has not. I do not think it is over simplistic to state that the reason the Pathway works is because midwives want it to and the reason it does not work is because midwives do not want it to. That is freedom to practise, but is that what we want?

Some critics complain that the Pathway is restrictive and that it de-personalises birth. I disagree with this opinion. The Pathway is an honest tool. We should talk with women about the Pathway and its aims and, what their wishes are. If women would like to aim for a normal birth then the evidence base used in the Pathway will maximise their opportunity. It is not a guarantee of a normal birth but the steering group considers it to be best practice. A clinical framework cannot de-personalise birth. It does not have to be followed in its entirety and there are many good reasons for not doing so. All that is asked is that midwives justify any deviation from the Pathway. The question we should be asking is: should we give midwives the freedom to choose not to use it and whom does that freedom best serve?

# Conclusion

It is time to attempt to answer the question posed at the beginning of the chapter. That is, 'Does being a principality with an assembly government help midwives in Wales to be free to practise?'

During the period under scrutiny midwives in Wales have practised in every way described in the literature. There have been teams of midwives, core and cluster midwives, continuity of carer, and caseload holding midwives. In the early days there were domino schemes set up and wound down. The conscientious manager kept abreast of the guidance starting with the 'little booklets' after the *Short Report*, and used other publications with checklists to see how midwives in their patch measured up. Returning to the analogy of the orchestra it would seem that the main tune being played throughout the past three decades has had much of the hospital-based, medical model, little or no choice midwifery as its theme. However, the small twiddles and sub-themes that are heard from time to time have encompassed all that is good in woman-centred care.

If it were not for the introduction of the NLP I would answer that midwives in Wales are no more, or no less free to practise normal midwifery than their colleagues in other parts of the UK. However, the single innovation of the NLP has made an impact on midwifery care all over Wales. If only for this, I would say that being a principality with our own self-determination, has made a positive difference in our freedom to practise.

## Reflective questions

Some midwives think that there is a need to regain confidence, skills and enthusiasm. Do you agree with this? Whatever your answer, it may help your reflection to write down the reasons why you have answered in this way.

Multi-professional inter-working, planning and respect are important aspects of maternity care and demonstrated in this chapter in the use of the clinical pathway for normal labour. What other ways of real team working can you think of?

Please consider this question again: 'Should we give midwives the freedom to choose not to use it [the clinical pathway for normal labour] and whom does that freedom best serve?' What do you think?

# References

Albers L 1999 The duration of labour in healthy women. Journal of Perinatology 19(2):114–119

Association of Radical Midwives 1986 Vision for the Future of Maternity Services. Ormskirk, Association of Radical Midwives

CESDI I 2001 All Wales Perinatal Survey and Confidential Enquiry into Stillbirths and Deaths in Infancy. CESDI, Cardiff

DoH 1993 (Chaired by Baroness Cumberlege) Changing Childbirth: Report of the expert maternity group. HMSO, London

DHSS 1982, 1984, 1985 Maternity Care in Action, Parts 1, 2 and 3. First, second and third reports of the Maternity Services Advisory Committee. HMSO, London

Drayton S, Rees C 1984 They know what they're doing. Nursing Mirror (Midwifery Forum) 159(5):4–8

Drayton S, Rees C 1989 Is anyone out there still giving enemas? In: Robinson S, Thomson A (eds) Midwives Research and Childbirth, Vol. 1. London: Chapman Hall, pp 139–153

EEC 1993 Council Directive no 93/104/EC 23 November 1993 concerning certain aspects of the organisation of working time. EEC, Brussels

House of Commons Social Services Committee 1980 (Chaired by R Short) Perinatal and neonatal mortality; Second report from the Social Services Committee 1979–80. HMSO, London

House of Commons Health Committee 1992 (Chaired by Sir Nicholas Winterton) Second Report, Maternity Services, Vol 1. HMSO, London

Flint C, Poulengeris P, Grant A 1989 The 'Know Your Midwife' scheme – a randomised trial of continuity of care by a team of midwives. Midwifery 5:11–16

Francis JG, Turnbull AC, Thomas FF 1970 Automatic oxytocin infusion equipment for the induction of labour. Journal of Obstetrics and Gynaecology of the British Commonwealth 77(7):594–602

Jones PL, Molloy MJ, Rosen M 1971 The Cardiff Penthrane inhaler. British Journal of Anaesthesiology 43(2):190–199

Lester C, Farrow S 1989 An evaluation of the Rhondda 'Know your Midwives' scheme: The first year's deliveries. Unpublished report. Institute of Healthcare Evaluation. University of Wales College of Medicine, Cardiff

Maternity Coalition Australia, AIMS (Australia, Australian Society of Independent Midwives and Community Midwifery, WA) 2002 National Maternity Action Plan for the introduction of community midwifery services in urban and regional Australia. Maternity Coalition Australia, Sydney

McNiven P, Williams J, Hodnett E et al 1998 An early assessment program: a randomised control trial. Birth 251:5–10

Ministry of Health 1970 Domiciliary midwifery and maternity bed needs: the standing maternity and midwifery advisory committee. Sub-committee chairman J Peel. HMSO, London

National Assembly for Wales 1999 An Introduction to Clinical Pathways. Putting patients first. NHS Wales, Cardiff

National Assembly for Wales 2004 The All Wales Normal Labour Pathway (HOWIS access). National Assembly for Wales, Cardiff

National Assembly for Wales 2004 Survey of Agricultural and Horticultural Census 3 June 2004. National Assembly for Wales, Cardiff

National Assembly for Wales 2005 Designed for life. National Assembly for Wales, Cardiff

Oakley A 1992 Measuring the effectiveness of psychosocial interventions in pregnancy. International Journal of Technological Assessment (8)Suppl 1:129–138

O'Driscoll K, Foley M, MacDonald DC 1984 Active management of labour as an alternative to Caesarean section. Obstetrics and Gynaecology 63:485–90

Royal College of Midwives 1988 Towards A Healthier Nation. Royal College of Midwives, London

Sleep J, Grant A, Garcia J, et al 1984 West Berkshire perineal management trial. BMJ 289:587–90

Stapleton H, Kirkham M, Thomas G 2002 Qualitative study of evidence-based leaflets in maternity care. BMJ 324(7338):639

Tew M 1992 Safer Childbirth? A Critical History of Maternity Care. Chapman and Hall, London

Thomas J, Paranjothy S 2001 National Sentinel Caesarean Section Audit Report. RCOG Press, London

Thornton JG, Lilford RJ 1994 Active management of labour: current knowledge and research issues. BMJ 309(6951) 366–9

UNICEF 1991 Baby Friendly Hospital Initiative. UNICEF, Geneva

Welsh Assembly Government 2002 Realising the potential: briefing paper 4. Delivering the future in Wales: a framework for realising the potential of midwives in Wales. Welsh Assembly Government, Cardiff

Welsh Office 1991 Protocol for investment in healthcare gain: Maternal and Early Child Health. Welsh Health Planning Forum, Cardiff

Welsh Office 1996 Welsh Maternity Services Review. Welsh Office, Cardiff

Welsh Office 1998 Health Evidence Bulletins Wales: Maternal and Early Child Health. Welsh Office, Cardiff

# CHAPTER SEVEN

# Between a rock and a hard place: the situation of the Finnish midwife

ROSEMARY MANDER

The situation in which the midwife in Finland finds herself may bear comparison with that of midwives in many other countries. What makes the Finnish situation unique, though, is the paradoxes with which it is imbued. These paradoxes serve to highlight crucial issues influencing the midwife's freedom to practise. These are issues which apply not only to the Finnish midwife practising in Finland, but to any midwife practising anywhere throughout the world.

To analyse the situation of the Finnish midwife and her practice, first of all it is necessary to give an outline of the background. The relevant context includes the geography and the culture of this country, together with an account of the system of maternity care and the midwife's history. After this I attempt to outline the paradoxes of the Finnish midwife's situation and the practice-related issues to which they point. To do this, I draw on the funded research project which I undertook in Finland and New Zealand (Mander 2005). In this chapter I draw mainly on the data collected from midwives during the Finnish phase of the study.

## Background

Although it is sometimes difficult to separate the two, it may be helpful to the reader if I explain the geography of Finland before moving on to its culture. This is because it is possible that the culture may be influenced, or even moulded, by the country's geographical features.

# Finland

Finland, or Suomi to give it its Finnish name, is a narrow and long country at the eastern end of the Baltic Sea, largely wedged between Sweden and Russia (Figure 7.1). The Finnish archipelago lies off the south-west coast. Inland from the coast are plains, to the north-east of which is the well-known lake district; this area is widely forested and extends to Finland's eastern border with Russia. The northern part of the country comprises arctic wastes.

Of Finland's population of just over five million, the majority (61%) live in urban areas (Sosiaali-ja terveysalan tutkimus-ja kehittämiskeskus (STAKES) 2002); these tend to be in and around the major cities in the south and south-west of the country. Thus, the coastal areas are generally more heavily populated, with the arctic wastes being least populated. For the vast sparsely populated areas away from the cities and coasts, remote and rural issues arise in the provision of healthcare in general and of maternity care in particular. The country's northerly latitude brings with it long dark winters to the extent that at the 70th parallel there are 51 days of uninterrupted night in winter. This may aggravate the Finns sense of isolation and, possibly, seasonal affective disorder.

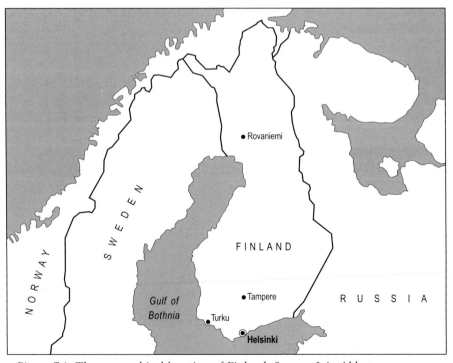

*Figure 7.1* The geographical location of Finland. Source: Iain Abbot

# The Finns

Finland has, for much of its history, been colonised by one or other of its powerful neighbours. From about 1155 to 1809 the ruling power was Sweden. Russia then took over, until 1917. It was in 1919 that the Finnish republic's constitution was signed. This means that Finland has been independent for less than a century. Obviously, being a colony for the largest part of a millennium has left its mark on Finland in many ways. The Swedish influence is most easily apparent in the country being bilingual (Finnish/Swedish). Tsarist Russia, on the other hand is said to have left the Finns with an obedient streak and a reluctance to speak out against authority.

Finland has a strongly egalitarian culture. This is exemplified by women having been given the vote as early as 1906. It is difficult to assess whether this history of women's rights has affected subsequent political activity. Perhaps coincidentally, though, the Finnish president and prime minister are, at the time of writing, both women. In spite of the current equality, until the nineteenth century Finnish women's status was lower than men's (Helsti, personal communication, 2005). The agrarian nature of Finnish society meant that women were important more for their skills with farm animals than for any other reason. This work ethic was a source of pride to Finnish women. They were expected to contribute fully and equally to the work force and took minimal time off, even for childbearing. In such an agrarian society belief in magic was strong and sorcerers were powerful, although they were quite distinct from midwives. The sorcerers' existence made medical practitioners superfluous. Superstitious beliefs persisted well into the twentieth century, with the 'evil eye' causing anxiety until the time of the Winter War (1939–1940) and Continuation War (1941–1944) (Stark-Arola 1998). Women's pride in their work waned with the increasing urbanisation of the twentieth century. The result was that the status of women's work declined and, reciprocally, motherhood became idealised.

The egalitarian nature of Finnish society is said to extend to its ethnic minority populations. The largest minority group are the Swedish-speaking Finns, who constitute 6% of the population (Hyyppä and Mäki 2001). The other traditional minorities, Saami, Roma and Tatar, together make up about 0.25% of the population. While Finland has traditionally been quite homogeneous due to restrictive immigration policies, this is changing; in 2000 as many as 2.7% of the population had been born outwith Finland.

The Finnish language, being unrelated to any European languages other than Hungarian, has aroused much speculation about Finns' racial origins (Singleton 1989). The complexities of this language may have served to isolate Finns; but Finland became central to the electronic communications industry in the late twentieth century, and there has been a national enthusiasm to learn English.

A crucial aspect of Finnish life, and one of which Finns are justifiably proud, is their health and welfare system. This pride is reflected in a European Commission survey (Eurostat 2001) which showed that Finland has the highest proportion of its population expressing satisfaction with their health system in the European Union. The European average satisfaction rate is 41.3%, whereas 80% of Finns are satisfied with their health service. This satisfaction may relate to the effectiveness of services such as maternity which results in a perinatal mortality rate as low as 5.7 in 2000 (STAKES 2002). The equivalent for England was 8.3 (Confidential Enquiry into Maternal and Child Health (CEMACH) 2005). The Finns' enlightened family policies not only permit, but actually encourage both parents to build relationships with their small children. These policies extend to full-time leave for child care if the child is younger than 3 years. This is followed by part-time leave until the child is in year two at school (Ministry of Labour 2003). After the initial maternity and paternity leaves, the parents are able to decide which of them will take the subsequent parental leave and how it will be shared.

## The midwife's story

Midwifery in Finland demonstrates a long history of power struggles. They happened at both a personal or clinical level as well as at organisational and educational levels.

Traditionally births in Finland have been at home, attended by a lay midwife, who had no formal education, known as a '*paarmuska*' (Helsti 1995). For ordinary people, the arrival of the trained midwife or '*kätilö*' in each municipality, in the late eighteenth century, brought many conflicts. The midwife was in conflict with both the childbearing woman and the *paarmuska* (Helsti 1995). The conflicts derived from the midwife's incomprehensible and unrealistically high standards of cleanliness. Unfortunately for the midwife, because there were so few and distances were so great, she was obliged to rely on the co-operation of the *paarmuska*:

> If two confinements came at the same time, the midwife could not be in two places at once. So the use of the paarmuska was still in a way dictated by necessity.
>
> *Helsti (1995:107)*

Helsti maintains that the acceptance of the midwife, and the practices which she brought with her, was complete by the 1930s. Thus, a midwife recounted a first time mother, stating her preferred position for the birth:

'On my back of course'. At that time no one could even imagine any other way.

*Helsti (1995:107)*

In terms of midwifery organisation and education, attempts had been made in 1688 to resolve child mortality problems by bringing the more educated midwife or '*kätilö*' under the 'Collegium Medicum' (Oinas et al 1999:116). Following this legislation, further proclamations defined the midwife's characteristics, abilities and, in 1859, her education. Even before the national trauma of the 'Winter War' against Russia (1939–1940) which served as Finland's defining moment (Singleton 1989), moves were afoot to stabilise the position of the 'municipal midwife'; simultaneously maternity care was being re-orientated towards preventive medicine. By cementing nationalist feeling and decimating the population, the Winter War accelerated moves towards family policies which, although not explicitly, were implicitly pronatalist.

After a series of educational reforms, the maternity and child health care systems were re-organised in 1944 to incorporate the midwife and the public health nurse (PHN). Under the world-famous paediatrician Arvo Ylppo, the *neuvola* system of free maternity advice centres became established as an institution which is somewhat more than the health centre with which we may be familiar; the midwife was required to provide more family-oriented care. These developments, aimed to strengthen the fledgeling nation through the family's wellbeing. With the rationalisation of the hospital system in the 1950s and 1960s, the woman was encouraged to give birth in hospital. Hence, the midwife's situation was further weakened. This process was exacerbated by another reform of midwifery education in 1968 which abolished the 'direct entry' route. 'Since that time only qualified nurses have been trained as midwives, and then to work exclusively in hospitals' (Oinas et al 1999:117). This limitation of midwifery practice may be significant for the midwife in view of home birth being her only truly distinctive sphere of practice. The woman's home is the one setting in which the midwife is both required and able to assume complete autonomy. In the same way as home birth is the only situation in which the midwife is able to practise unhindered, it may be that the midwife is the only childbirth attendant willing to practise in the woman's home (Brown 1994). Thus, it may be argued that home birth is, effectively, the midwife's 'unique selling point'. If this capacity is removed, or if she chooses to dispense with it, then that characteristic which defines her being as a midwife will have disappeared.

Finland's health policy has continued to develop its family-centred focus. The rate of change escalated, though, with the passage of the Finnish Public Health Act of 1972 (Kansanterveyslaki 1972). In many ways this legislation was extremely enlightened. Among other things, it required every municipality to provide its population (regardless of age) with free access to general health counselling, school health services, contraceptives (at low or no cost) and contraceptive education, sex education and easy access to abortion services (Kosunen and Rimpelä 1996). The authors of this legislation clearly took the view that holistic family health should be prioritised. This ethos, however, ignored the midwife's specialist role in pregnancy and the postnatal period and limited her contribution in antenatal care (Wrede et al 2001); her community title was changed to 'public health nurse'. Specialised nurse-midwives have continued to be educated to work in maternity and gynaecology wards as well as in the community. Because the 1972 legislation was drafted at governmental level, midwives, their managers and representatives were powerless to prevent what was, effectively, the coup de grâce to Finnish midwifery practice. The upshot is that some midwives continue to work in the *neuvola* system alongside PHNs. The majority of midwives, though, practise only within the confines of hospital labour wards.

## The research project

Having become aware of some of these developments in the Finnish maternity services, I enthusiastically welcomed an opportunity to investigate them by comparing them with the fundamentally different developments in New Zealand (see Chapter 14). The main aims of this study were to examine the roles of the various participants in the maternity scenario by focusing on decision-making processes at three levels:

- national policy
- organisational or unit
- clinical or interpersonal.

Because of the significance of home birth (see The midwife's story, above), place of birth decisions served as an example when needed. These aims required access to:

- managers and policy makers
- consumers of care
- care providers (i.e. practising midwives and PHNs in Finland).

The research questions sought to address how decisions are made at the three levels and how the different participants contribute. Because little is known about decision making in this context, qualitative research methods and a woman-centred approach were adopted.

A 'snowball technique' was the major strategy used to access a suitable sample. Thus, initial contact was made with a few 'experts' in each country, through personal and occupational links, professional literature and websites. On the basis of their recommendations I approached other potential informants. In Finland one 'expert' was able to assist recruitment through a call for volunteers on the 'Active Birth' website (2005). The process of making contacts began in advance of my departure to the countries and continued right through the data collection period. While the snowball technique is recognised as ensuring that the informants are suitably knowledgeable, its major weakness is that it is not possible to ascertain whether the field is comprehensively covered (Renzetti and Lee 1993). For example I was not given the names of any Saami in Finland, or of any Maori in New Zealand. As far as I am aware, I interviewed only one Swedish-speaking Finn. Thus, I neither intended nor claim that this sample is representative of the population. The recruitment was largely by email.

The sample, which totalled 34, comprised approximately equal numbers of consumers and healthcare providers (Table 7.1). Unsurprisingly, the number of managers and policy makers was smaller. Data were collected using semi-structured, one-to-one, face-to-face interviews. As usual in qualitative research, the interviews developed more structure as the research progressed and themes developed. The venue for the interview was chosen by the respondent at a mutually convenient time. For many professionals,

Table 7.1  The sample of informants in Finland

| Informants | No. |
|---|---|
| Consumers | 12 |
| Midwives | 5 |
| Public health nurses | 6 |
| Public health nurse/midwife | 1 |
| Policy makers/managers | 8 |
| Midwife/consumers | 2 |
| Total | 34 |

their place of work was selected. This carried the advantage that I became acquainted with the environment in which decisions were taken. For the consumer, she was able to choose whether I should come to her home, the place where I was staying or a local health facility. In the opening sequence of the interview I reiterated the structure of the research, explained informed consent, sought agreement to the interview being tape-recorded and outlined its format. Demographic data were collected by the informant's self-introduction. The tape recording was transcribed in full and data analysis began concurrently with the interviews. Common themes and concepts were sought which determined the direction of the questions for subsequent interviews.

All ethical conventions were scrupulously followed throughout this research. There were no specific benefits to the informants of being involved and no payments were made. Some of the informants said that they were glad to have had an opportunity to reflect on aspects of their experience or their work which they had not considered previously. Others, whose experience was isolating, said that they valued the chance to talk about it to an interested person. There were no serious risks involved as these interviews involved no physical intervention and were not psychologically threatening or traumatic. Often an informant would thank me for giving her an opportunity to talk about her experience.

# Paradoxical findings

A number of paradoxes emerged from this study, which inform the position of the midwife in Finland and her practice. In order to demonstrate the role of the Finnish midwife I address, first, the more general considerations, gradually moving towards the more personal or clinical matters. In this way a picture emerges of the nature of the relationship between the midwife and her raison d'être, the childbearing woman.

## Being strong

The Finnish characteristic which is known as '*sisu*' is so widely known that it verges on being stereotypical. The literal translation is 'grit, guts, pluck, spunk' (Sovijärvis 2005:363). According to Goodrich (1960), this is a characteristic which emerges in challenging situations. The most significant, he maintains, was the Winter War, when Finnish forces were outnumbered by 50 to 1 by the Russian invaders. Yet they still acquitted themselves honourably.

'*Sisu*' is not a sex-linked characteristic, so the Finnish woman shares a reputation for being strong. As an oral historian of the early twentieth century, Helsti identified the Finnish mother's strength:

> My mother was born in 1888. She told me about the wife of Leppälä farm . . . She gave birth to her baby there in the field, wrapped it inside her hem and took it into the house and came back to cut the rye. There were mothers like that in the olden days. In times of poverty and shortage the women were like iron.
>
> *Helsti (1997:506)*

The Finnish woman's current reputation for emotional and psychological strength relates to two main factors. The first is educational status, which derives from the nineteenth century tradition of the younger daughter in the family going to school, while her siblings laboured on the family farm. The second factor derives from the disproportionately great loss of young men during the wars of 1939–1945 (Singleton 1989:169). These two factors combined, so that when required, the woman was able to become the family breadwinner and mainstay of the Finnish workforce, until a normal sex-ratio was restored.

The informants told me, however, that this is not how they perceive their position. They felt that those who are most affected are relatively weak in matters of maternity policy decision-making:

> *F18*: Because they are all men making these decisions, then they are not young men. They are more like grandfathers – so they don't have so much experience. Maybe the situation would change if they were young ladies.

The woman's perception of her limited input was aggravated, even though the health care system is organised on a municipality basis, by the large centres exerting an unduly strong influence over policy decisions:

> *F27*: the big cities. And then there are some representatives from the smaller cities and the smaller communities. But, for instance, from [here] there is only one sitting in this government.

As well as in policy-making, Finnish women thought that they were too weak to speak out in more personal situations. This inability of the woman to take advantage of the opportunities which present themselves was clearly a source of regret:

> *F25*: On the whole, though, Finnish people tend not to challenge what they see as authority figures. A few are able to challenge, though.

For a consumer representative, the lack of information available to the woman compounds her inability to speak up. But information per se was insufficient to put the woman in a stronger negotiating position:

> *F06*: [mothers] do just like they are told in the hospital. They don't have any information to make a decision, but if they have information, they have to be very strong to make decisions.

As well as this general perception of lacking strength to question authority, this also pertains in the clinical situation. The midwife appears to be sub-servient to her medical colleagues in the context of decision-making, as reported by a midwife:

> *Rosemary*: Who else contributes [to decisions]?
> *F02*: Yes, there's the gynaecologist. She's the one who gives the orders. Of course we can speak about if the lady wants to go home in the latent phase or things like that. If it's about oxytocin infusion or breaking the membranes the decision is mostly the doctor's.
> *Rosemary*: Do you have experience of woman declining rupture of the membranes?
> *F02*: Then we can wait for some hours. If there is everything OK with the fetus, then we try to give some information to her. She can make her decision and informed consent. But I have to admit that sometimes a doctor just comes and breaks the membranes. The doctor comes and breaks the membranes [*sic*]. And then it's the midwife who has to explain to the mother what's happened and why.

The midwife's seriously weakened position was most obvious at the time of the drafting of the Public Health Act 1972, as was recounted to me by a midwifery policy maker/manager:

> *F12*: But in that law, midwives were forgotten. There is nothing about – in the whole law there is not one word about midwives, about preg-nancy. It's included in the health education – it's part of that. All pregnancy care is part of that.
> *Rosemary*: Just the public health nurse?
> *F12*: Yes, of course. That was the whole point of the law. And they had good connections [laugh] good connections. No one really realised.

Thus, the relatively powerless situation of Finnish midwives was outlined by another professional midwifery policy maker/manager:

> *F31*: And if they are in the hospital and there are no midwives who are strong in midwifery, they are waiting for doctors – [softly] 'We

are waiting for what he's saying about what we have to do'. And I
don't like that system. They – we midwives have our own area of
normal birth and to support women and if we need doctors or obstetricians we ask. But no, they want to visit in the labour room very
often. They want to take – they want to be boss. And what is needed
is very strong midwifery directors so that they can discuss with obstetricians how we work together. And that's very difficult now in
Finland.

By way of summary of the paradox of strength, a policy maker articulated
the sorry state, reflecting the weak position of the Finnish midwife:

> F33: Yes, and this makes me a little sad, that midwifery is kind of
> dying in Finland.

The Finnish midwife's position bears comparison with that of her Scottish
counterpart in the mid-late twentieth century (Askham and Barbour 1996).
Her lack of strength may be closely related to fear of certain pathological
outcomes, according to a midwife, who appeared confident in many aspects
of her role:

> F04: Well, usually the placenta comes in about ten or fifteen minutes,
> but I'm still a little bit pressing and pulling. And I know that's not
> perfectly natural, but I'm afraid that they start bleeding if I don't get
> the placenta out.

Such fears appear to be crucially important in determining the midwife's
attitude to home birth:

> F02: Of course as a midwife I'm afraid of the risks, like massive
> bleedings, placental ablations, problems at the second stage. And in
> this example I told you before, this mother came [to the hospital with
> her] cervix fully dilated, started to push the baby and then there was
> a [spontaneous rupture of membranes] and it was dark green
> porridge.

Clearly, fear of untoward outcomes makes the midwife reluctant to attend
home births. Such reluctance to undertake this quintessentially midwifery
role may serve to further threaten the midwife's already weakened
position.

## Choosing the place of birth

The fear of poor outcomes is not alone in disempowering the midwife by
reducing her enthusiasm for home births. Other influences also operate

through the anxiety of her medical colleagues, as articulated by an obstetrician/policy maker:

> *F27*: Somehow I understand that some women would like to have [the baby] at home but, as a doctor, so I must say that I'm a little bit afraid of the complications anyway. You know, it can be the umbilical cord complications; it can be something that you have to vacuum them, or even a [caesarean] section. What do you do if you are at home and you have to take a mother to an ambulance and going to the clinic which can be far away? So I must say that I prefer clinic or hospitals.

This medical anxiety was reported by a policy-maker to take the form of adamant opposition by two groups of practitioners:

> *F34*: And there is a very strong rejection of home births by obstetricians and paediatricians. So I think this – we are not going to have official support for home births in Finland.

The major reason for this medical opposition was spelt out by a midwife clinical manager:

> *F23*: then of course our doctors – obstetricians and paediatricians – they think it's dangerous if they don't have any technical equipment. For example the heartbeat monitor – the CTG [cardiotocograph].

The results of this medical antagonism to the Finnish midwife attending a birth at home was explained by midwives:

> *F04*: And I tried to ask our doctors' opinion about home birth. And it was so, so hard and dominating that 'never, never a midwife would go to a home birth' from our hospital midwives.

The penalty which would be applied for any midwife who chose not to follow this medical diktat also became clear:

> *Rosemary*: What would happen . . . ?
> *F23*: Aah. I don't think that you could work as a midwife. Everybody wouldn't understand. They would say how can you do this? This is not your work you're not allowed to do this.
> *F02*: Here the official opinion is that it is not allowed to go to someone's home to assist the birth if you want to work here.

The risk to the Finnish midwife who chooses to attend a home birth was mentioned by a number of midwives, but most explicitly by one:

> *F30*: And midwives that do homebirths or attend homebirths are very scarce. I know one hospital where the head OBGYN has said that if

he finds out that any of his hospital's midwives attend home births he will see that they will be fired.

Paradoxically, the Finnish Federation of Midwives has adopted a somewhat ambiguous stance on the midwife attending a home birth. It has produced guidelines for the midwife undertaking this supposedly forbidden activity. Unfortunately my Finnish does not extend to reading official documents, but I was informed:

> *F12*: We have in our federation – we have a paper. It came out last year. It's more like a statement. I hope it's on the web, although it's in Finnish, of course. We had a little group of midwives working together and trying to write down everything about home birth. What kind of equipment does the midwife need and everything like ethics, law, insurance. In order to help midwives who want to do that.

> *F23*: In our midwives federation we have [drawn up] home birth information, to check up the laws, rights, securities – insurances and then we made a list of those things. But midwives have to think before they go to help with a home birth. That was just a list. That was not an opinion about what we *should* have. Somehow it's just there to help those midwives who want to go.

> *Rosemary*: Was this list to support midwives attending home births?

> *F23*: No. I don't know. [Laugh] I don't know yet. It was just a list of things you have to remember if you go, but it's also to help the midwives.

## Being healthy, but . . .

As mentioned above, unlike some 'national illness services' (Scottish Executive Health Department (SEHD) 2000), the exemplary Finnish system focuses steadfastly on health, especially preventive health. When I asked the healthcare providers about the model or ideology which guided their practice, it invariably related to the healthy nature of childbearing. A PHN clearly expressed her healthy, social orientation:

> *F14*: I see it as healthy and that everything is OK, if her situation in life is good and goes well, unless she has some problems such as problems with her husband or with the family.

This philosophy was reiterated by a young mother with two small children:

> *F13*: I think if my friends and people my age, when we are pregnant and our mums or grannies or someone like that can say how can you

do that . . . because you're pregnant? And I say well I'm not sick – I'm only pregnant! So I think it's a very natural part of life.

This confidence in the healthy nature of childbearing, though, was shared to only a limited extent by a midwife clinical manager:

*F23*: I think it's a healthy process. It's a normal thing in the life of a woman who gets pregnant and has a baby. And that's normally, but I work in the antenatal section. There, some days, you think it's not – it's nothing normal in their life in pregnancy [laugh]. It goes so wrong.

This paradoxical view of the healthiness of childbearing was articulated consistently by midwives and PHNs. This view may be summarised as a 'healthy, but' model of childbearing:

*F14*: It is healthy without question – if everything goes well of course!

*F22*: I think the hospital is the right place to have the labour. But pregnancy or the birth is not an illness. I don't think – it's not very good to have the baby in the home. That's what I think. [Laugh].

*F20*: I think that most of our mothers are normal, healthy, and there are only a little such mothers who have some form of disease problems. Like diabetes. I think we have such mothers who have diabetes. Or something – some other long term disease, but it's the [tip of the iceberg]. [Laugh].

*Rosemary*: If they're healthy, why do they need to attend hospital?

*F20*: Because we midwives don't want to take the responsibility for her giving birth at home.

This 'healthy, but' model of childbearing may reflect the medicalisation of childbearing in Finland and, equally, part of the reason for the midwife's relatively weak position.

## Working with others

In many ways the organisation of the Finnish health system is determined by its powerful orientation to preventive medicine. This orientation demands that staff should work as a team, which pleases the PHN:

*F19*: But we have two doctors and we have such teams. I think I make a team with my doctor.

For the midwife in the labour ward working as a member of a team may be perceived as bringing different advantages. They may include limiting her autonomy and her accountability:

*F02*: And [in the hospital] we have the doctors and the multiprofessional team. But if we go to someone's home as an individual, it's our own problem.

Relations with other members of the 'team' may not always be so congenial. Such inter-professional issues relate largely to the midwife's interaction with the PHN and with the paediatrician; the obstetrician has been mentioned already (see above).

## The public health nurse and neuvola

It is well nigh impossible to separate the PHN from the ideological and physical environment in which she practices – the *neuvola*. To many Finns the origins of the concept and institution which are *neuvola* are shrouded in welcome antiquity:

*F30*: everyone knows about it because at first pregnant women go there and the children go to these child clinics to the age of six. And the neuvola is something so utterly traditionally Finnish. So I don't – I'm not surprised that 99.9% of women go to neuvola because it is such a traditional part of your pregnancy that you go to neuvola.

To other mothers, though, this concept and the form of 'care' which it offers is less satisfactory:

*F09*: And it should be the place where you are advised, but somehow mothers are afraid to go to neuvola because they can be told 'Stop eating candy' [smack], 'Now you have gained too much weight', and things like that. It should be really the place where you can go with your worries and then you are given advice and not orders. 'You will do that!' It's not very nice.

*F32*: And also the neuvola maternity advisory system is a bit behind. They live in the seventies with their knowledge . . . The neuvola is not interested in you – only the baby. So I got a lot of back problems when her weight – she gained weight very fast. And I said, 'Can you help me?' 'No we . . . blah, blah . . . we only deal with the babies.'

The concept itself was also criticised by a policy maker:

*F33*: The woman is expected to make a large number of visits to the neuvola, probably about twelve or fifteen. These are maternity visits, but their focus is on the formation of the family. The focus is not on the woman, it is about preparing her and the others in her family for the new family relationships. The neuvola looks out particularly for problems relating to the woman's alcohol intake or signs that there is a fear of motherhood. If there are any problems at all she is sent straight to the hospital. In this way the neuvola serves to screen the women, rather than providing care for them. And the education is focussed very much on the care of the baby, rather than the mother's care of herself.

Since their inception, the primary role of the *neuvola*, and the PHN when she arrived there, has been the provision of advice about the development of family relationships. This basic function, though, was unsatisfactory to some informants:

> F09: When breastfeeding my daughter during the pregnancy, I felt OK. I wasn't tired at all. And I knew that this was [right] for us. Then I was told that 'You should really wean her'. And I – when I said that I had no reason then they told me, 'You are tired'. 'I am not'. Then, 'You'll have a jealousy problem when the child is born and the toddler is not breast fed any more'.
>
> F25: Public health nurses just teach a couple of hours childbirth education. They are not able to teach the women 'cos they don't have the knowledge.

The relationship between the PHN and her midwife colleague was also reported by some to be less than satisfactory. This conflict relates partly to clinical changes which permit the PHN to perform midwifery functions:

> F34: Based on this new kind of education, these public health nurses can take care of postnatal check-ups of mothers.
>
> F12: They gave short further education for [public health nurses] to provide care; for example doing vaginal examinations – in order to know if there is a risk for premature labour.

While these changes may appear to be little more than substitution for labour force purposes, they may be far more significant than that for the midwife's future.

Also in employment, the position of the midwife is weak compared with that of the PHN:

> F34: It's the municipalities who are able to choose whether to employ public health nurses or midwives to provide antenatal care. The municipalities tend to choose public health nurses because they are more versatile in labour force terms, in that they can follow up the child to school age.
>
> F12: According to the law it's possible that communities take a midwife to work. It's OK. But they don't. Because all head nurses there are [public health nurses], of course. The basic health care

system in Finland is based on doctors and [public health nurses] working together. That's why. With this problem we have been working a lot.

At the level of professional organisations, the midwife is also in a relatively weak position:

*F34*: It's political somehow. The national association of public health nurses is much more powerful than midwives. The number of midwives is much lower than the number of public health nurses. And, you know, if somebody has gained something, it is very difficult to take it away.

The relationship between the two occupational groups is summarised by a policy-maker:

*F12*: Finnish nurses wanted to kill midwives.

## The paediatrician

Just as the PHN focuses on the fetus and baby at the expense of the mother, it is no surprise that the paediatrician shares this focus. The orientation of these personnel clearly has the potential to conflict with the tendency of the midwife to adopt a more balanced, woman-centred view. The conflicts with paediatricians related, first, to vitamin K administration to healthy babies. Sometimes the conflict was with the mother:

*F29*: When the birth was so natural, I just thought that there would be no vitamin K – nothing would be needed. It was not given and I thought that that was my decision. But then I think two days afterwards or three days after I gave birth, the child doctor checked us. She was really outraged that we hadn't given it. She was really angry with us and blamed us for being unthoughtful parents and risking our child's health. And I think that was really unnecessary and [nervous laugh] and that was weird and strange because no-one ever told us that it – I thought it was optional and then suddenly the doctor gives us pressure that we have not taken it, that we have made a mistake. She even threatened us with the police and that was strange for me.

Similar conflicts were reported by midwives:

*F04*: We've had some problems with the children's doctors. They insist that every baby should have this vitamin K. Some parents who live naturally, they don't want their babies to have it. We have had quite a problem with this. They have to sign a paper. And then we have problems – if a couple have a polyclinic birth it means that they have to stay six hours after delivery here in our labour ward. And the children's doctor comes to see everything's OK. And the children's doctor insists that the children's nurse has to take sugar blood in six hours. And we have really big problems with this because some mothers – and we see that the baby's doing fine and it's suckling the mother – it's just a healthy normal baby. And there's no reason to take the sugar blood. And the children's doctors say, 'We have to take this baby from you. And you can go home, but we will take care of it'.

And then the mother said, 'If you do this – I will NEVER COME to this hospital to have any babies. I will have home births'. And the children staff said, 'Give the baby to her,' and said, 'OK have the baby and go home'. [Laugh].

Other conflicts with paediatricians which were reported to me related to the feeding of healthy babies and children, largely in the context of the Baby Friendly Hospital Initiative (World Health Organization (WHO)/UNICEF 1989).

*Rosemary*: You've not yet achieved Baby Friendly status here?

*F31*: We started in 1996. But the paediatricians – yes. They don't trust the midwives. And they want that almost all babies get formula.

*F06*: Baby Friendly status is a very good thing, but here in [. . .] the doctors have said that they can't have Baby Friendly status because they treat very small and sick babies and these babies need to have formula as well as breast milk. And because of that they can't have Baby Friendly certification.

*F30*: The Finnish paediatricians association very strongly feels – and it has appeared as articles in their own journal – that the six months exclusive breast feeding and breastfeeding up to two years are just for underdeveloped countries – that in western countries babies don't have to have breast milk.

The Finnish midwife and mother are working tirelessly to improve Finnish breastfeeding rates. Their endeavours, though, appear to be threatened by the complacency of paediatricians:

*F31*: [At a breastfeeding conference] we had also paediatricians there. And breast feeding fully for four months, and half full breast feeding, it was 55% in Finland, 86% in Sweden and 87% in Norway. And the [Finnish] paediatricians said that this is OK. This is good. It's enough!! It's enough.

It is for reasons like these that a consumer representative made the damning observation:

*F06*: Paediatricians are the worst doctors in Finland.

From the comments made by midwives, it appears that due to inter-professional conflicts, she would support this observation. It is paradoxical that, while the Finnish health system is founded on teamwork to maintain health, the membership of that team is questionable. In addition, a major health maintenance activity, breastfeeding, is poorly supported.

## Subverting the system

Although Finns have a stereotypical tendency to respect authority, are proud of their fine healthcare system and seem convinced that institutional birth is preferable, there are certain inconsistencies which verge on the paradoxical. These paradoxes relate to issues mentioned already and may comprise tactics to subvert the system.

### Breastfeeding

Occasionally a mother would criticise the advice which she was offered at the *neuvola*. One mother in particular (F15), while commending the system in general, was unhappy at the poor support and outdated advice which she was given when breastfeeding her two children. The PHN's recommendations of early weaning of the older child, then the provision of scales for test-weighing resonate with the findings of a Scottish study (Chalmers 1991). This research identified the varied advice from the health visitor and midwife. This mother recounted the tactics she was forced to use to ensure that her younger child was fed appropriately while maintaining her relationship with the *neuvola* staff:

*F15*: And my son was very happy and he was ... and urinating and everything was functioning well and he was eating. ... [Laugh]. But [the public health nurse] said that I should give him extra formula. But I knew – I didn't at that moment know that much about this, except what I had learned from the clinic. So I contacted – what do you call it – an organisation which is interested in breastfeeding. They have a person to help and also my cousin – she is a psychologist. She seems to be very good at this [laugh]. And I got good support from her. So I trusted myself. Even though I was very confused 'cos when it's your first child and you want the best for him [laugh]. But I didn't give any extra milk. And I said to the nurse I was going to. 'Cos I had extra ... at that time. And then I told her that I had given him extra even though I hadn't 'cos in a way I felt that I was the authority, also, on what he wanted [laugh]. But when I next went to the clinic I found that his weight is starting to come up.

## Securing the optimal birth experience

Another example of a mother resorting to subterfuge in order to achieve her wished-for experience involved the help of a sympathetic obstetrician; thus, she subverted the system to 'book' for a particular hospital:

> *F11*: I called the hospital in [. . .] and they said, 'No you can't come here because what would happen if everyone went to where they want to go to? It would be chaos if every one just went to where they want to go to. So, no, you can't come here.' But then I called around to different private clinics to find a doctor who works at this hospital [. . .] in [. . .]. So I found this one doctor and he said, 'Oh yes, you can come. I will take you as a patient. So just come and you can say that you are my patient.' So I went to see him once before the birth at the hospital. It was one week before [baby] was born and he said that 'I'll write in these papers that I have [examined] you because of suspicions that the baby is too big.' Even there was no such suspicion, but he said, 'I'll write here that it was suspected that the baby is too large. And that's why I have consulted you here and then you can come here to this hospital.' So I went to this hospital in [. . .] and I liked it. It was a good experience.

This woman was clearly satisfied with her more 'natural' birth experience. The midwife, though, may encounter difficulty in facilitating the birth which the woman seeks in a medicalised setting. This difficulty is aggravated by the medical assumption that they have a right of entry (see Being strong, above):

> *F31*: They want to visit in the labour room very often.

A midwife told me, though, of how she excludes medical staff, who might threaten the woman's achievement of her sought-after experience:

> *Rosemary*: How would you facilitate a natural birth in hospital?
> *F04*: In hospital I try to keep the doctors away from the mother [laugh]. And I – the doctors respect me. Because I've been working here so long. And I can tell them that there is no reason to come to see the mother. I know where we are going. I will have everything in control. But everybody cannot do it.

Perhaps unfortunately, this midwife clearly recognised that not all of her midwifery colleagues would have the assertiveness skills to demonstrate such strength. It is clear from these two examples, though, that the midwife and the woman may adopt similarly robust strategies to defeat the 'system' in order to achieve what they know is appropriate. These strategies resonate with those identified as being used by midwives in Scotland to 'circumvent medical staff when it was felt that inappropriate decisions had been made' (Askham and Barbour 1996:45).

## Home birth

Whereas the last two examples related to ensuring the desired birth experience in a medicalised setting, some women told me of how they subverted the system in order to achieve a home birth. Unlike woman F11 (see above) who deliberately lied to *neuvola* staff, another woman simply omitted to mention that she intended to give birth at home:

> F24: I was about seven months pregnant when I came [back from abroad] to live here. And then I thought, 'OK, well I just carry on with my [home birth] plans,' y'know. But then I realised Oh it wasn't so easy as I thought. Cos suddenly everybody was 'Oh my God'. 'Oh it's not possible.' So then I actually refused to tell the neuvola. So in the first place I told but they were totally like – being so horrible to me. Like say, 'Oh my God. D'you want to kill your children?' And stuff like this. Like, 'You're not really being a responsible woman,' and everything like this. So I then I moved area in Finland where I was living – I moved to another place so I changed my neuvola place. And in the new place I didn't tell, 'cos I knew I was going to get so much criticism.

Another woman, whose wider family included many medical practitioners, found herself obliged to lie about her home birth plans, to achieve a less stressful pregnancy:

> F28: (Field notes) She was encouraged by [husband and a friend] and she lied to her parents and most of her friends, as they would not have been comfortable with the idea of a home birth.

## Keeping midwifery secrets

It is becoming apparent that a number of more or less devious strategies are employed to circumvent maternity conventions. Although the Finnish system is universally applauded, there are clearly occasions when this stereotypically direct people are forced to resort to subversive behaviour to achieve their desired outcomes. In one setting, I learned from a number of midwifery staff about the deceptions employed to permit one particular midwife to attend home births. These tactics were perpetrated in full knowledge of the potentially dire consequences if apprehended (see F30 above). Because of the sensitivity of this material, I have removed any identifying material.

(Field notes from interview with midwife who attends home births)

She explained the secret nature of her practice. A few of her midwife colleagues and manager know, but the medical staff are not supposed to know. She says that she has to follow the hospital line of recommending hospital birth; but if the women who phone her at home decline to come in, she says that she will go to them, rather than have an unassisted birth. I suppose that this is quite a pragmatic reason for attending home births.

(Interview with a midwife colleague of the Midwife who attends home births).

I know two midwives, one working here and one who is retired, and they can be called to assist a birth at someone's home. And one midwife in this town who is working in the private sector at an out patient clinic, she can be called too. These are informal. That mothers know people and the Active Birth society know people and therefore home births [happen]. But nobody knows about it, y'know, officially. We don't have any instruments and material because the society doesn't have any. They have to borrow them from [the maternity unit] here. And this is why we have to do it in secret.

*Rosemary*: The Midwife attending a home birth would come here for her cord clamps?

Yes, and all the instruments. I think that she has got something from here . . . If all the instruments and medications are not needed, they bring them back. And, of course, the instruments are brought back anyway. And then we have to carry those back in secret. I have done it because this Midwife who had to go to someone's home. She was working on night shift and I came here in the morning and the mother came here too. They didn't get anyone 'cos all the Midwives were working in that night. And then the father gave me those instruments back. And I carried them in to my cupboard where I change my clothes, to give them to the other Midwife when I see her. Everything in secret. It's very unofficial. Our boss is aware of it now, she is aware that this Midwife is available if someone wants her. But we don't speak about it – for good reason.

(Interview with these midwives' manager)

There are a couple of Midwives in Finland who go to help women to give birth at home. But it's not official. We haven't got that. Now I think here in [. . .] you – if someone asks you to come and help her birth you can't say it out loud. You have to hide it. And you have to say little. I know it's a little naughty, but we have to steal the equipment somehow out of the hospital if you are going to attend someone [who] wants to give birth at home.

It is apparent that these midwifery personnel were working strenuously to maintain the pretence that they are obedient to the system within which they are employed. At the same time, though, they are endeavouring to provide a much-needed service for the childbearing woman.

## Conclusion

As a relatively young country, Finland is greatly influenced by its history. A crucial feature of this history comprises strong, well-educated women working at least as equals alongside the menfolk. The history also comprises repeated colonisations by the then world powers, first from the west of Finland and then from the east. This colonial past has left its mark in the tendency towards obedience to authority. In the same way, the Finnish midwife's role in practice has largely been 'colonised' by the relatively recent arrival of the PHN. The national stereotype of being 'systems obedient' results in the midwife's acceptance of this reduced role, together with an acquiescence to medical authority in her main sphere of midwifery practice – the hospital labour ward.

The research project outlined in this chapter suggests that this picture may be in the process of undergoing changes. The women consumers of maternity care, being supremely well-informed, are seriously critical of the baby-centred and outdated *neuvola* system of maternity care. These criticisms are also levelled at paediatricians, who threaten women's confidence in their ability to decide about feeding their babies, and put pressure on them to accept other interventions. Partly in response to the demands of women, Active Birth is beginning to become established. Policy makers are questioning why the Finnish midwife is accepting her diminished role. Midwives are responding with increasing confidence to these changes, although they find themselves working with women surreptitiously to subvert the omnipotent healthcare system.

Thus, like the geographical position of her country, the Finnish midwife finds herself positioned between two major powers, the PHN and medical personnel. It is possible, though, that like this young country, Finnish midwifery may yet re-establish its independent identity.

> ## Reflective questions
>
> As we have seen, power struggles can be evident at differing levels and situations. Can you think of any power struggles in your situation?
>
> How would you deal with colleagues or clients who you felt were preventing you from offering 'best practice'.

## References

Active Birth 2005 Aktiivinen Synnytys Ry (Active Birth website) Online. Available: http://www.lapsiperhe.net/aktiivinensynnytys/etusivu.php3 (accessed 19 August 2005)

Askham J, Barbour R 1996 The negotiated role of the midwife in Scotland. In: Robinson S, Thomson A M (eds) Midwives, Research and Childbirth, Vol 4. Chapman and Hall, London, pp 33–59

Brown D J 1994 Opinions of general practitioners in Nottinghamshire about provision of intrapartum care. BMJ 309(6957):777–779

CEMACH 2005 Stillbirth, neonatal and post-neonatal mortality 2000–2003. England, Wales and Northern Ireland. RCOG Press, London

Chalmers JWT 1991 Variations in breast feeding advice, a telephone survey of community midwives and health visitors. Midwifery 7(4):162–166

Eurostat 2001 Key data on health 2000. Office for Official Publications of the European Communities, Luxemburg

Goodrich A 1960 Study in SISU: Finland's Fight for Independence. Ballantine Books, New York

Helsti H 1995 Midwife or paarmuska? The conflicts surrounding home confinements as reflectors of the cultural differences prevailing in the agrarian community. In: Korhonen T (ed) Encountering Ethnicities: Ethnological Aspects on Ethnicity, Identity and Migration. Suomalaisen Kirjallisuuden Seura, Helsinki, pp 105–117

Helsti H 1997 'Once were the mothers of iron': Countrywomen, birth and work during the first half of 20th century. Finland IX International Oral History Conference, Gothenburg, Sweden

Hyyppä mt mäki J 2001 Why do Swedish-speaking Finns have such longer active life? An area for social capital research. Health Promotion International 16(1):55–64

Kansanterveyslaki, Suomen asetuskokoelma 66/1972 (Finnish Public Health Act) 1972

Kosunen E, Rimpelä M 1996 Improving adolescence sexual health in Finland. Choices: Sexual Health and Family Planning in Europe, 25:18–21

Mander R 2005 Perceptions of decision-making in relation to maternity care organisation and place of birth in New Zealand and Finland. Unpublished report to funding body (British Academy). Based in University of Edinburgh, Edinburgh

Ministry of Labour 2003 Family leaves – a matter for both parents. Online. Available at: http://www.mol.fi/english/working/familyleaves2003.html (accessed 19 August 2005)

Oinas E, Nikkonen M, Pietila A 1999 A midwife-public-health nurse's work in northern Finland, 1950–87. International Journal of Nursing Practice September 5(3):116–122

Renzetti CM, Lee RM 1993 Researching Sensitive Topics. Sage, London

SEHD 2000 Our National Health: A Plan for Action, a Plan for Change. NHS Scotland Edinburgh

Singleton F 1989 A Short History of Finland. Cambridge University Press, Cambridge

Sovijärvi S 2005 Taskusanakirja. Söderström, Helsinki

STAKES (2002) Facts about Finnish Social Welfare and Health Care 2002. Sosiaali-ja terveysalan tutkimus-ja kehittämiskeskus (STAKES)(National Research and Development Centre for Welfare and Health), Helsinki

Stark-Arola L 1998 Gender, Boundaries and 'Fitting Together' in Finnish-Karelian Everyday Magic. In: Apo S, Nenola A, Stark-Arola L (eds) Gender and Folklore: Perspectives on Finnish and Karelian Culture. Studia Fennica Folkloristica 4. Finnish Literature Society, Helsinki, pp 31–62

WHO/UNICEF 1989 Protecting, promoting and supporting breastfeeding: The Special Role of Maternity Services. A joint WHO/UNICEF statement. World Health Organization, Geneva

Wrede S, Benoit C, Sandall J 2001 The State and birth/the state of birth maternal health policy in three countries. In: DeVries R, Benoit C, van Teijlingen E R et al (eds) Birth by Design: Pregnancy, Maternity Care, and Midwifery in North America and Europe. Routledge, London

# CHAPTER EIGHT

# Midwifery-led care

LIZ STEPHENS

A Royal College of Midwives (RCM 2001) position paper describes 'woman-centred care' as a philosophy of maternity care that gives priority to the wishes and needs of the user, emphasising the importance of informed choice. The RCM goes on to state that true woman-centred care must encompass midwifery-led care of normal pregnancy, birth and the postnatal period. Midwifery-led care is described as care where midwives act as the lead professional with good liaison and referral links to medical colleagues. It is popular with women, cost effective and delivers good outcomes.

I believe the two concepts of midwifery-led care and woman-centred care go hand in hand. Women in the UK value good midwifery care and midwives want to give midwifery-led care. Do we have the freedom to do so within the constraints of the modern day National Health Service (NHS)? This chapter will explore what we mean by midwifery-led care, using examples from practice to identify ways in which we can promote midwifery-led and woman-centred care, and ways in which the use of this philosophy of care might reveal problems in practice. The practices around birth in twenty-first century Britain will be critiqued. In addition, the chapter will discuss the question: Are we positioning ourselves with woman or with institution?

The RCM position statement (2001) goes on to state that effective implementation of woman-centred care requires the development of innovative models of service delivery. In today's NHS how realistic is this? We work in an era of recruitment and retention crises complicated by, in the southeast of England at least, a rising birth rate. Midwives have experienced the expansion of their role and increasing demands from women, in staffing establishments that are based on tradition and frequently have not changed for decades. The report of the Healthcare Commission (2005) raised serious concerns regarding maternity services, which are under-resourced and understaffed. In addition, professional dominance is rife, and midwives are leaving the profession due to an inability to work in the ways they want to (Ball et al 2002). Labour ward management is increasingly governed by policies and guidelines demanded by the Clinical Negligence Scheme for Trusts, meaning that midwives feel increasingly that they are unable to provide individualised, woman-centred care. Birth centres or midwifery-led units are promoted in the midwifery press and the *National Service Framework* (NSF) (DoH 2004); yet few women have access to them and admission criteria vary considerably (Hall 2002). This chapter will ask whether or not midwifery-led care out of hospital, either at home or in birth centres gives midwives freedom to practise.

During training, student midwives learn to practise in the ways of midwifery practice of the twenty-first century, in which:

- medicalisation is so widespread and pervasive that we no longer notice it (Gould 2002)
- epidurals are almost the norm and caesarean section rates keep rising
- midwives are positioned lower in the hierarchy than obstetricians.
- midwives all too often don't get to see a home birth throughout their training and learn to look after more than one woman at a time in labour and to depend on technology. They learn to conform, not to argue and so, eventually to perpetuate the system (Bosanquet 2002).

At the point of qualification current practice in most maternity units is to have a period of 'consolidation' within the hospital before a midwife can move to community practice if that is their wish. Yet during this consolidation period they learn to look after the most complex and high risk cases, depending on the technology of monitors, epidurals, augmentation, on the buzzer that calls help instantly and on the system that encourages women to conform to the hospital way of birth. They learn to believe in policies and protocols rather than women's bodies and women's ability to give birth. The result of all this is rising rates of intervention and subservience to the medical model.

*Changing Childbirth* (Department of Health (DoH) 1993) suggested that approximately 75% of women should have the midwife as lead professional. Yet there are units where the caesarean section rate is over 30% and rising. Taken along with other forms of intervention does this mean that there are now 65% of women who are low risk and suitable for midwifery-led care? Twice in my career to date I have been involved in establishing a birth centre away from the labour ward. It has surprised me how many doctors and midwives consider that it is dangerous to have a baby away from the labour ward. I believe that this demonstrates that the technocratic model of birth dominates all care and demands that care is 'with institution' rather than with woman.

# The technocratic model of birth

Birth today predominantly takes place within maternity units surrounded by the trappings of the medical profession and all that it stands for: science, power and knowledge (Henley-Einion 2003). The technocratic model of birth has become the norm in most Western cultures. This places heavy reliance on technology such as continuous electronic monitoring, induction, forceps and vacuum deliveries (Davis-Floyd 1992). Yet a World Health Organization (WHO) perinatal study group reviewing the scientific litera-ture and routine obstetric procedures concluded that only approximately 10% had an adequate scientific basis (Wagner 1997). Wagner (1997) describing how the medical establishment attempted to discredit this infor-mation, states that to discredit technology is tantamount to discrediting progress: with a strange dichotomy existing in which if you are not in favour of all technology you are therefore against all technology. This is coupled with an assumption that technology always means progress.

Foucault (1973) suggested that modern societies use surveillance and monitoring to discipline the activities of citizens. This surveillance can be at both an institutional and a personal level as he describes the doctor–patient relationship as a field of scientific investigation. Within Foucault's (1973, 1977) power knowledge analysis, discipline is crucial, not just as discipline in order to punish, but as disciplines in terms of theoretical knowledge, such as the discipline of medicine. In Foucault's analysis people work hard at their discipline which enables them to achieve power and status according them a rank and a space within an institution. In the maternity unit obstetricians have long periods of training and are thus accorded power, rank and status. The lesser length of training undertaken by midwives accords them less status and power.

This critique shows us ways in which medical dominance is perpetuated. Foucault's study of prisons suggested that they were a form of micro society where prisoners were coerced into conforming: it had its own experts, hierarchies and ranks as well as codes of conduct, protocols and proce-dures. This societal form of organisation is mirrored in other institutions such as hospitals. The panoptic or all-seeing eye is a metaphor taken from prison design to show how surveillance in modern society is pervasive to such an extent that we monitor ourselves and others in order to conform to society's norms. This carceral analysis can be used to look at the mater-nity service with its procedures and protocols that are used, not only to regulate bodies and events, but also as a form of surveillance: not following guidelines can be a reason for being reported to risk management for both doctors and midwives and to supervision for midwives. In our labour wards women and their unborn babies are monitored observed and examined. If they don't fall within the boundaries of 'normal' they are subject to technological interventions to ensure that they do. Surveillance, however, continues away from the institution: for instance, even home births where woman have made a choice of an alternative to hospital practices and policies, are subject to these, for example, the imposition of time limitations. The midwife is stuck in the middle trying to keep the woman happy yet constantly aware of the all-seeing eye of hospital policy and the judgements that will be made on her management.

The technocratic model of birth is the model that dominates childbirth in the twenty-first century (Davis-Floyd 2001, Kitzinger 2005). This model stresses mind-body separation, seeing the body as a machine and treating the woman as an object. Within this model the caregiver is a professional, distanced from the woman and practising within a hierarchical institution (Davis-Floyd 2001). Mander (2002) suggests that this is a model within which the majority of doctors work; however many midwives work within this model as well.

Science and technology are valued above all else within this model. The woman's first encounter with the maternity services is often a nuchal fold scan at 12 weeks. This highly technological screening is for Down's syndrome, for which there is no 'treatment' other than termination of pregnancy. Ultrasound scanning is used increasingly but yet there is no proved benefit to the unborn child or the woman (Foster 1995). On labour wards women are increasingly subject to interventions such as continuous electronic fetal monitoring and epidural anaesthesia, despite the frequent lack of evidence to support their efficacy. The widespread use of continuous electronic fetal monitoring followed its introduction without evaluation by any form of trial; the only proved consequence of its introduction has been a rise in the caesarean section rate (Enkin et al 2000).

Other interventions on our labour ward are even more subtle and insidious. Kitzinger (2005) critiques the presence of the clock, the chair and the bed, all seen as benign but each has the ability to undermine normal birth. Indicative of the way the technocratic model has become all pervasive is the way women's language has changed over the years. Kitzinger (2005) describes how language both expresses and reflects the way we think, and can make reality. I was recently in conversation with a midwifery friend who pointed out how women in transition, the stage of labour that marks passing from the first to second stage, used to say, 'God help me' or, 'I want my mother' or, 'I want to go home'. All too often recently this has changed to, 'I want an epidural'. I think that this demonstrates a society that no longer believes in God and where families are no longer an accessible form of support. Thus, society has turned to technology instead. I believe that

that this demonstrates that birth is such an important part of culture it both reflects and shapes it. Midwives working within this culture feel they have to respond to the request for an epidural in case they incur a complaint; yet they do not feel they have to respond to 'I want to go home'. This then gives technology the privilege of being rational, and fits in with the dominant understanding of the service, whereas to go home would not be acceptable.

Midwives working within the labour wards where the technocratic model is dominant, learn to conform and become 'good girls' (Bosanquet 2002). This is demonstrated by the attitude of midwives to waterbirth. Waterbirth has been shown to be as safe as birth out of the water for both women and their babies and is highly evaluated by women (Alderdice et al 1995). When I took up my current post there was a waterbirth service, supported by a small group of committed midwives, whereas other midwives did not 'do' waterbirth. To support the service I had a birthing pool put into the labour ward, I have run waterbirth workshops for midwives and I offered to be on call to support midwives new to waterbirth. Nevertheless, women are frequently refused waterbirth on spurious grounds such as, the midwife is not trained in waterbirth, or, the pool is out of action, among others. Midwives who do not 'do' waterbirth however will happily 'do' epidurals with the increased level of work required, the increased levels of side effects and the increased risks of further intervention. I believe this is because waterbirth is viewed as not being technological enough to fit in with the dominant belief system. Kitzinger (2005) believes this is an expression of the way power is used to manipulate women in childbirth to conform to what is valued by the institution. Waterbirth has become subject to research, education and guidelines which, instead of making it more mainstream, have made it seem something inherently dangerous. Midwives who do support waterbirth are seen as 'other' and can be marginalised within the work culture. Equally, midwives who support home births, in some areas are marginalised to the extent that it has been called a global witch hunt (Wagner 1995). Scientific 'objective' knowledge is valued above all other yet its basis is frequently not that scientific. The power of knowledge used by those in authority within our institutions is not that it is correct but that it counts (Jordan 1997). Within our hospitals it is the power of obstetrics that has become the authoritative knowledge.

The story of a recent incident demonstrates this. A midwife working on the labour ward was caring for a woman who had had a previous caesarean section. The woman was in early labour and wished to mobilise in labour. On speaking to the woman it was obvious that she was not in fully established labour. The midwife discussed the incidence of scar rupture with the woman along with the reasons for continuous monitoring. She informed the woman that it was her body and her choice to make as long as she was informed of, and understood the choices she had. The woman was informed and articulate and the midwife was willing to support her in her choice. Following a lengthy discussion the woman decided she did not want continuous monitoring at this stage of her labour but might decide to have it as the labour progressed. This plan was documented in the notes. She was seen on the consultant ward round, and it was decided that she should have a vaginal examination. The midwife questioned the need for this at this stage stating that the woman was not in fully established labour. Both the midwife and woman were over-ridden: the woman was told that the scar could rupture at any time and the baby would be at risk. Without medical intervention the risks of this happening in early labour are minimal, and increase with both medical interventions and labour progress.

The vaginal examination revealed that the woman was in the very early stages of labour. The consultant insisted that she be continuously monitored, which would not prevent scar rupture but might possibly identify it slightly earlier. The woman was effectively silenced by the threat to her baby's wellbeing, and the midwife silenced by the power of the medical model. To challenge this model within the locus of power, the labour ward, can lead to marginalisation. When this was discussed with the consultant obstetrician he acknowledged that midwives' knowledge of labour was different from that of an obstetrician as midwives observe women throughout the labour continuum. This gives them the ability to form an opinion regarding whether or not a woman is in labour. Obstetricians rarely if ever observe a complete labour and therefore do not have this observational knowledge and use vaginal examination to judge whether or not a woman is in labour. However, vaginal examination is a subjective measure.

This scenario demonstrates how midwifery knowledge is devalued and ignored. In this case it resulted in the woman's having a procedure that is unpleasant, undignified, increases vulnerability and is unnecessary. This led to further interventions in the form of continuous monitoring and sedation. These in turn can lead to augmentation of labour and an increased risk of scar rupture.

# Home birth

Within midwifery there is currently much debate around the issue of normality. The Royal College of Midwives (RCM) is running a normal birth campaign to raise the profile of normality. For low-risk women home birth has been shown to result in less intervention (Northern Region Perinatal Mortality Survey Coordination Group 1996, Wiegers et al 1996, Davies J

1997, CESDI 1999, Chamberlain et al 1999, Wickham 1999). Why then do midwives not champion home birth to a greater extent? Home birth is almost always physiological or at the very least low intervention. Midwives as experts in normal birth should logically be actively promoting home births. True freedom to practise, where midwives care for a woman throughout her childbearing period, planning, implementing and evaluating care, and using the full range of her skills and knowledge (Sargent 2002) is most likely to be at home births. A woman wanting home birth rarely sees an obstetrician, or general practitioner (GP), and the midwife makes any decisions around referral or transfer.

My observation of home births over the years has led me to believe that home birth positions childbirth in the heart of the family and empowers women to believe in their bodies and to rely on their social networks. In addition, home birth introduces the baby into the home and the family from the beginning and starts the relationship off on the right basis. Hospital makes birth clinical (Davis-Floyd 1992) yet it is the miracle of new life and the extension of a family. Hospital birth often leads to a range of interventions that women find distressing and traumatic. These might undermine their belief in their own bodies and their ability to mother the new baby (Oakley and Rajan 1990). Birth is a universal part of female physiology and biology but as it is shaped by societies and cultures, it is more than a simple biological fact (Davis-Floyd and Sargent 1997): it is a rite of passage. How we manage birth is a reflection on our society as a whole.

The current Government agenda is towards increasing normality and a higher home birth rate (DoH 1993, 2004). Also, it stresses the importance of user choice and involvement. Services need to be based within the community setting. This creates a climate that is supportive of home birth, yet since the publication of *Changing Childbirth* (DoH 1993) the home birth rate has hardly increased at all. The current rate nationally is around 2% (BirthChoice UK 2004). Why should this be? If women were offered true choice the home birth rate would be around 8–10% (DoH 1993). My own experience as a community midwife supports these figures: when offered home birth as a realistic option, around 10% of women in my caseload chose to have one.

Within midwifery in recent years there have been problems of chronic recruitment and retention. These mean that there is the constant problem of having enough midwives to provide a safe home birth service. There is anecdotal evidence of women booking for home birth and being told at 37 weeks, or when they go into labour that there is no midwife available to look after them at home. This puts both women and midwives in an impossible position. It cannot be right to offer women an option that they want and look forward to and then withdraw it at the last minute. Midwives are left feeling guilty and frustrated that they have not been able to provide this service. Midwives on our busy labour wards are left to look after women who arrive upset and unhappy with what has happened to them, if indeed they choose to go into hospital rather than have their baby at home unattended. Such a policy of withdrawing a home birth service I believe to be inexcusable, not only for the reasons given above, but also that once more it means privileging hospital over home and intervention over physiology. Such decisions are made by managers, no doubt with the best of intentions. However such a decision is putting the service and women under further stress. The midwives who practise home birth by and large do not want to practise on labour wards; therefore they leave (Ball et al 2002). This then perpetuates recruitment and retention problems. In addition, midwives who want to practise midwifery-led care are unlikely to be attracted to such a unit.

Other ways of dissuading women from giving birth at home have been documented. It is interesting to note that the Association for the Improvement of Maternity Services (AIMS 2004) website discusses 'home birth bullying' and describes tactics used to persuade women wanting home births into hospitals. Home birth is virtually completely the domain of the midwife, yet some midwives are colluding in persuading women to go into hospital where they are subject to higher rates of interventions and dissatisfaction with their birth experience. Lorna Davies (2004) used a midwifery group to obtain midwives' and student midwives' experiences of ways in which women are dissuaded from having home births. Her findings showed that there are midwives who prevent women from having home births for completely invalid reasons, often physical and spurious such as: you have an untested pelvis; too much amniotic fluid; too little amniotic fluid. One woman was told she could not have a home birth because she was partially sighted, a condition that would not interfere with the physical process of labour, but would have significant psychological impact in knowing her surroundings and feeling able to relax. Social factors are also cited such as living in a terraced house (neighbours might hear) and living in a council flat. One woman who lived on a barge was told that she could not have a home birth because the midwife might fall from the tow path into the canal if she had to attend at night. Midwives talk about being practitioners in their own right and experts in normality, yet home birth is where they are truly the lead professional, with physiological birth being the norm. Discouraging women from home birth in this way, as well as increased trauma and dissatisfaction being expressed by women about their birth experiences lead me to believe that some midwives have no interest in the promotion of normality. It also seems to indicate that the medical model of birth is the norm: Gould (2002) describes subliminal medicalisation, where the medicalisation of childbirth is so widespread and embedded that it is no longer noticed.

In a recent home birth story (Madden 2005) a midwife with 25 years' practice described how she thought she knew birth after practising in the labour ward for many years. However, being present at a home birth made her challenge the way she had known and practised birth. Yet some midwives are obviously practising within community settings and facilitating home births against their wishes (Madden 2005). To be cared for by a reluctant midwife at a home birth must have an impact on women. My personal training for home birth included only an expectation that I would get on with it. This was after years of practice within high technology labour ward settings. I believe this is the reality for most community midwives. This must have implications for the way in which they practise in out-of-hospital settings.

The hospital way of managing birth is about monitoring. Midwives are taught to monitor progress, blood pressure, fetal wellbeing, and, less overtly, they learn to monitor behaviour. When such monitoring is used at home births, women describe it as intrusive and question its necessity (Edwards 2004). Edwards (2004) suggests that midwives are so afraid of not adhering to routine practices such as vaginal examinations that they continued with them when women were expressing pain and requests to stop. Without education and support it is not surprising that many midwives are fearful of, and therefore not supportive of home birth. I recently attended a woman having a home birth. She had had her previous baby at home. Afterwards, she commented on the completely different nature of the births. At her previous birth she had felt constantly pressured to transfer into hospital, and felt she had given birth at home despite the midwives. With this birth she had the labour and birth experience that she wanted and felt supported in that. This woman was a strong and assertive woman with a fully supportive partner who had felt that he was 'patrolling the boundaries' with the first birth. Women less committed and without such support may well have transferred in to hospital.

There is evidence that some midwives are trying to change the ethos of home birth. Jean Robinson (1996) believes we have 'modern home births' where midwives take hospital practices and interventions into the woman's home. Jennifer Hall (1999) describes a home birth where the midwives spent a lot of time and effort transforming the woman's home into a mini hospital with much rustling of paper packs and setting up of equipment, again to the detriment of the woman's birth experience. If we want freedom to practise, we need to ensure that we pass on the skills of home birth to midwives who want to practise in this way. In our hospitals we have built a model of practice development that maintains this status quo, where 'development' has become all about suturing, topping up epidurals, analysing cardiotocographs (CTGs). These are all important, but not to the detriment of low-risk midwifery practice, where the midwife's skill lies in doing nothing or watchful expectancy.

The Birth Trauma Association website (2004) is a sad indictment of current maternity care practices. It contains stories of women who have been so severely traumatised by their birth experience that they suffer from depression and post-traumatic stress disorder (PTSD). The majority of these concern hospital births and intervention. However, there is one story of a home birth where the midwife was uncaring and unsupportive, resulting in the woman's transfer into hospital and a subsequent range of interventions.

Not all women are unhappy with their hospital birth experiences. Nevertheless, in my current practice I tend to have women referred to me who have had previous traumatic birth experiences. Their evidence has led me to believe that dissatisfaction with hospital experiences is more widespread than is acknowledged within the profession. The hierarchical nature of hospitals places obstetric knowledge as authoritative and above that of midwifery knowledge and women's knowledge of, and belief in, their bodies (Davis-Floyd and Sargent 1997). In addition, it leads midwives to seek approval from the institution thereby withdrawing from her role as women's advocate. In a recent book chapter (Stephens 2004) I wrote advocating a with woman model of midwifery. Such a model of practice positions the midwife 'with woman'. and enables the midwife to work with her to protect her from institutional bullying: where evidence or the wellbeing of her baby are used to coerce her into having interventions she does not want.

Evidence is usually based on some form of research. However, within the current state of knowledge the randomised controlled trial is seen as the only reliable evidence. To prove anything, large numbers need to be involved and results tell us if a benefit is there for a statistically significant majority. If this benefit means having an intervention that a woman does not want, we do not know whether she is in the group that would benefit or not. Within our society we take risks on a daily basis, crossing the road, going skiing, doing extreme sports: such risks are down to individual choice. Yet women who choose to take a relatively small risk, such as not having continuous monitoring after having had a previous caesarean section are subjected to censure and bullying by the rational power of science. The paradox of this is that such 'scientific' power is sometimes used to the detriment of women, and is based on scientific rational ways of knowing. Belenky et al (1999) show that women's ways of knowing are different and include emotional and psychological factors as well as physical. Belenky et al describe five epistemological perspectives from which women know and view the world. One of these perspectives is silence, where women experience themselves as mindless and voiceless and subject to the whims of external authority. This seems to be particularly pertinent to the maternity services where women are frequently unable to express their needs and choices in a service that is provided for women but where key decision makers are frequently men; and where midwives work from the perspective of received knowledge rather than constructed.

# Birth centres

With the possibility that midwives may have largely lost the freedom to practise home births, what then of birth centres? Birth centres or midwifery-led units have had a chequered career. Sometimes called maternity units, general practitioner units or peripheral units they used to be widespread. Many were closed over the years to conform with centralisation. Some have survived in the guise of midwifery-led units but are under constant surveillance and pressure to close, especially if they are not alongside a maternity unit. In addition, they are seen as expensive to run. More recently, following the successful establishment and evaluation of the Edgware Birth Centre there are more birth centres being opened throughout the UK (Saunders et al 2000). Birth centres are homely out-of-hospital facilities that provide care for women who want and can safely choose to have a non-interventionist birth (Rosser 2001). There is no accepted definition of what a birth centre is; however a review by the National Perinatal Epidemiology Unit (NPEU) uses the definition:

> A birth centre is an institution that offers care to women with a straightforward pregnancy and where midwives take primary professional responsibility for care. During labour and birth medical services including obstetric, neonatal and anaesthetic are available should they be needed, but they may be on a separate site, or in a separate building, which may involve transfer by car or ambulance
>
> *NPEU (2005:8)*

Birth centres are run by midwives skilled in supporting women through normal birth without the use of technology and intervention. Crucially, women's needs are at the centre of the organisation and their influence on care is apparent (Rosser 2001). Birth centres can be freestanding, sited away from a site that provides high risk maternity services or sited alongside a maternity unit. An alongside unit may be sited adjacent to a labour ward or on the same hospital site but physically distant from the labour ward.

Those that are geographically distant from the labour ward appear to enable midwives to develop practice that is not influenced by labour ward practices, and in particular minimise transfers 'for an epidural' (personal communication, consultant midwife group, 2003). Within labour wards women are frequently seen as the 'work' to be moved along a production line (Hunt and Symonds 1995), whereas the philosophy of midwifery-led units is one of working with women, enabling them to relax and supporting physiological birth. Evaluations of birth centres to date, show that they reduce the need for interventions such as pharmacological pain relief, episiotomy, forceps and caesarean sections (Waldenstrom et al 1997, Saunders et al 2000, Hodnett 2004). Women report high levels of satisfaction with birth centre care and midwives enjoy working in them (Saunders et al 2000, Gould et al 2004, Hodnett 2004).

Birth centres do not currently have a standard philosophy of care, guidelines or audit tools. Transfer rates reported by birth centres vary widely, influenced by differences in eligibility criteria, transfer procedures and midwives experience and confidence in working in out of hospital settings. Without nationally agreed criteria and audits it is difficult to assess the success of birth centres, yet the evidence so far would suggest that midwives enjoy working in them and have the freedom to practise midwifery-led care. The danger for such units is that as they proliferate, more midwives will transfer from labour ward practice. We need to ensure that midwives have the skills, education and support to enable them to be competent and confident to practise in such settings.

We also need to address the issue of continuity of care for women using birth centres. Many include antenatal clinics which are run on site as part of their responsibility. Some welcome the involvement of community midwives who wish to care for their own women in labour. Many, however, provide birth services only. This is often due to geographical problems but the limited provision of care denies women and midwives the opportunity of building a trusting relationship that improves the experience and outcome for both parties. Birth centres may be the way forward for midwifery care, but we must ensure that we provide continuity, maximising both the outcomes and the experience for women.

# Caseload holding and continuity

The notion of continuity is an important one in the midwife–woman relationship. Continuity itself is a complex issue as it can mean continuity of care from a team of midwives, or continuity of carer by a single known midwife. The Cochrane review (Hodnett 2002) includes trials of care given by a small number of caregivers throughout pregnancy, labour and birth. When compared with women who have multiple carers, women cared for in this way are less likely: to have antenatal hospital admissions; to have pain relieving drugs in labour; to have perineal trauma. And, they are more likely to have babies born in better condition. These advantages are not inconsiderable and therefore care needs to be organised in a way that offers women continuity.

One reasonable way of offering women continuity of care is through caseload practice. Within caseload practice women are usually looked after by two midwives from booking through pregnancy. In labour they will be cared for by at least one of these midwives. This type of care is highly regarded by women (Allen et al 1997, McCourt and Page 1996), but requires a heavy on-call commitment for the midwives. Midwives who choose this type of practice report high levels of satisfaction as well as a supportive and enabling relationship with women (Sandall 1997, McCourt and Percival 2000). My own experience of caseload practice was that it gave me freedom to practise in the way I want to practise: in an equal partnership with women, enabling the building of a mutually beneficial relationship.

Not all midwives want, or are able to practise in this way. However, there is an increasing trend to address the needs of disadvantaged women, such as in Sure Start areas with caseload teams (Hutchings and Henty 2001). Such schemes appear to achieve higher normal birth rates as well as increased home birth rates (Hutchings and Henty 2001, Reed 2002). Given that the most vulnerable women in our society are 20 times more likely to die in childbirth than those in social class 1 and 2 (CEMACH 2004), this would seem to be a viable and realistic way of attempting to address some of these inequalities, and worthy of further evaluation.

## Freedom to practise midwifery-led care

How then are we to achieve freedom to practise? Is freedom to practise achievable or indeed desirable? For me the answer is in the title 'midwife': mid-with, wife-woman. The only way we can have freedom to practise woman-centred midwife-led care is by positioning ourselves alongside women. To do this, we need to subscribe to a with woman model of care. Such a model would incorporate five key principles, which underpin a feminist model of healthcare delivery (Foster 1989). These principles include the sharing of all knowledge with the woman in a way that will give her greater control. Healthcare providers should work in open egalitarian and democratic ways, which will enable the sharing of knowledge expertise and other types of medical power. Healthcare should be holistic, treating the woman as an individual and listening to her needs. Midwives should share themselves as well as their expertise, empathising with women rather than taking a professional stance. The final principle is that healthcare must be equally accessible to all women regardless of class, race, or sexual orientation (Foster 1989).

These key principles depend upon two main factors. First, as midwives we need to ensure that we are positioned 'with women'. As previously noted, all too often in today's health service midwives are positioned 'with institution'. Second, we need to employ best evidence to give women good reliable information taking into account their individual, personal and social preferences. This will enable them to take control. Yet, giving information that is truly unbiased can be difficult. The problem may be compounded if a woman then makes a choice that the medical establishment does not approve, such as choosing to have a vaginal breech at home. In cases like this the midwife can feel trapped between the two sides. Many healthcare professionals will advise a woman in this situation to have a caesarean section. If the midwife chooses to join with them, is this participating in institutional bullying? Yet, if she supports the woman in making choices regarding her body and birth then she risks disapproval and marginalisation from the establishment. The key to such a situation lies with the midwife: she has to be with the woman, ensuring that she has the information, treating her as an individual, listening to her needs, documenting her choices and the information given, using supervisory support, but always ensuring the woman is supported and informed. Midwives need to be educated and informed and able to read and analyse the evidence, and present it to women in a supportive and non-judgmental way.

Within such a with woman model of care, childbirth is a social event. Walsh and Newburn (2002) describe a social model of care contrasting it to a medical model. Within the social model they describe childbirth as a life event within a safe place: home as opposed to hospital; where support is from friends rather than professionals; nature is opposed to technology; women are enabled to let go rather than be controlled. Although I believe that this is the ideal for many women, medicalisation and hospital birth have become so pervasive in our society that many women are not convinced of the safety of home birth; and many midwives have not been trained or supported in obtaining the skills to support such a model. Within the with woman model the woman is supported in the way she chooses and in the place she chooses. A key feature of the with woman model is continuity of carer. Within such a model women's voices become legitimate voices within the system. They work in partnership with midwives to achieve safe satisfying birth experiences in the place of their choice.

A further key feature of this model of care will be its community base. The philosophy will be primarily one of following women, or being with woman, rather than staffing the institution. It is possible that if midwives continue to train and work within the hospital they will not be able to free themselves from its political and ideological forces (Bosanquet 2002). Yet we still have a system that socialises student midwives into the hospital way of birth and insists on a consolidation period on qualification. Midwife education and training needs to be community based, rooted in normality and based in community, ideally one-to-one schemes, and birth centres. A midwife who has built up a good relationship with a women during the antenatal period will want to help her achieve the birth she wants and will support that woman to realise her goal. When working within the hospital environment midwives feel pressured to conform to hospital times, norms and guidelines, with covert policing by peers, managers and other professional groups (Kirkham 1999, Bosanquet 2002). By moving the emphasis to out of hospital birth the technological model of birth will be less dominant and midwives will be able to work in ways that meet the needs of women. Many midwives are not able to work in continuity of care schemes. Nevertheless, they can still adhere to the with woman model, where birth is a physiological family life event and a rite of passage for that woman and her family.

As midwives we need to be prepared to support women and support each other. Mavis Kirkham (1999) shows how midwives fail to support each other and are left in the position of doing good by stealth. Such concealment makes concerted action impossible. The way midwives treat each other is fundamental in defining and maintaining the culture of midwifery (Kirkham 1999). It must be a central tenet of the with woman model that midwives support each other, and through supporting each other, support women.

# Conclusion

This chapter has considered what we mean by midwifery-led care and whether it gives us freedom to practise. It suggests that we are most likely to achieve freedom to practise by positioning ourselves alongside women. In the current configuration of maternity services this is most likely to be achieved in out-of-hospital settings. Current belief systems consider such settings appropriate for approximately 75% of women; yet more than 90% of women are giving birth within the highly technological context of labour wards. Over the long term the planning of maternity services needs to take this into consideration. However, in the short term many women and midwives have no other choice available. Within hospital settings it can be difficult for midwives to promote normal birth and woman-centred care. Yet it is crucial that we are able to do this within such technological environments or we do women and childbirth a disservice. If we are to achieve freedom to practise then we need to ensure we have the skills to provide individualised care based on the best available evidence, taking into account the wishes and beliefs of each woman and supporting her on her journey.

Yet, I believe we need as a profession to do more than this: we need to be childbirth activists. If we see midwives as experts in normal childbirth we need to fight for that normality as it is increasingly under threat. We need to demand services that support normality: if you do not have a midwifery-led unit where you work, you need to start questioning why and working towards establishing one. If you have no continuity of care schemes, even if you are unable to work in one yourself, you need to start suggesting ways in which it could work, and supporting those midwives who are able to work in this way. If you work in a unit that does not support home birth you need to question why not, and work with other midwives to find out how the service can be provided.

Midwives are predominantly women. Therefore we need to position ourselves alongside women and support them rather than the system, and that means supporting each other. We all criticise the service at times, yet we are that service and therefore we need to be a part of its organisation and policies. We have the powerful example of New Zealand where women who were dissatisfied with the service worked alongside midwives to ensure services were changed. We all need to reflect on what freedom to practise means to us and how our own vision fits with woman-centred care and current service provision where we work. If you want freedom to practise you need to be aware that it comes with a price and that price is support, commitment and enthusiasm for women, for childbirth and for each other. There is no place for silence.

---

## Reflective questions

Interventions in and around our labour wards can be both subtle and obvious. What can midwives do to lessen the negative effects of even subtle interventions (like ticking clocks).

Some interventions are unnecessary and unkind. How can you ensure that your midwifery knowledge is not devalued or ignored and use it to improve this situation?

Can you say that you are truly 'alongside women' in your position as a student midwife or midwife?

# References

AIMS 2004 Home birth alert. Online. Available at: www.aims.org.uk/ homebirth (accessed)

Alderdice F, Renfrew M, Marchant S 1995 Labour and birth in water in England and Wales: survey report. British Journal of Midwifery 3(7):375–382

Allen I, Bourke Dowling S, Williams S 1997 A leading role for midwives? Evaluation of midwifery group practice development projects. Policy Studies Institute, London

Anderson T 2004 The misleading myth of choice: the continuing oppression of women in chidbirth. In: Kirkham M (ed) Informed Choice in Maternity Care. Palgrave MacMillan, Basingstoke, 257–265

Ball L, Curtis P, Kirkham M 2002 Why do midwives leave? RCM, London

Belenky M, Clinchy B, Goldberger N, Tarule J 1999 Women's Ways of Knowing: The Development of Self Voice and Mind, 2nd edn. Basic Books, New York

BirthChoice. 2004 Online. Available at: http://www.birthchoiceuk.com/ (accessed 22 December 2004)

Birth trauma. Online. Available at: http://www.birthtraumaassociation. org.uk/ (accessed 19 December 2004)

Bosanquet A 2002 Stones can make people docile: reflections of a student midwife on how the hospital environment makes 'good girls'. MIDIRS Midwifery Digest, 12(3):301–305

CEMACH 2004 Why mothers die 2000–2002. RCOG, London

CESDI 1999 5th Annual Report Part iv Place of delivery. The Practising Midwife 2 (1):38–39

Chamberlain G, Wraight A, Crowley P 1999 Birth at home: A report of the National Survey of home births in the UK by the National Birthday Trust. The Practising Midwife 2(7):35–39

Davies J 1997 The Midwife in the Northern Regions home birth study. British Journal of Midwifery 5(4):219–224

Davies L 2004 Allowed shouldn't be allowed. MIDIRS Midwifery Digest, 14(2):151–156

Davis-Floyd R 1992 Birth as an American Rite of Passage. University of California Press, Berkeley

Davis-Floyd R 2001 The technocratic, humanistic and holistic paradigms of childbirth. International Journal of Gynaecology and Obstetrics, 75: S5–S23

Davis-Floyd R, Sargent C 1997 Introduction, the anthropology of birth. In: Davis-Floyd R, Sargent C (eds) Childbirth and Authoritative

Knowledge: Cross Cultural Perspectives. University of California Press, Berkeley

DoH 1993 Changing Childbirth: Report of the Expert Maternity Group, HMSO, London

DoH 2004 National Service Framework for children, young people and the maternity services, Standard 11, HMSO, London

Edwards NP 2004 Why can't women just say no? And does it really matter? In: Kirkham M, (ed) Informed Choice in Maternity Care. Palgrave Macmillan, Basingstoke, 1–31

Enkin M, Keirse M, Neilson J et al 2000 A Guide to Effective Care in Pregnancy and Childbirth, 3rd edn. Oxford University Press, Oxford

Foster P 1989 Improving the doctor/ patient relationship: a feminist perspective. Journal of Social Politics 18(3):337–361

Foster P 1995 Women and the health care industry: an unhealthy relationship. Open University Press, Buckingham

Foucault M 1973 The Birth of the Clinic. Routledge, London

Foucault M 1977 Discipline and Punish: the Birth of the Prison eAllen Lanr, London

Gould D 2002 Subliminal medicalisation. British Journal of Midwifery, 10(7):418

Gould D, Lupton B, Marks M, et al 2004 Outcomes of an alongside birth centre in a tertiary referral centre. Midwives Journal, 7(6):252–256

Hall J 1999 Home birth: the midwife effect. The Practising Midwife, 7(4):225–227

Hall J 2002 Interfering or intervention? The Practising Midwife, 5(7): 4–5

Healthcare Commission 2005 State of Healthcare Report. Online. Available at: http://www.healthcarecommission.org.uk

Henley-Einion A 2003 The medicalisation of birth. In: Squire C (ed) The social context of birth. 173–187

Hodnett E 2004 Home-like versus conventional institutional settings for birth. Cochrane Review. The Cochrane Library, Issue 3. John Wiley, Chichester

Hodnett ED 2002 Continuity of caregivers for care during pregnancy and childbirth. The Cochrane Library, Oxford Update Software, Cochrane Library Issue 4

Home birth campaign. Online. Available: http://www.aims.org/homebirth

Hunt S, Symonds A 1995 The social meaning of midwifery. MacMillan Press, Basingstoke

Hutchings J, Henty D 2001 Caseload practice in partnership with Sure Start: changing the culture of birth. MIDIRS Midwifery Digest, 11(3) Supp 2:538–540

Jordan B 1997 Authoritative knowledge and its construction. In: Davis-Floyd R, Sargent C (eds) Childbirth and Authoritative Knowledge: Cross-Cultural Perspectives. University of California Press, Berkeley pp 55–80

Kirkham M 1999 The culture of midwifery in the National Health Service in England. Journal of Advanced Nursing, 30(3):732–739

Kitzinger S 2005 The Politics of Birth. Elsevier Science, Philadelphia

Madden E 2005 A birth vision. RCM Midwives Journal, 8(2):68–71

Mander R 2002 The midwife and the medical practitioner. In: Mander R, Fleming V (eds) Failure to Progress: the Contraction of the Midwifery Profession. Routledge, London, pp 170–189

McCourt C, Page L 1996 Report on the evaluation of one-to-one midwifery. Centre for Midwifery Practice, Thames Valley University, London

McCourt C, Percival P 2000 Social support in childbirth. In: Page LA (ed) The New Midwifery: Science and Sensitivity in Practice. London, Churchill Livingstone, pp 245–268

Northern Region Perinatal Mortality Survey Coordinating Group 1996 Collaborative survey of perinatal loss in planned and unplanned home births. British Medical Journal 313:371–375

NPEU 2005 Report of a structured review of birth centre outcomes. National Perinatal Epidemiology Unit, Oxford

Oakley A, Rajan L 1990 Obstetric technology and maternal emotional well-being: a further research note. Journal of Reproductive and Infant Psychology 8(1):45–55

RCM 2001 Position Paper Woman-Centred Care. RCM, London

Reed B 2002 The Albany midwifery practice. MIDIRS Midwifery Digest 12(1):118–121

Robinson J 1996 Delivered at Home: Comment on Book. British Journal of Midwifery 4(5):274–275

Rosser J 2001 Birth centres – the key to modernising maternity services. MIDIRS Midwifery Digest 11(Suppl 2):522–526

Sandall J 1997 Midwives' burnout and continuity of care. British Journal of Midwifery 5(2):106–111

Sargent L 2002 Practice and autonomy. In: Mander R, Fleming V (eds) Failure to Progress: the Contraction of the Midwifery Profession. Routledge, London, pp 39–63

Saunders D, Boulton M, Chapple J et al 2000 Evaluation of the Edgware Birth Centre, North Thames Perinatal Public Health

Stephens L 2004 Pregnancy. In: Stewart M (ed) Pregnancy, Birth and Maternity Care: Feminist Perspectives. Elsevier Science, London, pp 41–57

Wagner M 1995 Global witch hunt. The Lancet 346(8981):1020–1023

Wagner M 1997 Confessions of a dissident. In: Davis-Floyd R, Sargent C (eds) Childbirth and Authoritative Knowledge: Cross Cultural Perspectives. University of California Press, Berkeley, pp 366–397

Waldenstrom U, Nilsson CA, Winbladh B 1997 The Stockholm birth centre trial: maternal and infant outcomes. British Journal of Obstetrics and Gynaecology 104(4):410–418

Walsh D, Newburn M 2002 Towards a social model of childbirth: part 1. British Journal of Midwifery 10(8):476–481

Wickham S 1999 Home birth: what are the issues? Midwifery Today 16–18

Wiegers T A, Keirse M, Vander Zee J, et al 1996 Outcome of planned home birth and planned hospital births in low risk pregnancies: a prospective study. BMJ 313:1309–1313

## Additional resources

Kirkham M, Stapleton H 2004 The culture of the maternity service in Wales and England as a barrier to informed choice. In: Kirkham M (ed) Informed Choice in Maternity Care. Palgrave MacMillan, Basingstoke, 117–147

Squire C 2003 Women and Society. In: Squire C (ed) The Social Context of Birth. Radcliffe Medical Press, Oxford, pp 1–21

Walsh D 2004 Feminism and intrapartum care: a quest for holistic birth. In: Stewart M (ed) Pregnancy, Birth and Maternity Care: Feminist Perspectives. Elsevier Science, London, pp 57–71

# CHAPTER NINE

# The impact of war on the practice of midwifery and the wellbeing of women and children in Iraq

BARBARA KUYPERS

I have written this chapter following a visit to Basrah in the southern region of Iraq. I made this visit on behalf of the Royal College of Midwives (RCM) to make an assessment of the maternity services in the sector. Funding was made available to send a representative to Iraq alongside a Multi-Agency Faculty. The Faculty's remit was to instruct Managing Obstetric Emergencies and Trauma (MOET) courses for local Iraqi healthcare professionals.

The visit occurred in June 2004 during a time of transition. I had hoped to interview staff at work. However, due to the circumstances connected with the worsening security in Basrah, site visits and interviewing of staff within their place of work were not possible. As a result the professionals approached to be interviewed were Iraqi staff attending the military base at Basrah during a MOET training programme. In addition, midwives from two of the local Basrah maternity units also made themselves available for discussions.

The chapter is a composite of the original report of the visit written for the RCM (Kuypers 2004) and further discussions within the theme of 'freedom to practise'. These will outline how conflict impacts on the infrastructure of a country's healthcare provision and how this influences the choices that clinical practitioners have regarding their practice in both public and private sectors. Due to the post-conflict circumstances of the country the chapter will also outline a series of influences that have affected and continue to have an impact on the delivery of care for women during pregnancy and birth. This will assist in adding context about the culture of pregnancy and birth and the profession of midwifery in Iraq.

Various drivers govern the work of any clinician and so the emerging public health scenarios will also be detailed. Iraq is a large country and the regions often have very different public health needs. The issue of 'freedom to practise' can be interpreted differently in different situations:

- Do health service providers in a country at war have fewer freedoms given the constraints on the safety movements of personnel?
- Or, do they have more freedoms with regard to the collapse of both provider and professional regulatory structures?

The discussions of this chapter deal in general with the impact of war on public health. More specifically, the chapter addresses the effects of war on the health of women and children and the practice of midwives. In the main, the discussions have been informed by interviews made in Iraq in 2004 and by relevant documents (Medact Report 2003, Ryan 2003).

# Terms of reference of the visit

The primary purpose of the mission was to build on the previous project of providing two MOET programmes for local obstetricians, anaesthetists and midwives organised by the MOET in IRAQ Group and supported by the Leonard Cheshire Centre of Conflict Recovery. The mission that departed from the UK on 16 June 2004 hoped to train the local delegates to become trainers for future MOET programmes. The Leonard Cheshire Centre of Conflict Recovery invited the RCM to participate in its second mission with a view to scanning the midwifery horizon in southern Iraq. The role of the RCM representative during the mission was to:

- explore the current state/position of midwifery in southern Iraq
- acquire maternity statistics, e.g. maternal and perinatal mortality and morbidity, place of birth, number of births by midwives, etc.
- assess the provision of and access to midwifery education
- role and status of the midwife
- role and status of the traditional birth attendant (TBA)
- assess the scope of RCM contribution to midwifery in Iraq and identify what role the RCM might play in supporting and assisting midwives in supporting women and families during the childbearing process.

# The public health picture

To give a comprehensive public health picture, the geography, demography and politics of Iraq need to be taken into account. Iraq has a population of 25 million and it is estimated that 50% of the population is younger than 18 years of age (Table 9.1). The major cities are Baghdad, the capital, Arbil, Basrah, Diyala, Kirkuk and Mosul (Figure 9.1). Iran, Saudi Arabia, Kuwait, Jordan, Syria and Turkey border the country. Arabic is the main language; Kurdish is also spoken; many professional groups speak fluent English.

**Table 9.1  Iraq: demographics (WHO 2003)**

| | |
|---|---|
| Population | 25 million |
| Growth rate | 2.8% |
| Population below 18 years | 50% |
| Population above 65 years | 3.1% |
| Dependency ratio | 84% (50–70% unemployed) |
| Crude birth rate | 36.4% per 1000 |
| Crude death rate | 7.6% per 1000 |
| Females 15–49 years | 24% (of population) |
| Fertility rate | 4.9 per woman |

The geography of the country is mainly desert with low fertile plains particularly in the Kurdish regions. Many of the cities are built along the Tigris and the Euphrates rivers. The temperatures vary considerably with damp rains in the north and dry arid conditions in the south. Basrah, where this Review took place, basks in temperatures between 45°C and 65°C during the summer months.

The Ba'ath party came to power in Iraq over 35 years ago. Historically the health services were financed by central Government and provided freely to all Iraqis irrespective of income. However, there was evidence of reduced resources allocated to various hospitals contrasting with other institutions which received handsome amounts of funds. Often hospitals attached to universities did very well since they could have budgets allo-

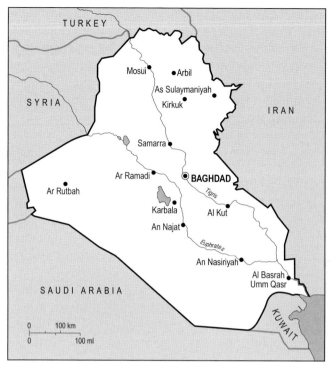

*Figure 9.1* Iraq: country map. Source: Medact Reports 2003, 2006

cated from both the ministries of education and health. Conversely, hospitals in areas with limited allegiance to the Ba'ath Party had reduced access to funds and became increasingly dependent on contributions from local mosques or other local charities. Additionally, the practice of 'charging' for care provided by individuals in the hospitals was not unknown. This is still a custom that the new ministry is attempting to reverse. The south of the country, and Basrah in particular, suffered from loss of funds: Basrah is far from Baghdad geographically and politically. This meant that often overall public services, not just in health, were severely restricted in relation to resourcing.

In 1991 the first Gulf War took place. Its impact and the following decade of sanctions seriously damaged the infrastructure of the services and many public health programmes became compromised with a subsequent drastic decline in services. Hospitals as well as the wider communities suffered from poor sanitation. Open drains and stagnant water pools caused waterborne diseases in children and adults already in poor health.

In the more rural communities problems occurred with maintaining essential provisions in particular, power and clean water. Some hospitals had fractured water and electricity supplies. This led to a dependency on fuel generators to ensure continuation of operating theatre sessions or intensive care facilities. In addition, medical equipment and pharmaceutical procurement was seriously impeded. Many hospitals developed workshops that enabled facilities to lengthen the productive life of medical kits that would have been condemned in other healthcare services. Iraq was also required to build many of its own pharmaceutical generic drug production plants. Due to the nature of this work the plants were often the targets of United Nations (UN) weapon inspections. By 1997, the Iraqi Government was only able to meet 10–15% of the country's medicine needs and only a quarter of medical equipment was considered operational. Laboratory services were also compromised. Thus, it can be seen that a whole chain of health provision from diagnosis to treatment was seriously impaired as a result of the increased isolation and sanctions against the country.

The first Gulf War also affected clinical personnel. With an intellectual embargo resulting in a reduction in teaching and academic provision, many senior clinicians felt that they personally were at risk and that their professional capacity to function was compromised. Reluctantly, they sought refugee status overseas. In Britain for instance, in 2003, there were over 700 Iraqi medical doctors working with the National Health Service (NHS), all of whom would have been educated from primary school through to postgraduate status in one of the Iraqi universities.

# The impact of war and conflict on public health (2003)

As shown below the state of people's health in Iraq was already poor when the 2003 war started (World Health Organisation (WHO) Country Office in Iraq, UNICEF at a glance: Iraq 2005):

- Life expectancy at birth: 59 for men and 63 for women.
- Deaths of children under 5: 133/1000 or 1 in 8.
- Maternal mortality: 294 for every 100000 births.
- 1 in 4 children under the age of 5 are chronically malnourished.
- A quarter of children are born underweight.

For an interim time following the 2003 war, these figures would have deteriorated although there are no current data demonstrating this formally. This conclusion is further consolidated by the visible collapse of basic services such as the provision of water and power, safe schooling and public spaces and increases in poor sanitation with piling of rubbish heaps within residential areas.

Civilian facilities damaged by the coalition weapons included schools, hospitals and public health centres, several power and water facilities and many homes. Other public spaces, for instance, markets, farms and hotels were also hit. All of these cause significant short- and long-term health risks for civilians in the aftermath of the war. The health services show signs of being under particular strain and subsequently there is a slowing down of the reconstruction process.

The impact on families and communities of loss of men folk and the abrupt widowhood of women has far reaching consequences. For women, loss of husbands, brothers and sons in the war isolates and reduces their ability to advocate for themselves and their families particularly if they are not in paid employment. For many women, there is also the dilemma of 'missing' menfolk. There were reports by women of male members of the family being taken by both military or police personnel with no indication of their destination. In addition, the Medact Report describes Iraq as a place of 'social breakdown' where criminal elements in Iraqi society have had almost free rein in a number of cities. Professionals in high public office are frequently reported as kidnapped and held for ransom: this is an element that has been recognised since the immediate aftermath of the war (Medact Report 2003, 2006, Dispatches 2006).

Some of the effects of war have had more positive outcomes. Many women suffer from untreated depression. Yet, as a result of continued morbidity, there is a growth in informal (some underground) women's networks, and shared households to enable greater support and shared food for women and their families (up to one million households) who have no men in the family. Another positive example deals with employment. It is estimated that immediately after the war less than 50% of the population was employed, many in the public sector whereas others found work in small businesses. Many living in small rural communities are subsistence farmers. In recent years, however, there has been a massive recruitment campaign both into public sector jobs and significantly in the building trades.

When the 2003 war started, the state of people's health in Iraq was already poor. Since then there has been an increase in waterborne diseases such as gastrointestinal diseases, typhoid and cholera. Malnutrition and hospitalisation of children increased from 4% to 8% and 7 of 10 children had diarrhoea (UNICEF 2005). In addition, due to the frequency of power cuts, there has been a demand for the use of kerosene to provide light and cooking gas. This has resulted in substantially more hospital admissions of victims suffering from burns.

The war also affected what was known as the 'cold chain'. This was the term used to cover a system of production and cold storage of vaccines. During the war, power supplies broke down, the cold chain was broken and an estimated over 200 000 children missed their vaccination dates. This opened a window of opportunity for preventable diseases such as measles and tuberculosis. However, in April 2004, the WHO ran a very successful measles vaccination campaign led by the public health doctors in the sector. This is a key achievement and raised morale and confidence in the communities.

War affected the home birth figures: these increased during and immediately after the conflict. During the recent war and in previous times of conflict, many pregnant women birthed outwith hospital, either at home with a midwife or TBA or in a midwife's home organised for the purpose. Women appeared to see the home of a licensed midwife as a place of safety. Hospital medical, nursing and midwifery staff continued to work at their local hospitals. Some midwives worked in hospital and in their homes. Sara, a senior midwife recalls:

> I had more women arriving to my home than I had expected, to have their baby near to where they lived, rather than travel to the hospital. I would leave the hospital after a whole day and arrive home to find women waiting for me there . . . my home was not my own for months . . . Sometimes I needed to call other midwives to help me or they would call me if they needed help . . . usually one of our children would run out with a message if the phones were down
>
> *Personal communication (2004)*

The above quote indicates that some midwives worked in the hospitals and in their homes. This led to very long hours. There were also problems getting home from hospital when there were roadblocks. Some midwives even had to phone another midwife to stand in for them until they were able to make their way home where women were waiting. Getting to and from work in hospital was a difficult business. Halame, a midwife based at the Basrah Maternity Hospital highlighted some of the dangers:

> Working was difficult during the early part of the war when we were first attacked . . . getting to work involved waiting at road blocks and your vehicle being searched. You had to set out sometimes two hours or more before the time you were expected by your colleagues . . . When you were at work you worried about your family at home, when you were at home, you worried about your friends at work . . . whereever you were you worried . . . It is better now . . . travelling is still dangerous though . . . you may have been told a route is clear and then find

it closed and you need to divert through an area that you do not feel safe in . . . the main roads are still the safest as you are not likely to get ambushed

*Personal communication (2004)*

If necessary, women were referred to hospital in a taxi or private car. However referral was not without problems. The travelling problems Halame described above were also very real for pregnant women. News reports at the time of the war showed women who required planned hospital care for the birth of their babies waiting to be let through road blocks. Some women birthed with military personnel in attendance due to the delays experienced at checkpoints. The danger of the situation was emphasised recently when a pregnant Iraqi woman was shot dead by 'mistake' by US troops at a road-block north of Baghdad. The woman and her cousin were travelling by taxi to the maternity hospital (Williams 2006). This incident highlights some of the difficulties of: Iraqis possibly not understanding instructions to stop; nervous soldiers; crowds of people around the roadblock; and the extreme heat and not enough water, exacerbating an already dangerous situation.

Because of the war, not all maternity units remained open. For example, one of the maternity departments in a general hospital in Basrah closed and wards were converted to emergency admission areas for casualties. Midwives were either transferred to the remaining maternity units or remained as extra nursing support. Many of the public health clinics were also required to close due to lack of supplies and personnel being called to assist to the main university and general hospitals. In addition hospitals closed elective activities so that their wards were ready for casualties. Fazal, an anaesthetist said:

It was a stressful time. Doctors, midwives and nurses from the public clinics came in to the main city hospitals so you were working with staff you had not met before. The hospital had closed down the theatre lists so there was no elective work at all. I have never been busier as I was working between the emergency room, the maternity wards and then the theatres for urgent operations. We were forever running out of supplies and asking people to run errands to collect equipment from other departments. If the electricity was down we were operating with generator supplies; on occasion we boiled up instruments as we needed them . . . It felt chaotic and disorderly and all the time you had crowds at the hospital entrances bringing in injured or taking them home. Women coming in to the maternity wards had an entrance of their own but we had some babies born in the emergency rooms too.

*Personal communication (2004)*

War also affected the procurement of items which tend to be taken for granted in day-to-day life. In general, nurses and midwives do not have access to sustained supplies of basic equipment. The replacing of items such as thermometers, sphygmomanometers and stethoscopes that have high usage and are easily damaged proves very difficult. The reusage of disposable items such as syringes and needles, gloves and aprons is not unusual. Handwashing facilities such as gels and the limited issuing of uniforms means that infection control is a key problem in the hospitals. Sometimes, patients bring in their own medical supplies such as dressings or syringes and needles if they can afford this.

# Maternal and child health

For this aspect of the chapter, as well as maternal and infant data, I shall include public health data such as demographic information (see Table 9.1), children's mortality rates and communicable disease and cancer statistics as they have an impact on the general health and wellbeing of women of childbearing age.

## Maternal health and mortality

According to the Maternal and Under 5 Child Mortality Survey conducted in 1999 maternal mortality rates had reached 294 per 100 000 live births. However, the rates across Iraq are inconsistent; this is due to the variable health status of women and also what can be described as the 'micro climates' of practice within the hospitals, midwives and TBAs in the regions. While some regions have had much higher maternal death rates of over 300/100 000 others have a much-reduced rate from the national average of 294/100 000. For instance, in the Kurdish region of Mosul, there has been a reduction of maternal mortality down to 50/100 000. Thus, it can be demonstrated that within each sector there are indicators of practice and public health knowledge that can directly influence maternal outcome. Increased mortality can be attributed to a high rate of malnutrition with some areas in the country totally dependent on the Oil for Food Programme. Since the war there has been decreased access to public health centres: many have been damaged and rendered to rubble; also, many of the staff have been called to the city hospitals to assist with emergency admissions that currently dominate the hospital workloads.

An escalation in the maternal mortality rate (MMR) can be chronicled over the past 15 years (Figure 9.2) and there are similar patterns for rates of death among infants and children under 5 years of age (Figure 9.3). The

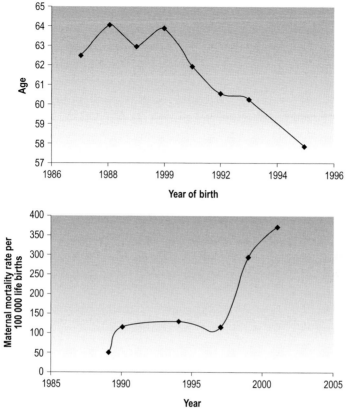

*Figure 9.2* (a) Life expectancy at birth. (b) Maternal mortality rates in Iraq. Source: van de Fliert WM 2003 Iraq 2003 – an analysis of the health system: A complex humanitarian emergency or a post-conflict reconstruction

significance of the critical state of the health service and the impact of the 1991 Gulf War and the following sanctions can clearly be demonstrated (Tables 9.2 and 9.3). As stated earlier, the caesarean section rate at the Basrah Maternity and Child Hospital was approximately 20% whereas in a more northern unit the rate was as high as 45%. The variability between Basrah, Baghdad and the more northern cities of Mosul and Tigret in regard of its maternity and obstetric practice is likely therefore to have an impact on the mortality and morbidity of women.

## Child mortality rates and health status

A UNICEF global childhood mortality survey conducted in 1999 demonstrated that the possibility of dying before reaching a fifth birthday was at

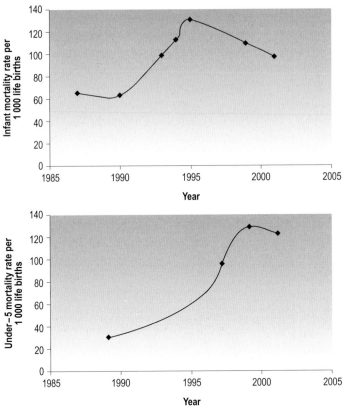

*Figure 9.3* Infant and child mortality rates in Iraq. Source: van de Fliert WM 2003 Iraq 2003 – an analysis of the health system: A complex humanitarian emergency or a post-conflict reconstruction

| Table 9.2 Direct causes for maternal death (WHO 2003) | |
|---|---|
| Massive obstetric haemorrhage | 28% |
| Post abortion | 19% |
| Eclampsia | 17% |
| Post-partum infection | 15% |
| Post anaesthetic deaths and other medical | 14% |
| Obstructed labour and ruptured uterus | 7% |

Table 9.3  Maternal health indicators for Iraq 2000/2003 (WHO 2003)

| | |
|---|---|
| Maternal mortality rate | 294/100000 |
| Low birthweight infants born | 25% |
| Prevalence of anaemia in women | 50% |
| Percentage receiving antenatal care* | 68% |
| Percentage delivered by trained personnel* | 81% |

*With an obstetrician, midwife or traditional birth attendant

the level of 130 deaths per 1000 live births or 1 in 8 children (see also Figure 9.3). Of this number, 108 were infants dying in the first year of life (UNICEF 1999). More specifically, in Iraq, in the same way that the MMR varies across the country, the child mortality rates (CMR) are also variable. In the Kurdish regions, during the same year of survey, the infant mortality rate (IMR) was 59 per 1000 births with the deaths of children under 5 years of age standing at 72 per 1000 live births.

Malnutrition is a serious chronic disease state exacerbated by sanctions imposed on Iraq. Before March 2003, over 16 million Iraqis, half of them children, were 100% dependent on the Oil for Food Programme and rations distributed by the Government. Later studies completed by UNICEF indicate a rise of 11% in malnutrition rates in children since 2003. Poor nutrition has a direct effect on morbidity and the body's ability to fight disease. In Iraq, the three major killers among children are acute lower respiratory infection, diarrhoeal diseases and measles; together, these diseases account for 70% of the deaths. The 2003 war also affected the ongoing vaccination programmes. By 1999, these programmes were considered to be successful with over 90% of children vaccinated against diphtheria, 94% against measles and 85% with bacille Calmette Guérin (BCG) vaccine against tuberculosis. However, there has been a sharp decline in vaccination take-up against preventable diseases during and since the 2003 war: nearly 270000 infants were not vaccinated in their first year of life.

The Ministry of Health also set up a National Cancer Register to monitor the impact of the various diseases that affect the population:

- The Iraqi Cancer Register was set up in the 1990s with, for instance, over 25000 cases registered from 1995 to 1997.
- Childhood cancers are reported as 8–10 times more common than in the West: they amount to about 8% of the total registered cancers in Iraq

whereas in developed countries, childhood cancers represent only 0.5–1% of the total.

- The Cancer Register reports a significant increase in childhood cancers, particularly leukaemias in the southern region in and around Basrah since 1993; 58% of cancers are diagnosed at an advanced stage and therefore incurable.

# Pregnancy and birth in Iraq: choices for professionals and for women

Iraq is a strongly Arabic and Muslim society and the social world is unequivocally divided into male and female. The strong socialisation of boys and girls from an early age means that there are particular expectations of girls and women in relation to reproduction. Boys and girls are educated to have different expectations of life and to develop emotionally and intellectually in particular ways. In addition, in their daily lives, they are expected to conform to different norms of dress and behaviour.

However, it is easy to assume that women have their lives informed and dictated to by the male leaders in the family and that women do not challenge or stretch the boundaries of the cultural norms. In reality for example, the practice of medicine in Iraq has as many women choosing this profession as there are men. In addition, the choice of profession may also be strongly influenced by the class and economic status of family and this is particularly the case where families have supported children through higher education colleges to enable them eventually to enter a medical school.

Iraq has a whole spectrum of healthcare services for women from which to choose to receive care during their pregnancies. Maternity care can be provided in modern hospital environments or in more peri-urban or rural public health centres. Women can choose to be cared for privately by an obstetrician with a full package of antenatal care and choice of delivery, or cared for privately by a licensed midwife either in the home of the midwife or in the home of the mother with her family. Women may also choose to be cared for by a licensed TBA and for women in peri-urban areas or in the countryside this is the most usual choice of carer. Lastly, 15% of women in Iraq give birth without the attendance of anyone qualified but with a lay matriarch of the community. This is a woman who has had no formal training but has acquired her knowledge by being present at any number of births before being the principal carer at births in her community.

During discussions to gain information for the Review, it was clear that many services have been working with high clinical competency but in deprived and compromised hospital facilities. For young doctors establishing their practice and developing competencies in new skills, difficulties occur due to lack of modern pieces of kit and equipment. This is exemplified by the limited nature of the procurement policies which, due to cost, have historically been very restrictive For instance, during an interview with a consultant anaesthetist working in a hospital with a caesarean section rate of over 45%, the consultant explained how he has tried to introduce the use of epidural anaesthesia but has been frustrated by the inability of the hospital to provide higher gauge needles. However, the tools of midwifery remain the same as a good pair of hands and a fetal stethoscope. The use of battery hand-held fetal heart monitors and cardiotocographs hardly exist as routine pieces of equipment in hospitals or clinics.

# Being a midwife: educational pathways, pay and practice

This section describes the educational pathways for women in Iraq who aim to make midwifery their career. It also examines aspects of payment for midwives and discusses midwifery practice in the public health and private sectors.

## Educational pathways

Children attend primary school from 8 to 12 years and then senior primary until 15 years of age; they can then proceed to secondary education from 15 to 18 years. Primary, secondary and university education responsibilities lie with the Ministry of Education as do the education pathways for doctors, nurses, midwives and other professions allied to health. For instance, young adults can also enter a health institute at 15 years of age to begin their nurse training.

Nursing and midwifery health institutes are attached to hospitals whereas medical training rests with university institutions. However, since the 2003 War there have been discussions about bringing nursing and midwifery education under the auspices of the universities. One important point to be considered is that since 2003, a number of graduates from universities and colleges had not been allocated to their place of work by June 2004. Thus they could not consolidate their training at the appropriate time.

The pathways to becoming a midwife are varied:

- Three years' nursing and one-year midwifery degree education at a nursing and midwifery college.
- Three years' nursing with one-year midwifery diploma education at a health institute.
- Three years' direct entry midwifery attached to a health institute.

The majority of nurses and midwives take the diploma of education. For midwives, this qualification provides them with registration and a licence to practise as a midwife. This licence is renewed annually with the Ministry of Health.

Interviews revealed that many midwives are dual qualified. Work in the public health centres particularly uses both nursing and midwifery competencies for adult and child health requirements. However, the number of direct entry midwives, who can begin their training from 15 years of age, appears to be increasing. There are concerns regarding this: many of the older dual qualified midwives are nearing retirement or will reduce their working hours. Also, too many direct entry midwives would limit the numbers with dual qualification who can support the public health centres. There are also training courses for TBAs; these are usually based at the health institutes. The duration of these courses is variable but seem to be predominantly 12 months. Again a certificate and licence is provided but it is not clear if a central register of TBAs is kept in the same detail as for diploma midwives.

The midwifery courses are approximately 50% academic teaching with 50% of the time working clinically within the hospital to which the health institute is attached. Tutors at the health institutes are either senior nurses or midwives, and obstetricians. The language of use in university education is English whereas in the health institutes it is either Arabic or Kurdish. When midwifery education is brought under the umbrella of the universities the use of English as the only language of teaching and learning will have consequences for the midwives as it limits opportunities of combined professional teaching. However, this aspect of gaining access to shared learning between physicians, nurses and midwives was something the midwives particularly referred to as a positive learning environment. It was, for instance, the teaching methodology used by the MOET Group during this particular visit and was well received by all attendants.

## Midwifery pay and conditions with the Ministry of Health

The Ministry of Health allocates the nurses and midwives to their place of work and this is dependent on vacancies and establishments. These are held centrally by the Ministry of Health rather than by the hospitals themselves. Staff can be allocated anywhere within the region or sector and have limited opportunity to request to transfer or to remain where they are if they should want this. It is not unknown for some to offer money to influence their allocation. If staff should want to transfer for personal circumstances they are required to put this in writing to the regional offices of the Ministry of Health. If long leave is needed (say over 14 days) again a request should be made to the Ministry of Health. Short leaves of a few days can be made to the hospital director.

Midwives working in the public sector are paid by the Ministry of Health. Midwives with, say, over 20 years of service were earning similar salaries to midwives only just becoming licensed. Thus, the qualification, length of service and competency as a practitioner do not necessarily increase a salary significantly. Salaries for nurses and midwives prior to the 2003 War were minimal: the range was between US$1 and US$3 per month (US$1 = 1460 Iraqi dinars). Salaries might be augmented by a further fee. Prior to the recent war, hospitals had a minimal fee basis for families to pay to the services. The staff of the hospital received small amounts from this fund on a monthly basis and this could add up to another US dollar on top of their monthly salary.

The situation has improved since the 2003 War. Since then, the Coalition Provisional Authority (CPA) and Ministry of Health have agreed a substantial uplift of salaries for public health sector staff: nurses and midwives now receive from US$35 each month. As can be imagined this has lifted the spirits and status of healthcare workers and has reduced and in some instances dismissed the need for fee-paying requirements for the patients to the hospitals. The fees used to be a variable amount but usually were less than 10 000 Iraqi dinars (or US$5–7). However, again there remain reports of staff asking for monies directly from patients and it is expected that the assumption of this type of practice will continue for some while.

All primigravid women are encouraged and expected to give birth in hospitals or public health centres were there is access to both midwifery and either obstetric or general practitioner support. A woman may have had some antenatal care at the hospital or public health centre or may arrive unannounced at the hospital because she is unwell or as she begins her labour. Once admitted to the hospitals, the tradition is that they are unable to have a companion with them during labour and delivery. Another tradition affecting midwives is to do with 'standing orders'. In Iraq, midwives working in public hospitals have no prescribing or administrative 'standing orders' and so the obstetrician prescribes pain relief to each woman as required. However, standing orders do not affect the midwife working privately. Here midwives may ask their obstetric colleagues to write prescriptions for combined ergometrine and oxytocin (Syntometrine), which the women will buy from local pharmacies. Or simply, the midwives can be issued with ampoules from the hospital.

Epidurals in public health hospitals are few. Epidural anaesthesia is not routinely offered in any of the Basrah hospitals although one facility north of the sector has an anaesthetist who is offering epidural anaesthesia for caesarean sections – this is the exception. Traditionally, women expect to have a painful labour and the absence of pain is interpreted by them as poor progress in the labour. This may change as the hospitals re-equip and modernise.

## Private practice among midwives and traditional birth attendants

In Iraq, midwives appear to have greater freedom to practise when they are in private practice than within the constraints of a public hospital. Midwives are allowed to practise privately as soon as they are qualified and licensed. All of the midwives interviewed had a private practice alongside their public sector work. Over 50% of births in Iraq are with the private businesses of midwives and TBAs. Additionally, 25% of all births are in rural areas and mostly attended by a TBA or matriarch in the family.

On licence, the midwives receive a certificate, which can be displayed at the gate or door of their home. This enables women and families to know that it is a residence of a midwife. The plaque often indicates 'Licensed Midwife – Um Mohamoud' or 'Um Jalal'. The certificate should also display the licence number. TBAs may also practise privately as soon as they are qualified and licensed. The plaque at their door would indicate 'Licensed Traditional Birth Attendant'. Usually the midwife's private practice is carried out either at the midwife's home or the home of the client. Most women attend the midwife's address. In contrast with the 'no birth companion' policy in public hospitals, a woman will have her mother or a sister with her as birth companion.

As is often the case, midwives will acquire a substantial private practice by word of mouth. The client may have been delivered already by the midwife in the public sector as a primigravida. For subsequent pregnancies she may make private arrangements with the midwife: thus, the midwife and mother develop a business/professional relationship and understanding. Midwives may develop 'partnerships' or 'exchange in kind' as often clients booked privately may go into labour while the midwife is at work at the hospital or clinic. Midwives work together to arrange 'cover' for each other when this happens. It does not appear that midwives in private practice employ TBAs to assist them but they may have a lay assistant to help them, for instance, with housekeeping and laundry. Midwifery care outwith labour appears to be minimal. Women may have only one or two antenatal appointments with the midwife. Postnatally, it is usual to have one appointment about a week after the birth to assess the recovery of the mother and the feeding and wellbeing of the baby.

Midwives discourage women from having a private birth following a previous caesarean section. Some women, of course, do request a private or a home birth, as they feel that they will better accomplish a normal birth with a midwife rather than in the hospital. Women who have had more than one caesarean section, however, are likely to be booked at the hospital for an elective caesarean section and midwives would do their utmost to encourage this.

There remain situations where transfer of a woman to hospital is necessary. Grand-multiparity in Iraq is common and maternal exhaustion and failure-to-progress are frequent reasons for transfer. The average fertility rate in Iraq is 4.7. The impressions gained at these discussions were that midwives had accomplished competency and transferred to hospital those women who were not making progress or were symptomatic of deterioration. Catastrophic haemorrhage is a contributor to the maternal death statistics and when it was asked if midwives experienced sudden collapse of women at their homes resulting in death, the midwives indicated that this was unusual but that they had experienced it.

If complications arise during a private birth at home, transfer of the woman is made by taxi or private car. The midwife accompanies the mother to the hospital and is likely to remain with her. In the event of a sudden death at home, the body is transferred to the hospital (again by car) for death certification with the midwife giving a brief history of the event. Burial is arranged by the following nightfall. For TBAs, who mostly practise away from the hospitals and in the rural areas, the complication recognition and response rate may be much diminished and consequences for the mother therefore much more serious.

There is a recognised under-reporting of stillbirths or infant deaths particularly in the rural areas. Deaths are formally reported to hospital or public health bio-statistics offices. The Director of Public Health then receives these figures and he forwards them to the Ministry of Health. The framework for reporting deaths is currently under review and a new data gathering form has recently been issued to gain increased information in relation of causes of death.

## Aspects of conflict recovery

Since the end of the 2003 War there has been considerable work by the CPA and respective Ministries to reinstall the structures that will enable the public sectors to recover and eventually lead and implement the work of the health services. However, it should also be explained that this is not consistent across the country and that many projects are subject to sabotage due to insurgent activity or are damaged as part of military operations. There have been, however, some particular successes in the southern sector, which are worth reporting here.

- There has been a recognition of the requirement to assist with professional development among nurses and midwives and some programmes have already been put into place and facilitated by the CPA personnel to consolidate and develop enhanced skills. Particular areas targeted have been emergency care as the majority of hospital care has been emergency provision rather than elective work. Motivation is noted to have increased among clinicians.
- A rebuilding programme of buildings and infrastructure is underway to refurbish damaged clinics and public health centres.
- There is an established dissemination of medications throughout the key hospitals within the sector and this is slowly being extended to the public health centres. In addition, hospitals have functional laboratory and pathology services again.
- The cold chain after a period of collapse has been reinstalled. This was an early project for the CPA, as a considerable number of children in their first year of life had not received any vaccinations.
- Various rehabilitation services have become established for people who have experienced amputations. A limb-fitting centre in Basrah has recently reopened that provides physiotherapy services and limb assessment and fitting.
- A burns unit has also reopened and this is making an impact on the early and appropriate management of people who experience burns. This service is especially significant for children who have a high accident rate with fuels such as paraffin and kerosene.
- There has been an increase in the members of the community using public sector provisions. There is greater confidence in families sending their children to school and there has been a significant rise in the number of people using the hospitals since the financial charging for care has ended.
- New tools have been issued by the Public Health Department to gain more accurate reportage of communicable diseases, and adult, maternal and infant deaths.
- There is clear structure throughout the health governorates nationally, which will enable the health services to have a clear strategic and consistent way forward. This will end the isolation of particular towns and communities.

# Freedom to practise or constraint – issues of regulation

The current situation in relation to the professions of nursing and midwifery in Iraq reflects their isolation, which has come about due to the impact of conflict and years of sanction and subsequent neglect. The requirement to reinstall the high quality of nursing and midwifery operationally throughout the health services infrastructure is a key target. However, this will be against a backdrop of the current poor public image and status of the professions. The WHO has had a chief objective over the three years prior to the war of assisting nurses and midwives to set in place the mechanisms that will enable the advancement of the professions and so to care for the population of Iraq.

The strategic plan developed in 2002 targeted the areas of education, regulation, policy and planning and leadership development. There was also a concentration and focus on revision of the primary and secondary school curriculum to encompass more learning around family health. In addition there were plans to advance the development of the curriculum for the training of TBAs with the increased supply of educational materials to the health institutions involved. However, the recent 2003 conflict stopped any forward progress with these strategies and for the new Ministry of Health alongside other public sector ministries, there is the additional impact of the further damage and deterioration of the state of public health centres, hospitals and schools.

In August 2003, a group of health service stakeholders met to discuss the systems that required to be put in place to reconstruct the nursing and midwifery professions for the country's health services. From the debates and discussions the following Vision Statement for Iraqi Nursing and Midwifery emerged:

Competent Nursing Professionals will provide nursing and midwifery services of the highest possible standard and safety, founded on scientific principles and current research and knowledge in order to meet the present and future health service needs of the people of Iraq. The quality of nursing education and services will improve through curriculum revision in colleges and institutions and by upgrading nurses in service through continuing education. As valued team members, nurses will contribute to the development of health care in collaboration with other members of the health team and its related sectors with the ultimate goal of improving the health and quality of life of the Iraqi people.

*Physician Review (2004)*

The issues of professional regulation are paramount for nursing and midwifery and for the continued training programme for the TBA. In so many ways, Iraq is making progress with the re-establishment of public service infrastructure. Nevertheless, there are also catastrophic episodes when attacks by insurgents unravel the confidence and hope of the public as a whole, and nurses and midwives in particular, of reaching a countrywide stability.

Iraq has seen armed conflict now for over 20 years in various wars and insurgent activities. Civil conflict will most likely continue to blight the country for some time to come. Freedom to practise one's profession has to be put into the context of the history of the country. For some practitioners, all of their professional lives have been during times of war or constraint on practice. Balancing the demands of a public sector career with one of private practice to generate funds or services in kind for family or a community was integral for many of the clinicians interviewed as part of the visit undertaken in June 2004.

Freedom for many clinicians may mean working in the face of the challenges while still wishing to extend their scope of practice and expertise. It also includes pioneering new services against a backdrop of civil unrest and personal danger in which they are sometimes overwhelmed by the conflict. For others, it may just mean making a living and staying safe.

---

## Reflective questions

This chapter has highlighted midwifery practice within ongoing conflict and that 'freedom to practise one's profession has to be put into the context of the history of the country'. Do you know the history of your country and its relevance to the development of midwifery practice?

Consider other countries in conflict or post-disaster (e.g. tsunami), either currently or recently. Find out and compare how midwives practise in these countries/situations.

---

## References

Dispatches 2006 The Women's Story. Channel 4, 8 May

Kuypers B 2004 A review of maternity services in Southern Iraq 16–25 June 2004. RCM, London

Medact Report 2003 Continuing Collateral Damage – the health and environmental costs of war on Iraq. Medact, London

Medact Report 2006 Conflict fuels Iraqi health crisis – Iraqi Update. Medact, London

Physician Review of the Strategy and Action Plan for the Development of Nursing and Midwifery in Iraq 2004. Iraq Ministry of Health with the assistance of Associates

Ryan J (Leonard Cheshire Professor of Conflict Recovery) 2003 Health Assessment South East Iraq and Review of Humanitarian Assistance. Medical Branch Multi-National Division (South East)

UNICEF 1999 Iraq child and mortality surveys. Online. Available at: <http://www.unicef.org>www.unicef.org/infobycountry (accessed 28 November 2006)

UNICEF 2005 At a glance: Iraq – the big picture. Online. Available at: http://www.unicef.org/infobycountry/iraq.html (accessed 2 June 2006)

Williams D 2006 US troops shoot dead pregnant Iraq woman. The Daily Mail, 31 May. Online. Available at: www.dailymail.co.uk (accessed 1 June 2006 and 28 November 2006)

WHO 2003 The Health Situation in Iraq Prior to March 2003. WHO East Mediterranean Regional Office, Jordan

WHO Country Office in Iraq. Online. Available at: www.who.int<http://www.who.int>go to Country Iraq and this also brings you into the Jordan office details (Po Box 3044 Amman) (accessed 28 November 2006)

## Additional resources

CPA (South) 2004 (June) Part 1: Report

CPA (South) 2004 Part 2: Sector Details of Hospital and Public Health Centre Structure and Key Personnel

MOET Iraq Initiative and Training Courses held in Southern Iraq 2004 (April) Leonard Cheshire Centre of Conflict Recovery

MOET Iraq Initiative and Training Courses Phase 2 held in Southern Iraq 2004 (June)

Zakaria Muhannad 2004 (May) Report on the visit to Azadi Hospital – Duhawk City Kurdistan Region

Foreign and Commonwealth Office website: www.fco.gov.uk

Medact: Changing Barriers to Health website: www.medact.org
www.lc.ccr.org (accessed 28 November 2006)

# CHAPTER TEN

# Midwifery Irish style Government policy and its effects on midwifery practice

MARY HIGGINS

Midwifery, dedicated to providing maternity services for childbearing women, is grounded in a belief that pregnancy and birth are natural events set in a social context. Midwives are educated to practise autonomously: not in isolation from other health professionals but with freedom to practise and to make decisions 'on [their] own responsibility' (International Confederation of Midwives (ICM) 1992) with and for childbearing women and their babies. A midwife is there 'to accompany a woman on the journey through pregnancy and birth and be available as she adjusts to her new baby' (Robertson 1997:9). This implies mutuality in the midwife–woman relationship. This relationship is more easily achieved if midwives have freedom to practise and freedom to make decisions about their practice, either individually or collectively.

As this book demonstrates, the concept of, and rules for midwives' freedom to practise varies internationally. 'Midwives are . . . primary caregivers for normal, healthy, pregnant women' (Robertson 1997:5). Yet, it does not always work out like this: in some countries circumstances prevail to prevent or curtail midwives' practice.

The aim of this chapter is to explore the concept of freedom to practise midwifery in Ireland. A review of the recent history of Irish midwifery will illustrate factors that contribute to the limited freedom to practise experienced by midwives at the beginning of the twenty-first century. These aspects comprise the work of the Government including legislation, and attitudes of bodies appointed by Government. It is through acknowledging the history that we begin to see why midwives in Ireland today are not free to practise as the ICM (1992) has described.

A lack of understanding and communication between Government and the profession of midwifery remains today. This has contributed to the limitation of professional development of midwives in Ireland. To examine this more closely, the chapter also looks at midwifery in Ireland today and current factors that affect midwifery. It also offers some ideas for the future of Irish midwifery. A strong case in favour of midwifery as a distinct profession in Ireland is presented. This important aspect of the chapter links with a short section highlighting issues that will require consideration in the effort for Irish midwives to achieve freedom to practise. This, in turn, will be for the long-term benefit of childbearing women and their babies.

# Midwifery in Ireland today

The ICM endorses the concept of midwifery as described above (ICM 2005). The World Health Organisation has accepted the ICM's definition of the midwife (Higgins 2005). The European Union's description of the role of the midwife enshrines the rights of the midwife (80/155/EEC). This does not mean that all midwives have the freedom to practise according to the tenets of these bodies. In Ireland today, midwives have limited career opportunities within the provisions made for maternity care. The Health Act 1970 provides for women to have general practitioner (GP) and obstetric consultant-led care during pregnancy with birth taking place in hospital. As a result of the requirements of the Health Act and the Nurses Act 1950 Irish midwives have been disempowered. Today the majority of Ireland's midwives provide obstetrician-led maternity care in a hospital setting. In 2000 there were 55 166 births (Department of Health and Children (DoHC) 2004), all with midwives present and most of which took place in hospital settings. Midwives also provide care for women before and after birth. However, approximately 97–98% of maternity care is mediated through obstetricians and from a midwife's perspective the likelihood of practising as an autonomous professional is restricted. In addition, many midwives, who have gained their education and practice within the current system of maternity care, view autonomous practice with apprehension. Thus, we can see at the outset of this chapter, that although globally the theory of freedom to practise for midwives exists, in Ireland, midwives' hold on freedom to practise is tenuous.

In Ireland, the Health Service Executive (HSE) is responsible for managing maternity care as well as healthcare in general. Irish women have limited options in maternity care: most give birth in hospital under obstetrically organised care. For women who seek a home birth, the HSE Southern Area contracts with independent midwives in Cork and Kerry to provide an appropriate service. In the rest of Ireland, where available, a woman wishing a home birth contacts an independent midwife directly and applies to the relevant HSE for funding. However, at present independent midwifery services are only available in Cork, Galway, Dublin and Sligo. Elsewhere, women either accept hospital birth or make other arrangements: for instance, some women have moved to areas where home birth is available but clearly, this is not an option for most women.

Another maternity care option that is used in some areas is the DOMINO service. DOMINO stands for DOMiciliary IN and Out. Mothers using the DOMINO service are looked after antenatally by their midwife and come to the hospital when they are in labour where they are cared for by one of the DOMINO team midwives. Mother and baby remain in hospital for a number of hours after birth. Postnatal care continues at home from the midwives on the team. DOMINO care has the added bonus for the midwives in that they also give intranatal care (Murphy-Black 1992:115, Campbell and Macfarlane 1994:93). However, Ireland's facilities for offering a DOMINO service are limited, and this further affects midwives' practice. Two of the Dublin maternity hospitals – the Rotunda Hospital and the National Maternity Hospital – and the HSE Southern Area, through the Waterford and Wexford Regional Hospitals, currently offer a DOMINO service to women within designated areas.

Thus for most Irish women choice in maternity services is limited to opting for private or public care. This choice is further curtailed by the cost of private health insurance. Therefore limitations on midwifery practice have an impact on both women and midwives. To discover the reason for the current situation it is necessary to consider the history of Irish midwifery.

# An historical perspective

In 1902, when the Midwives Act became law in England and Wales, Ireland was part of the British Isles. Many of the tenets of the Act affected Irish midwives although the Midwives (Ireland) Act was not passed until 1918. Each country had a Central Midwives Board (CMB). The Boards, comprising doctors, midwives and laypersons, regulated the registration and practice of midwives. They oversaw the education and examination of pupil midwives (contemporary midwifery students) and provided post-registration education programmes. Reciprocal inter-Board arrangements ensured freedom of movement of midwives between jurisdictions and, if a midwife's name was removed from the register, prevented illegal practice elsewhere (Higgins 2005).

It is not unusual today to hear midwives and others criticising the CMBs, highlighting medical control of midwifery with little input from midwives themselves. However, others have argued that at the time in question – late nineteenth and early twentieth centuries – those who worked to ensure that midwifery would have legal standing realised that the support of the medical profession was important. In Ireland doctors and midwives worked tirelessly to protect the profession of midwifery (Higgins 2005). The Irish CMB (CMB(I)) had been in existence for 30 years when, in December 1948, it discussed a worrying memorandum from the Department of Health (DoH). This related to a draft Nursing Bill proposing to 'dissolve the General Nursing Council and the CMB(I) and set up a Body to control all nursing personnel under one Board'. Midwives across Ireland, in clinical practice and education, reflected the CMB(I)'s anxiety with the proposal (Higgins 2005).

The CMB(I) believed that those who drafted the Bill were unaware of the differences between the midwives and nurses and their respective regulatory bodies. The proposed new body, An Bord Altranais (An Bord Altranais (ABA): Nursing Board), would have 23 members of whom only two were to be midwives. The Bill made no reference to the midwife: the term 'qualified nurse' applied to all. As far as the CMB(I) was concerned, midwifery had always been a separate profession from nursing and this position must prevail; the decision to cease using the term 'midwife' was unacceptable; the level of midwifery representation on the proposed ABA was totally inadequate; and CMB(I) members argued that in the interests of both midwives and the public, midwifery should be properly represented. From their perspective, midwives in their practice had far greater responsibilities than the general nurse (Higgins 2005).

Change was also proposed elsewhere. One of the midwives on the Board reported that she had met English Working Party members at the National Maternity Hospital, Dublin. Apparently, a similar change was proposed for the UK. However, no change would be made in the UK at the time. The CMBs for England and Wales, Scotland and Northern Ireland would continue to act independently with no changes to their constitutions (Anonymous 1949). The CMB (I) decided to make a submission to the Minister of Health, Dr Noel Brown. This informed him of the Board's concerns and what the CMBs in the UK had done about a similar proposal; it highlighted the importance of the reciprocal agreements between the CMBs in Ireland and the UK and asked him to receive a deputation from the Board (Higgins 2005). The Minister met the CMB(I), listened to their concerns but offered no assurances.

By June 1949 the Nurses Bill was with the Senate (usually referred to as An Seanad; this is the Upper House of the Irish Parliament). The CMB(I)

Chairman reported that no response had been received from the Minister. After prolonged debate the members decided unanimously to submit the following resolution to the DoH:

> The Board having studied the Nurses Bill, 1949 consider that the dissolution of the Central Midwives Board is not advisable. The Board considers that the Bill in its present form would not be possible to administer.
>
> *Higgins (2005)*

In October 1949 the situation became more serious. The DoH informed the CMB(I) that some of its suggestions were under consideration. However, the Government now intended to use the term 'maternity nurse' instead of 'midwife', and despite the CMB(I)'s objections and plea for the retention of the term 'midwife' the Government continued to refer to the 'maternity nurse'. Nurses who had passed Part 1 of the midwifery education programme (up to the early 1970s midwifery education was divided into two separate sections) were already called 'maternity nurses'. Apart from anything else, would CMBs of other jurisdictions recognise certificates describing a person as a 'maternity nurse' (Higgins 2005)? At this time the Board learned how midwifery would be regulated in the proposed Bill: a Maternity Nurses Committee was to be set up and three of its members would sit on ABA. Such limited representation did not augur well for midwifery as a profession. However, the Board decided that its priority in relation to the Nurses Bill was to press for the retention of the term 'midwife' (Higgins 2005).

By November 1949 although the Government still preferred the term 'maternity nurse', the committee stage of the Bill had been postponed. This was because the CMB for England and Wales (CMB (E&W)) stated that the existing reciprocal agreements were with the CMB(I). When that Board was dissolved 'the reciprocal agreements now in force with the various Midwives Boards would cease to exist'. This would be a serious handicap for 'maternity nurses' who wished to work in any country of the UK as their employment opportunities would be limited if they were not recognised as midwives. To strengthen its case, the CMB (E&W) informed the CMB(I) that, 'the term "maternity nurse" meant something entirely different from "midwife" and that the term "maternity nurse" was universally regarded as denoting a person of lower status' (Higgins 2005). In addition, the change of terminology could affect the numbers applying for places at midwifery training schools. Midwifery tutors considered that potential candidates would not be interested in acquiring a certificate that appeared to give them a 'lower status' than midwives (Higgins 2005).

There was also a problem of, not only a lack of communication, but also a lack of openness. For instance, Senate reports suggested that the Government had kept the CMB(I) abreast of all developments. This was incorrect. The CMB(I), making the Government's lack of consultation clear and that it had not agreed to its own dissolution, wrote regarding the matter to the Taoiseach (Prime Minister of Ireland), John Costello (Higgins 2005). The Taoiseach's response was sympathetic. The CMB(I) succeeded in having the term 'midwife' retained in the Nurses Act but failed to retain a separate Midwives Act and the CMB(I). Instead, a Statutory Midwifery Committee (SMC) would regulate midwifery and all decisions would be approved by the new body, An Bord Altranais. The Nurses Act became law at the end of 1950.

The passage of the Bill through the Senate in July 1949 evoked mostly positive supportive discussion. There remained a lack of understanding of midwives and their role and, the use of the term 'maternity nurse'. During one of the debates, Professor Bigger (a doctor, Senator and General Medical Council member) stated, 'the general standard of maternity nurses is not as high as the general standard of general nurses' and 'the maternity nurse is not as well educated as the general nurse' (Anonymous 1949:3). This was an outdated view. It is true that at the beginning of the twentieth century in Ireland, while nursing was considered to be a respectable profession, midwives were not so highly regarded (Robins 2000:11,14). However, from 1918 onwards, the education and regulation of midwives had improved through legislative change: the Midwives Acts of 1918, 1931 and 1944. Also, the Irish Nurses and Midwives Union, a group of professionals working for improvements in midwifery and nursing, campaigned against 'handy-women' and named those practising illegally to the authorities. In addition, the Union organised education courses for registered midwives and nurses and recommended an increase in the length of the midwifery curriculum to the CMB(I) (Scanlan 1991:91). These measures noticeably raised the status of midwives in Ireland.

By the time that the Nurses Bill reached Committee Stage many senators objected to the proposed change of title from 'midwife' to 'maternity nurse'. This was particularly highlighted when Professor Bigger stated the concerns of all the relevant CMBs: that for full midwifery reciprocity between the countries of the UK and Ireland, Irish midwives had to be registered as midwives. When the senators realised this they suggested that the Bill be held in abeyance until the matter was resolved. Professor Bigger felt so strongly about the matter that he informed the Senate that he would vote against the Bill unless the term 'midwife' was retained (Anonymous 1949:3). The CMB(I) had its last meeting on Wednesday 30 May 1951, 33 years after the Midwives (Ireland) Act 1918 was passed (Higgins 2005). However, the Board, supported by a number of Senators, succeeded in having the title 'midwife' retained. In addition, the undoubted hard work of the CMB(I) over the years, supported by legislation, had resulted in an improvement in midwifery education and with the work of the Irish Nurses and Midwives Union created a base for midwifery to sustain the profession in the years to come.

ABA came into being on 7 June 1951. The first meeting of its SMC took place on 14 June 1951 (Higgins 2005). Of its eight members, five were doctors, one of whom was the President of ABA. There were two midwives who were also nurses and one direct entry midwife. The SMC dealt with the issues previously managed by the CMB(I) but, without power to decide on midwifery matters, it had to refer all decisions to ABA for ratification. The Committee members soon realised that they were in an untenable situation. Towards the end of 1952 an SMC submission to ABA stated: 'the Statutory Midwives Committee wish to have their functions defined by An Bord, as the present position is unsatisfactory' (Higgins 2005). There is no record of a response to the submission and the issue was not resolved. Nevertheless, the SMC continued to work on behalf of Irish midwives according to the requirements of the Nurses Act. One important change was made at the December 1952 meeting: the classification 'Midwives Division of the Register' was substituted for the 'Roll of Midwives'. The actual name of this Division of the Register was and still is the 'Midwives Division of the Register *of Nurses*' (author's italics). It seems that the Committee avoided reference to nurses where it could (Higgins 2005).

During the ensuing two years problems continued to surface. One of the most important issues was that of regulation of midwives. Another was the issue of professional discipline. As the CMB(I) was no longer in existence, herein lay a problem. In the Midwives Act 1944 a special requirement provided for the summoning of witnesses to give evidence in penal cases. The 1950s legislation did not repeal this section of the Act. However, the 'Rules for Nurses' now included midwives and ABA decided that the 1944 provision did not apply. Conflicting rules and the way in which the various Acts were interpreted made it difficult for the SMC to carry out its business. This is exactly what the former CMB(I) had predicted would happen (Higgins 2005).

A further contentious issue surfaced in October 1956. ABA showed its new badge to the SMC. During the 1950s, the issue of wearing badges was considered to be very important: the badge carried the registration number of its owner; midwives and nurses had different badges and thus members of the public could recognise the difference between the two professions. Now, An Bord planned a new badge, common to all divisions of the Register. However, the section of the Midwives Act 1944 relating to the midwives' badge had not been repealed. Thus midwives and nurses wearing similar badges would constitute an offence and SMC members asked ABA to approve a separate badge for midwives. Their case was strengthened when An Bord's legal adviser concurred with the SMC's interpretation of the law. However, notwithstanding the legal advice, ABA requested the Minister of Health to amend the Act to allow the same badge to be worn by all nurses (which in An Bord's eyes included midwives) and the Minister complied. As an additional slight, ABA applied to the Minister without discussing the matter again with the SMC. This is further evidence of how An Bord took little account of the SMC even though it had statutory status. A further nail in the coffin for midwifery was hammered home when the battle for the badge was finally lost in the Nurses Act 1961. The Act decreed that midwives and nurses were to have the same badge (Higgins 2005).

With the benefit of hindsight the Nurses Act 1950 was a poorly thought-out piece of legislation. The Government of the day appeared uncomprehending of the differences between the professions of midwifery and nursing and started a series of changes resulting in adverse effects on midwifery and maternity care up to the present day. Indeed, the Minister of Health, Dr Noel Browne, demonstrated a lack of understanding when he said to the Senate, 'The problem of ensuring an adequate supply of *nurses* must, in the main, be attacked by the body or bodies responsible for the control of professional nurses. *These two bodies at the present moment are the General Nursing Council and the Central Midwives Board*' (author's italics) (Anonymous 1949).

The CMB(I) fought to maintain the distinction between midwifery and nursing. Later, its successor, the SMC tried – and failed – to have its views taken into account. As the CMB(I) members warned, the small midwifery representation on ABA could not ensure that midwifery decisions were carried. Three midwives out of a total membership of 23 could not ensure that midwifery in Ireland was recognised as a profession distinct from nursing. The SMC continued, but its limited powers led to an enfeebling of its work. This led to a further removal of power and recognition: the Nurses Act 1985 disbanded the SMC and permitted the fitness to practise committees of ABA to judge midwives without any midwifery representation. The Chief Executive Officer of ABA responded to SMC members' concerns by informing them that a submission from An Bord to the Minister had not mentioned the issue. A meeting took place between the SMC and the Midwives' Section of the Irish Nurses Organisation (INO) (Ireland's main Union and professional body for midwives and nurses). There is no trace of the relevant minutes in An Bord's archive, the INO minutes were lost and the meeting was not reported in the *World of Irish Nursing* (the title of the INO journal at the time) (Higgins 2005).

The Nurses Act 1985 reiterated the approach of the 1950 Act in its attitude towards midwives. First, it stated that the term 'nurse' includes the 'midwife' (Nurses Act 1985). This stance adversely affects the efforts of today's midwives in Ireland in their quest for professional recognition. Second, the Act removed the last mark of difference between midwives and nurses. Until that time midwives, working in hospitals or the community, had a statutory requirement to notify their intention to practise to the appropriate health board. After the implementation of the new Act, the only midwives required to notify their intention to practise were and are independent midwives (Nurses Act 1985). This was important: by removing midwives' statutory obligation to notify their intention to practise, the Act removed not only a token of the difference between midwives and nurses, but also an element of the identity of midwifery. Third, there was, and is, a continuing lack of governmental regard for the consultative process. This was evident in an examination of the minutes of the CMB(I) meetings of 1949 (Higgins 2005). At the time, the Government omitted to circulate the draft Nurses Bill to the CMB(I) before it went to the Senate. The CMB(I), set up as a result of government legislation, should have been kept fully informed and given the opportunity to discuss any future changes affecting the Board.

More recently, in the mid-1990s, following industrial action by midwives and nurses, the Government set up the Commission on Nursing (*Report of The Commission on Nursing*, Government of Ireland 1998). Midwives seized every opportunity to impress upon the members of the Commission the need for legal recognition of the difference between midwives and nurses. The Commission therefore recommended that the Nurses Act 1985 should be amended to recognise the distinct character of the midwifery profession (*Report of the Commission on Nursing*, Government of Ireland 1998:3,9). In 2000 the DoHC invited the Midwives' Section of the INO to give its views on this amendment. Following discussion among midwives, the Midwives Section suggested a Midwives Act rather than an amendment to the 1985 legislation. The DoHC did not acknowledge the Midwives' Section's submission; there has been no consultation and midwives are still waiting for the promised amendment to the Act.

It can be argued that midwives themselves are, in part at least, responsible for the weakening of their profession. Numerically midwives make up only a fraction of the membership of the INO. This, however, is not an adequate reason for accepting the term 'nurse' when it is applied to them. Many maternity hospitals still have nurses' dining rooms, nurses' changing rooms and nurses' homes. Many midwives refer to each other as nurses and do not object when other health professionals refer to them as nurses.

This acceptance of inappropriate nomenclature is not new. Throughout 1949 and 1950 the *Nurses Magazine* (the title of the INO journal of the time) provided comment on the proposed Nurses Bill. It also recorded that the Executive Council of the INO discussed the proposed legislation. Many of the reports referred to 'nurses' when they were, in fact, commenting on midwives and midwifery. The December 1950 *Nurses Magazine* editorial (reporting on the second reading of the Nurses Bill) describes midwifery as a branch of nursing (Anonymous 1950). No letters of protest against such descriptions appeared in any edition of the magazine.

The history of Irish midwifery and nursing legislation reflects a situation beset by lack of understanding of midwifery on the Government's part, and a subsuming of a smaller professional group (midwives) into a larger one (nurses). It is likely that nurses in Ireland, and, perhaps some midwives, did not have a problem with this. If the views expressed in the editorial of the December 1950 INO magazine reflect those of most members of the INO then the belief that midwifery should remain a separate profession was not an important issue for the majority (Anonymous 1950). However, there is no doubt that the 1950 legislation affected midwifery and midwives' freedom to practise in Ireland today. Many midwives believe that the Nurses Act 1985 is the legislation responsible for this (anecdotal evidence). However, the Nurses Act 1985 only reinforced the Nurses Act 1950 which seriously weakened the profession of midwifery by removing the CMB(I) and replacing it with the almost powerless SMC.

# The future for Irish midwifery

It is clear that if midwifery in Ireland is to survive as a distinct profession, serious consideration must be given, at both national and local levels, to a number of issues in the maternity services in Ireland (Devane 2003 e-list discussion). First, midwives in Ireland could examine midwifery in other countries such as New Zealand, Scotland, England and Australia. Examples of midwifery practice in other countries could be incorporated into aspects of Irish midwifery practice and developed where appropriate. Second, the establishment of a national collaborative body in Ireland would push maternity care forwards. The group's task would be to reach a consensus on the future of maternity services (Devane 2003 e-list discussion). Such a body would have wide representation including childbearing women, health service providers, midwives, policy makers and professional organisations. The main aim of the group would be to develop a framework for implementing a collaborative approach to midwifery and obstetric practice in relation to models of care and the needs and choices of childbearing women. Other important issues relate to the human resources aspect of the maternity services. These include recruitment and retention of midwives, education, insurance for independent midwives and the development of links between the relevant professional groups (Devane 2003 e-list discussion). However, at the time of writing, the question of how such a body could be developed has still not been addressed.

When discussing the future for Irish midwifery it is appropriate to look briefly again at the *Report of the Commission on Nursing* (Government of Ireland 1998). The report was instrumental in raising many midwives' hopes: that they might have more freedom to practise and have greater control of their profession. In 1998 midwives in Ireland who campaigned for midwifery's professional recognition in its own right had reason to be optimistic. The *Report of the Commission on Nursing* accepted the importance of the submissions of midwives. It recommended that the Nurses Act 1985 should be amended: to take cognisance of the fact that midwifery and nursing are separate professions; to re-establish a SMC within ABA; and, to return the handling of midwifery fitness to practise issues to midwives (*Report of Commission on Nursing*, Government of Ireland 1998). Following industrial action by midwives and nurses the government set up a monitoring committee 'to oversee the implementation of the Commission on Nursing's recommendations as part of the full implementation of the strike settlement' (Anonymous 1999/2000). At this time midwives were confident that very soon midwifery would have legal recognition.

At the time of writing (2006) midwives are struggling to maintain their enthusiasm in the face of many setbacks. The amendments to the Nurses Act 1985 have not yet been made. Midwives are tired of hearing that the expected changes are imminent. Efforts to procure comment on the proposed changes have been unsuccessful with DoHC civil servants giving non-committal responses to the INO's requests for clarification concerning timing.

In addition, midwives campaigning for change in Ireland have realised for a long time that there is still much to do to convince others of the benefits of stronger midwifery input into maternity care.

- Midwives themselves need encouragement and support.
- Obstetricians and general practitioners need to be convinced that midwives are competent to take on the role of lead professional in the care of many pregnant women. This also includes inter-professional trust.
- Education of the general public will be necessary – of the role of the midwife and encouragement to embrace the opportunity offered.
- Women and their families will have to be informed of the advantages and safety of midwife-led care.

If the Government had implemented the recommended changes to the Nurses Act 1985, the efforts of campaigning midwives for recognition of midwifery as a distinct profession would have been greatly enhanced.

# Factors that impact on midwifery

Other ongoing issues in Ireland have had an effect on midwives' ability to have freedom to practise, on midwifery's status as a profession and, ultimately, on the care which childbearing women in Ireland are offered. This section explores some of these issues.

First, midwives numerically comprise a small professional group. The INO has a membership of 33 000, of which midwives make up less than 7%. Midwives have tried hard and failed to persuade the INO to recognise their presence within the union by using the term midwife in the title. The issue of the name change was again on the agenda for the INO's 2006 Annual Delegate Conference. However, on Wednesday 3 May 2006 the delegates to the Conference voted to reject the motion to change the name. Thus, it remains the INO.

Second, there is an issue concerning the nursing register. In 2005 ABA commissioned University College Dublin to conduct research on the feasibility of having a single point of entry to the nursing register. *The Report on the Commission on Nursing* (Government of Ireland 1998:80) considered a generic approach to pre-registration education but recommended that general, psychiatric and mental handicap nursing continue as separate entities. It noted that in countries using a generic approach to education, midwifery was excluded. However, An Bord decided to include midwifery, as a 'branch of nursing', for consideration in the study. This decision suggests that the governing body for nurses and midwives remains obdurate in its attitude towards midwives as a separate professional group and ignores the recommendations of the Commission on Nursing.

Third, there is the issue of acceptance of what might be seen as a decline in midwifery. Approximately 40% of women utilising the maternity services in Ireland have private health insurance and most of them want obstetric-led care. Many women do not even know about midwives (personal observation). Should midwives accept that a decline in midwifery in Ireland is inevitable? A pragmatic view suggests that in most Irish maternity units the role of the midwife resembles that of an obstetric nurse. In Chapter 2 Reid discusses models of childbirth. For the vast majority of midwives in Ireland there is only the medical model. In general, the Irish health service has followed the American approach to healthcare: it could be argued that to have obstetric nurses instead of midwives would be a rational and economically sound proposition.

A fourth current issue sounded encouraging for midwifery at its outset. In 1999 the DoHC appointed a part time Midwifery Adviser. This was a positive outcome to the *Report on the Commission on Nursing* in response to the recommendation regarding the separate nature of the midwifery profession. In addition, to assist the Adviser, a Midwifery Advisory Forum was appointed. It included representatives from midwifery management, practice, independent midwifery and from midwifery schools and third level institutions. Forum Members and the Midwifery Adviser met regularly; issues relating to midwifery and the maternity services were brought without delay to the attention of the Chief Nurse and departmental civil servants. However, the Midwifery Adviser's contract expired in January 2005. The DoHC promised that the matter of renewing the contract would receive attention. In late autumn, a letter from the Minister's office advised that advertisements would shortly appear in the national newspapers for nurse/midwife advisers (DoHC 2005). Once again, the DoHC demonstrated its lack of understanding that midwifery and nursing are separate professions.

# The case for midwifery

Given the difficulties that midwives in Ireland have in acquiring freedom to practise and achieving something more akin to a midwifery or social model of childbirth for women, it would be understandable if midwives felt like giving up, or at least questioning what they are fighting for – questions like:

- Is there any value in fighting to retain midwifery and all that its retention entails?
- Is 'normal birth' worth protecting? In a technological age perhaps women should be encouraged to use every technical aid available to assist them during pregnancy and childbirth.
- Why experience any pain during labour if it can be eliminated by the use of drugs?

This section offers a brief discussion of the worth of continuing to aspire towards the aim of a more normal child-birthing model, freedom for midwives in Ireland to practise and the establishment of midwifery in Ireland as a distinct profession.

The twenty-first century is an age of 'high-tech'. In the past 100 years care of childbearing women has progressed greatly. However, 'high-tech care' with its emphasis on the medical model of care and the efficient use of beds in the birthing suites of our maternity units has interfered with the physiological progress of birth. For instance, Jacobson et al (1990) working in Sweden, followed by Nyberg et al (2000) in the USA, demonstrate a link between the use of opioid analgesia and Entonox during labour and development of drug addiction as an adult. Sepkoski et al (1992) found that women who had epidural anaesthesia demonstrated a lack of interest in their infants. Murray et al (1981) noted that mothers who had epidural anaesthesia during labour, interviewed one month after giving birth, described their babies as being difficult to care for. The use of such analgesia is less of an issue for babies born at home or in midwife led units because there these drugs are rarely used and epidural anaesthesia is unavailable. Thus, the use of analgesia in labour has an impact on an individual labour and, in the longer term, may be to the detriment of society as a whole.

In births where obstetric intervention has occurred, we sometimes see a 'cascade of events' leading from the initial intervention to increased risks of surgery, perineal trauma and mother-baby separation. If the initial intervention can be avoided and one-to-one support provided, the opportunity for spontaneous birthing is increased (Johanson and Newburn 2001, 2002). Pearce (1992:114, 115) describes another more positive cascade of events: when a newborn is allowed skin to skin contact with his mother, 'a cascade of supportive confirmative information activates every sense . . . Thus intelligent learning begins at birth'. In addition, the mother is affected by her baby's closeness: 'A major block of dormant intelligences is activated . . . the mother then knows exactly what to do and can communicate with her baby on an intuitive level'. Pearce believes that separation of mother and baby causes serious damage 'past the point of repair' – a worthy argument for midwives to have the freedom to practise the midwifery or social model of care and through that move towards achieving best practice.

There are other arguments for midwifery care: 'Many midwives have a special affinity with women during pregnancy and birth' (Robertson 1997:25). Robertson postulates that having insight and empathy for birthing women is easier because the midwife – almost always a woman – has the same reproductive instincts. This can allow the development of 'easy alliances and deep understanding'. However Robertson is also aware of how the environment in which the majority of midwives work today affects their ability to give the kind of emotional and psychological care that protects natural birth.

The last argument I should like to put forward here in the case for midwifery is simple but strong: midwives are the best people 'to accompany women on the journey through pregnancy and birth' (Robertson 1997:9).

It is important for those who believe in midwifery to continue to campaign for its retention as a separate profession dedicated to the health of society through its care for mothers and their babies.

## Freedom to practise midwifery in Ireland: issues to be considered

Thus, there is a good case for midwifery and freedom to practise. Yet, when the Nurses Act 1985 obtains its amendment in favour of midwives, this will not be the end of the story. Irish midwives will be acknowledged as midwives rather than nurses but there will still be a considerable task ahead. For instance, in Ireland there has been no state supported community midwifery service for many years. It is in the context of birth at home and in midwife-led units that midwifery students learn to appreciate the benefits of births that happen without technological intervention and where there is ample opportunity to learn about normal birth. Nevertheless, Ireland has only two midwife-led units that opened in the summer of 2004. As stated earlier there are also a number of small-scale home birth and DOMINO services throughout the country. However they cannot meet the needs of all women who wish to access such care. Neither can they provide the necessary experience of physiological birth for all student midwives.

Then there is the issue of clinical governance and safeguarding high standards of care. Elements of clinical governance have been a part of the midwifery code and rules since early midwifery legislation in Great Britain but this is not currently the case in Ireland where *Guidelines for Midwives* (Midwifery Sub Committee 2001) is used. Clinical governance can be looked on as a framework for constantly improving quality and promoting excellence. There is an important link between clinical governance and statutory supervision of midwives. However, such supervision is an alien concept for Irish midwives: there is no statutory supervision for midwives working in maternity hospitals and units; for independent midwives supervision is there, in theory. So, this is one more issue to be grappled with if it is included in the proposed amendment to the Nurses Act 1985. There are benefits there for midwives and, ultimately, childbearing women.

And, education will be an issue. In the autumn of 2006 (Anonymous 2005) pre-registration midwifery education programmes commenced in Ireland. These are open to those who wish to become midwives but who do not have a nursing qualification. It could be argued that pre-registration midwives have an advantage over their colleagues who study midwifery at postgraduate level. They come to the maternity services with a view of birth as a natural life event and are not imbued with an illness model of care learned during a nursing programme. However, unless there is a radical change in maternity care these pre-registration midwives will be no different from their postgraduate colleagues. They will get most of their practical experience of midwifery in large maternity units that have high rates of intervention in pregnancy and childbirth. In a service that refers to pregnant women as patients and where the caesarean section rate is running at 25% it is difficult to appreciate that birth can be a normal event.

# Conclusion

This chapter has explored the concept of freedom to practise midwifery from the point of view of midwifery in Ireland. This has been done through: a brief review of midwifery in Ireland today; an exploration of the recent history of midwifery in Ireland; some ideas for the future of Irish midwifery; current factors that affect midwifery; the case for midwifery; and, issues to be considered for Irish midwives to achieve freedom to practise.

Freedom to practise midwifery is a particular issue for Irish midwives. The first Midwives Act in Ireland was implemented in 1918 and oversaw the setting up of the CMB(I) in Ireland. In the late 1940s discussions took place to pass a Nurses Bill that would to a great extent, subsume into nursing the profession of midwifery in Ireland. The CMB(I) fought for midwives, for their identity and for their status as a profession distinct from nursing. Although the Irish Government eventually permitted midwives to retain their title – rather than its preferred term 'maternity nurse' – the events surrounding the passing of the Nurses Act 1950 demonstrated its lack of understanding regarding midwifery. It took pressure from the UK CMBs finally to achieve the retention of the name 'midwife' in Ireland. Yet, lack of understanding and communication is ongoing and has contributed to the limitation of professional development of midwives in Ireland.

With the current provisions made for maternity care in Ireland today midwives have restricted career opportunities and feel disempowered. Most births take place in hospital under obstetric-led care. There is limited home birth and DOMINO provision. Government legislation, with the collusion of ABA, disbanded the SMC and allowed non-midwives to decide on midwifery fitness to practise cases. The DoHC offered a ray of hope by setting up a midwifery advisory post but did not renew the post when the contract ran out in 2005. Repeated requests for the promised amendment to the Nurses Act 1985 in favour of midwifery have been sidestepped (*Report of the Commission on Nursing*, Government of Ireland 1998). It can be seen that government policy in Ireland has had a marked effect on freedom to practise midwifery. This has a subsequent effect on childbearing women, the way they are cared for and the way that midwives are unable to achieve the 'best practice' to which they aspire.

When the long awaited Amendment of the Nurses Act 1985 is implemented, it will recognise midwifery in Ireland as a profession distinct from nursing and will mark the beginning of a long road to reclaim midwifery practice. One of the most important issues for Irish midwives will be the need to become politically aware so that they do not lose again an independence so hard won. In addition midwives must encourage each other to be free to practise and make decisions with and for the women in their care and to accept willingly the concept of best practice, individually and collectively chosen by midwives for midwives.

Many women in Ireland want to experience birth as a social rather than medical event. To help to achieve this, midwives must have the freedom to work with women to ensure maternity services that will give all women an empowering birth experience as they undergo this 'important life changing experience' (Gibson 2004: 183). The mutuality of the mother/midwife relationship is an essential component of a good mother/midwife relationship. It requires midwives to recognise that all women are born with innate knowledge about how to 'grow and give birth to a baby' (Robertson 1997:9). It perceives the midwife as 'with woman', supporting her as she makes choices and decisions about her pregnancy and birth: a powerful and satisfying experience for both.

---

## Reflective questions

Do midwives have legal recognition in your country? If not, why not? If yes, how and when did it come about?

Is there a national collaborative body or similar group/s in the country where you live, to work towards an ever-improving future for maternity services? The Irish proposal for such a body includes childbearing women, health service providers, midwives, policy makers and professional organisations.

How would you develop such a group?

---

## References

Anonymous 1949 Report of the Working Party on Midwives (UK). The Irish Nurses Magazine, 16(3):4–6

Anonymous 1949 Editorial. Report of Senate debate July 1949. The Irish Nurses Magazine 16(9):1, 3

Anonymous 1950 Editorial. The Irish Nurses Magazine, 17(11):1

Anonymous 1999/2000 (Dec/Jan) News Item. World of Irish Nursing :7

Anonymous 2005 News Item. World of Irish Nursing and Midwifery 13(5):10

Campbell R and Macfarlane A 1994 Where to be Born? The Debate and the Evidence, 2nd edn. National Perinatal Epidemiology Unit, Oxford, p 93

Council Directive of 21 January 1980, (80/155/EEC). Official Journal of the European Communities No L 33/8, 11280

DoHC 2005 Correspondence between Mary Higgins, Chairperson of the Midwives Section Irish Nurses Organisation and Mary Harney, Minister for Health and Children

The Economic and Social Research Institute 2004 Report on Perinatal Statistics for 2001. The Economic and Social Research Institute, Dublin

Gibson J 2004 Unrealistic expectations. In: Wickham S (ed) Midwifery Best Practice. Elsevier, Edinburgh, pp 183–185

Government of Ireland 1998 Report of the Commission on Nursing. A Blueprint for the Future. The Stationery Office, Dublin pp 3, 9, 80, 172–174

Higgins M 2005 The Effects of Government Policy on the Development of Midwifery in Ireland. Unpublished thesis, National University of Ireland, Cork

International Confederation of Midwives (ICM) 1992 Definition of the Midwife Position Statement, the Hague, Netherlands, ICM

ICM 2005 Definition of the Midwife Position Statement, the Hague, Netherlands, ICM

Jacobson B, Nyberg K, Gronbladh L et al (1990) Opiate addiction in adult offspring through possible imprinting after obstetric treatment. British Medical Journal 301:1067–1070

Johanson R, Newburn M 2001 Promoting normality in childbirth. British Medical Journal 323:7322:1142–1143; reprinted in MIDIRS Midwifery Digest 2002, 12(1):70–71

Midwifery Sub Committee Guidelines for Midwives 2001, 3rd edn. An Bord Altranais, Dublin

Murphy-Black T 1992 Systems of midwifery care in use in Scotland. Midwifery 8:113–124

Murray AD, Dolby AD, Nation RL et al (1981) Effects of epidural anaesthesia on newborns and their mothers Child Development 52(1):71–82

Nurses Act 1985 No 18/1985 Online. Available at: http://www.irlgov.ie

Nyberg K, Buka S, Lee L 2000 Perinatal medication as a potential risk factor for adult drug abuse in a North American cohort. Epidemiology pp 11:715–716

Pearce J 1992 Evolution's End. Harper, San Francisco

Robertson A 1997 The Midwife Companion: The Art of Support During Birth. ACE Graphics, Camperdown, Australia

Robins J 2000 Nursing and Midwifery in Ireland in the Twentieth Century. Fifty Years of An Bord Altranais (The Nursing Board) 1950–2000. An Bord Altranais, Dublin pp 11, 14, 16–18

Scanlan P 1991 The Irish Nurse: A Study of Nursing in Ireland: History and Education 1718–1981. Drumlin Publications, Manorhamilton

Senate Records Seanad Éireann Volume 37 1 December 1949 Nurses Bill 1949 Committee Stage. Online. Available at: http://www.irlgov.ie

Sepkoski CM, Lester BM, Ostheimer GW et al 1992 The effects of maternal epidural anaesthesia on neonatal behaviour during the first month. Developmental Medicine and Child Neurology 34(12):1072–1080

# A culturally diverse and disease-burdened environment: the effects on midwifery practice

CHERYL NIKODEM

Midwifery is certainly one of the oldest professions documented. Records that midwives practised independently go back to ancient times. A good example is when Rachel gave birth, 'when she was in hard labor, that the midwife said to her, "Do not fear; you will have this son also"' (Patterson 1995).

This chapter will discuss some issues that have an impact on South African midwives and their freedom to practise midwifery.

## History of midwifery in South Africa

There is no readily available documentation of who attended to births before 1652 in South Africa. Documentation shows that midwives (geswore vroemoere) assisted with births since 1652 in South Africa (Nolte 1998). These midwives held responsible positions in the community as they were licensed and certified and had the freedom to practise independently. There were very few certified midwives, especially in the rural inland areas and lay women started to assist women during birth. Shortage of midwives is still a reality in South Africa and lay women referred to as traditional midwives or traditional birth attendants (TBA) still assist with births today (Odendaal 2004). Traditional midwives are usually elderly women, who had no special training in midwifery but who learned the skills from other traditional midwives. Thus they learned their craft from practical experience and not from theoretical knowledge. Traditional midwives formed a crucial part of midwifery during the Great Trek as reflected in Trichardt's diary where he wrote that Mrs Botha assisted with the birth as the old wise women were not present (Nolte 1998).

It became apparent that midwives needed some training or guidance. The first known guidelines for midwives were published by Dr Johan I Häzer in 1793 vs Huislik Geneeskundige Handboek voor de Ingesetenen van Nederlands Afrika (Nolte 1998). The first professional school to educate midwives was established around 1809 in the Cape under the guidance of Dr Wehr, a qualified male midwife. These midwives underwent a three-month course which included theory and practice. They graduated after an official examination and were allowed to practise independently (Nolte 1998).

Sister Henrietta Stockdale campaigned for state registration for midwives. This was accomplished in 1891 via the Medical and Chemist Act 34 of 1891. This act gave midwives the freedom to run a professional practice independently; it also protected the profession: only registered midwives were allowed to be referred to as a 'certified midwife'. In addition, this act was the first act in the world that gave official recognition to state registration of midwives. Sister Mary Watkins became one of the first state registered midwives in the world when she wrote and passed the Colonial Medical Council examination in obstetrics in 1893 and was entered in the Register of Midwives. She later opened a training school for midwives in Kimberley (Nolte 1998, Muller 2003).

The South African Association of trained nurses was established in 1914 and regulated training until the Nursing Act 45 of 1944 was promulgated. The South African Nursing Council (SANC) took over the regulatory powers of nurses and midwives and is currently still the professional regulatory body. The SANC is a statutory body and was constituted in terms of the Nursing Act. It is responsible for controlling affairs such as training, examination, registering and ethical conduct of nurses and midwives. The midwifery/nursing profession in South Africa currently is autonomous and self-regulatory. Thus the professional body set the professional and ethical standards to ensure quality services. It protects the public against unsafe practices and it confers accountability on the midwives. The freedom of midwives to practise is guided by the regulations set out by SANC and disciplinary measures are in place if conduct is unbecoming. SANC approves all the training and education programmes for midwives in South Africa; however, assessment of students is done at the education institute. In other words, although the basic training programme is approved by SANC, each institution assesses its own graduates and there is no uniform examination or uniform 'board exam' in South Africa (Nursing Act 1978, Muller 2003).

As stated above, TBAs are not obliged to undergo any official training and are not registered on any register. They have no midwifery training, and their beliefs and practices are not well understood; some may be beneficial and others are seen to be harmful customs. They attend to women during pregnancy, birth and the postnatal period using traditional methods such as herbs and other homeopathic medications to induce or enhance labour, relieve pain, stop bleeding and even to turn a breech presentation. Some midwives see the TBA as a hindrance to the professional midwife, as she is seen to practise without the needed knowledge, skills and expertise, but most agree that there is a definite place for the TBA in South Africa. The World Health Organization (WHO) recommends that people be within an hour of the nearest healthcare facility. This is not possible in many areas due to difficult terrain, no transport, and no financial means to pay for transport. A recent situation analysis done in the Western Cape showed that delays due to transport, even emergency transport such as an ambulance, can be as long as six hours (*Saving Babies*, Department of Health (DoH) 2003, Odendaal 2004). Therefore, TBAs, who look after women in their homes, provide essential services in the areas where transport, finances and midwife shortages are prevalent. It is suggested that the SANC takes responsibility to involve the TBAs in some form of education, as WHO recommends that every woman should have the right to birth in the company of a skilled attendant. Currently the medical health professional society is discussing the inclusion of traditional healers on an official register, but so far (2006) nothing has been done to recognise TBAs as healthcare givers.

# Impact of midwifery training and education

Training of midwives previously took place via nursing colleges associated with hospitals under the supervision of obstetricians, midwives and midwifery tutors. Originally, midwives could either enter into a direct entry qualification in midwifery or do a post basic diploma in midwifery after they had qualified as a general nurse. The SANC decided to change this system in 1968 and implemented an integrated course that could produce multi-qualified personnel. Thus, nurses who completed a three and a half or four-year course were qualified as nurses and midwives. In 1972 SANC stopped all direct entry midwifery courses and stated that all persons who want to become a midwife must be registered as a nurse. There are currently no training institutions in South Africa that are training persons as midwives only. The SANC register had only 802 persons registered as midwives in 2003.

The new democratically elected Government brought along several changes in the higher education system. One of the changes was that all colleges need to be affiliated with a university. Thus, colleges are no longer under the control of hospitals but are self-standing and affiliated with universities. All universities and colleges currently offer a four-year degree or diploma that allow the student to qualify at the end of the training as a registered nurse (general, psychiatry, community) and a midwife. Currently the registration list shows that South Africa has over 180 000 of all category nurses/midwives and about 82 213 registered nurse/midwives (http://www. sanc.co.za/press403.htm). The problem is that this number is not a true reflection of practising midwives or midwives practising in a maternal health unit. A further burden on midwifery practice is the decrease in the total number of nurse/midwives completing their training each year. The output of all nursing education institutions in South Africa providing the four-year programme leading to registration as a nurse (general, psychiatric and community) and midwife for 2005 has diminished by more than 1000 since 1996. Only 1533 persons completed the programme in 2005 versus 2629 who completed the course in 1996 (http://www.sanc.co.za/stats. htm).

Statistics therefore reflect the acute shortage of midwives in South Africa. This in turn prevents midwives from fulfilling their full role as professional midwives. Midwives in South Africa are a dying breed and South Africa needs midwives now more than ever. Not only are there few practising midwives but young qualified nurses no longer stay on to practise. The current SANC register shows that less than 3% of registered nurse/midwives are younger than 30 years, 24% are between 30 and 39 years, 36% between 40 and 49 years, 24% between 50 and 59 years and 12% older than 60 years (http://www.sanc.co.za/stats.htm).

A further hindrance is the issue of recognition of post basic qualifications. SANC recognised advanced midwifery and neonatal training as a post basic qualification. This was once a sought after qualification as it enhances midwifery skills and knowledge. The course is still offered as a post basic diploma or as part of a master's degree at several universities. The problem today is that few midwives enrol for this course and those who do complete the course do not stay in the clinical field. Statistics from the Western Cape showed that there are only eight midwives with an advanced midwifery qualification who are practising in the clinical field (Odendaal 2004). Currently, there is not one midwife with a PhD who works in the public services or private clinics as an employee. The biggest hindrance is that the state and private institutions do not recognise this additional training. Midwives who have specialised still receive similar salaries to those who have only a basic diploma in midwifery. A particularly important factor is that their professional classification stays the same. In other words they are not acknowledged as midwifery specialists or consultants in the clinical field. Medical doctors are recognised when they specialise and are known as registrars when they are busy doing their specialisation courses. Registrars get a four-year post in a government hospital where they receive status as a registrar, salary and paid time to attend lectures and study. When they qualify they are recognised as consultants, are appointed in specialists' posts and their salaries are adjusted to recognise their qualifications. Midwives on the other hand, have to pay for their own studies, have to put in leave to attend lectures, do not receive recognition as 'registrars' in the clinical field, and get no recognition whatsoever as a specialist once they have qualified. These 'specialist' midwives usually leave the clinical field immediately to take up an administrative vacancy as they can earn a higher salary and be professionally promoted to a senior professional nurse or chief professional nurse. Thus the lack of recognition of specialist midwives by the Government and private institutions is one of the biggest obstacles to experienced midwives who wish to practise midwifery. Retention of specialist midwives in the clinical field will not improve if the Government does not recognise the highly developed skills of the advanced, master's or PhD qualified midwife.

# Place of birth

Implications of education and training resulted in the change of place where women chose to give birth. Women used to give birth at home assisted by registered or traditional midwives. Somerset Hospital was established in 1818 and was the first civilian hospital for public and private patients. Until that time hospitals were purely military institutions. The first lying-in beds were made available for labouring women in the Albany Hospital in Grahamstown in 1858 (Muller 2003). As the theoretical knowledge of midwives increased they realised that there were advantages for certain high-risk women to give birth in hospitals. The problem was that the social demand for hospital confinements increased and fewer midwives were attending births at home. By 1960 the freedom to practise home births was completely undermined as most women delivered in hospitals. Women believed it was better to deliver in a hospital setting and neither the public nor the private hospitals supported independent midwives' access to their facilities. Midwives were forced to start working as 'obstetric nurses' under the guidance of obstetricians in these facilities.

A further restriction in freedom to practise was the issue that medical assurance companies did not recognise the midwife as a private practitioner and did not reimburse the client for any consultations with a private midwife. Few women made use of private midwives. The only women who still used midwives as principal care givers were those who could not afford medical assurance or women who had enough money to pay the midwife for services rendered without claiming reimbursement from their medical assurance. Many women who could not get to the hospital facilities still used traditional midwives to assist them during antenatal, labour and birth.

Thus between 1960 and 1986 due to societal pressures, professional private midwives lost their freedom to practise. Midwives were forced to work in hospitals or clinics, directed by obstetricians and they were not allowed to make any decisions regarding the care of the women they were looking after. Professional midwives who wanted to express their freedom to practise started to set up their own practices by giving antenatal preparation classes, postnatal home visits and acting as lactation consultants. This step forward was increased by a breakthrough in 1989: medical assurance companies agreed to start paying midwives for services rendered. Since then there has been a surge of midwives taking full responsibility for the women during antenatal, labour, birth and the postnatal period. In 1994 with the help of Justus Hofmeyr, an obstetrician, Cheryl Nikodem was instrumental in the establishing of the first midwifery unit in a private hospital, Garden City Clinic. She later participated in the design and commissioning of the first private clinic which caters mainly for private midwife practitioners: Linkwood birth unit at Linkwood Clinic in Johannesburg. Today midwives are again free to practise as independent practitioners as more and more facilities are opening their doors to welcome independent midwives to the use of their facilities if needed.

## Current scope of midwifery practice in South Africa

In South Africa a midwife functions independently, dependently and inter-dependently as part of the multi-professional health team. The role of the midwife is to assist the pregnant woman, her family and community to promote, maintain and restore health during the procedures surrounding childbirth by means of: prevention of ill health; promotion of good health; holistic healing; and, rehabilitation. A registered midwife is allowed to open her own private practice directly after qualifying. Currently there is no system in place to ensure ongoing updating of knowledge. As long as a midwife pays the yearly registration fee she may continue to practise.

Midwives' scope of practice concerning dispensing rights is limited (Nursing Act 1978). Midwives are not allowed to prescribe essential medication such as magnesium sulphate in case of severe pre-eclampsia, or oxytocin to prevent postpartum haemorrhage. They are also not allowed to prescribe antifungal medications to treat candidiasis or any other vaginal infection. They are fully dependent on the medical practitioner for the prescription of medications. As medical practitioners are not readily available, this is a very big problem in private midwifery practices and in midwifery obstetric units. As midwives' practice is required to be evidence based, as far as giving medication is concerned, they continue to take the risk on a daily basis to practise outside their permitted scope of practice in these units. Thus, they administer medication where appropriate, for instance, oxytocin to prevent postpartum haemorrhage, folate, iron, magnesium sulphate and anti-retrovirals.

## Public and private health facilities

South Africa currently has two different methods of organising its health services: the public health system and the private health system. Private clinics and hospitals are expensive and clients can choose who their main care giver is. Clients need to be members of a medical assurance scheme or pay the facility cash in advance. Public clinics and hospitals serve the majority of the population. Pregnant women and children under the age of six have free access to medical care; other clients pay a minimal fee.

The majority of pregnant women in South Africa use governmental health services to give birth. Most of the care is provided by midwives. Obstetricians usually provide care only for women who have been identified as being at a 'high risk'. There are midwives who have received additional training in advanced midwifery who are able to manage high risk women in emergency situations, but these midwives are few.

Obstetricians and midwives provide a shared care to their clients. These public services are overcrowded and understaffed and women in these facilities endure unpleasant experiences and practices (Brown 2004). Midwives who work in these public facilities are frequently exposed to unpleasant circumstances and difficult conditions. These contribute to a poor working environment and have an impact on midwives' freedom to practise. They include:

- Severe shortages of personnel. One midwife can look after up to four labouring and delivering women at the same time.
- Shortages of essential supplies such as gloves. Many times there are no gloves; other times the gloves are of such poor quality that they

break the moment you put them on. There is often no linen to change the bed when it becomes wet; women are now asked to bring their own sheets, blankets and pillows when they come to a public facility.

- Shortages of essential drugs. Shortages such as lifesaving drugs (oxytocin and magnesium sulphate) frustrates midwives as they cannot deliver essential care to the women.
- Shortages of equipment. Resuscitation equipment such as laryngoscopes, resuscitation cribs for neonates, incubators, Doppler apparatus (Doptone); cardiotocograph machines are not available at many of the midwifery obstetric units (Odendaal 2004).

The above factors are not conducive to good midwifery care and this is reflected in the clients' opinions. A study done by Matizirofa (2006) showed that 41% of clients who responded were very satisfied and 54% were moderately satisfied about the antenatal care that they had received. Fewer women in the study were very satisfied with the care during delivery (39.3%), which confirms the fact that women who deliver in the public services may experience unpleasant practices which have been shown to be ineffective or harmful, such as with-holding food and water during labour. Clients' views regarding postnatal care were the worst: only 25% of women rated the care as excellent.

Obstetricians in private facilities take care of low and high risk women. The clients choose their primary caregiver, either a midwife or an obstetrician and in rural areas a general practitioner. Midwives who practise privately are only allowed to look after low-risk women and need to refer high-risk women to a medical practitioner. The majority of women in the private sector receive their care from obstetricians or general medical practitioners. Midwives who look after their clients during labour in this situation are not allowed to make any decisions and work merely as obstetric nurses as they only follow orders. These women may not experience the same unpleasant practices as those who give birth in the public services but they are exposed to other issues such as high caesarean section (90%) and epidural anaesthesia rates. For instance when an anaesthetist is in the ward attending to one woman, another woman in early labour may be coerced into agreeing to have an epidural even if she is still coping well with her labour pains. She is quite likely to be told that the anaesthetist may not be available later and he is right here now, so she should agree to an epidural for pain relief.

Thus, we can see how midwives working in both the public and private sectors in South Africa face situations where their ability to have freedom to practise is jeopardised by the systems in place.

# Political and governmental issues that influence midwifery practice in South Africa

Historically, South Africa has had a turbulent past dominated by apartheid on the one side and the freedom fighters on the other side. Apartheid was legislated into force in the 1950s. This prohibited the mixes of races, and people of colour had to live in their own districts. There were different education systems and health systems for white people and people of colour. The Reconstruction and Development Programme (RDP) constitutes a policy framework that forms the basis of transformation in South Africa in order to overcome the legacy of apartheid. The population of South Africa is made up of a mixture of races. The majority is black South Africans (75%), whites comprise about 13%, Asian people 3% and other mixed races ('coloureds') 9%. There are 11 official languages and about 24% of the adult population is still illiterate (Muller 2003). Thus, taking into account all the different languages and legions of cultures, health education is not an easy task in South Africa.

However, the situation is improving for childbearing women. Since the end of the apartheid era in 1994, the provision of maternal healthcare has gone through a transformation. Through the enactment of legalisation and policies the democratically elected Government in South Africa has made a concerted effort to improve maternal and child health services for all.

Many of the new policies have affected the freedom of midwives to practise. Some of these policies are discussed below.

## 1994 – National Health Plan

A single, comprehensive, equal and integrated National Health System is planned. This will be co-ordinated under the leadership of the Minister of Health – the national authority – the Department of Health. The health plan promotes primary healthcare facilities. These facilities are mainly staffed by nurses and midwives only (Muller 2003).

Midwives are expected to take responsibility for their clients. However, because the health plan does not address their rights for instance, to pre-scribe essential medications, their decision making powers are not complete. This causes frustration in the caregiver: for example, she may be able to identify the problem, say, a candida infection, but cannot prescribe treatment and has to refer the patient to a medical officer for a prescription.

# 1995 – Free public health services for pregnant women and children under six years

On 24 May 1994, the State President declared that all healthcare for pregnant women and children under the age of 6 years would be free. The purpose of this policy was to improve access to healthcare for women and children by removing the barrier of health service fees by 2005 (http://www.hst.org.za/publications/109). This was a wonderful concept. The problem was that the facilities got flooded with clients and the facilities received no financial assistance to increase their staff numbers. Midwives got burnt-out due to the overload of clients and left the profession to seek employment in other countries or other employment sectors. This placed a further burden on those who stayed behind.

# 1996 – Choice on Termination of Pregnancy

The amendment to the Choice on Termination of Pregnancy Act 1996 stated that a registered nurse 'who has undergone prescribed training in terms of this Act' may perform termination of pregnancy. This act allowed for midwives to enhance their careers and quite a few midwives have completed the prescribed course and are now assisting with termination of pregnancies.

# 1997 – National Committee for Confidential Enquiry into Maternal Deaths

Despite the significant advances and efforts that have been made to improve maternal health facilities, midwives, women and their infants are still exposed to risks that contribute to the high maternal death rate and the high infant mortality rate. The maternal mortality ratio is reported as 230/100 000 live births and infant mortality as 53/1000 live births. The majority of women in developing countries lose their lives due to preventable complications (*Saving Babies*, DoH 2003). The confidential enquiries into maternal deaths identified the major causes that contributed to maternal deaths as failure to use health facilities, inadequacy of services and substandard care. Forty-four per cent of the women who died of hypertension-related problems delayed seeking help from health facilities. Midwives at primary healthcare facilities were not able to detect, for example, valvular heart diseases, or could not manage women with hypertension in pregnancy appropriately. Thus, with a shortage of resources and skills, coupled with a poor uptake of services, midwives struggle to take care of women (National Committee for the Confidential Enquiry into Maternal Deaths 1998).

# 1999 – Prevention of mother-to-child transmission (PMTCT) of human immunodeficiency virus (HIV) programmes (Doherty et al 2003)

The roll-out of this programme was extremely slow (Doherty et al 2003). At the time of writing (2006) many clinics especially in the rural areas still do not offer PMTCT to women as they do not have the resources available to test and treat the women and their newborns. The programme of the PMTCT is excellent, but has brought with it another burden for midwives. On the positive side, the roll-out supports the appointment of a new staff member at the facilities. The problem is that the Government has advertised this PMTCT post at a salary much higher than that which midwives would earn in a labour ward. A labour ward midwife requires many more skills and works in much more stressful circumstances than does a PMTCT midwife. So, once again we have lost practising midwives as many have joined the roll-out of the PMTCT.

# Freedom to practise suffers under the burden of disease

The first cases of HIV in South Africa were diagnosed in 1982. The first antenatal survey was done in 1990 and it was found that 0.8% of pregnant women were HIV positive. Ten years later research has shown that 24.8% of pregnant women who use public antenatal care facilities were HIV positive. Based on the antenatal data it is estimated that more than 6.29 million people in South Africa were living with HIV at the end of 2004, and about 600 people die of HIV-related illness each day (Berry 2004, Noble 2006). Today there is compelling evidence that infectious diseases such as HIV/acquired immune deficiency syndrome (AIDS) and tuberculosis (TB) are a threat to women in their reproductive health. The South African Department of Health did a survey on 16 000 antenatal women and estimate that 29.5% of pregnant women were living with HIV in 2004. The prevalence varied between the nine provinces from 19.3% (Limpopo province) to 40.7% in KwaZuluNatal (Noble 2006). Studies have shown that 54% of maternal deaths caused by TB were attributable to HIV-1 infections (Shisana et al 2003). HIV/AIDS is a fast growing epidemic in South Africa affecting up to 32.5% of childbearing women in some of the provinces. The Government initially was against the use of antiretroviral (ARV) treatment for people living with HIV. Medical practitioners were sentenced if they prescribed ARVs for women. The world AIDS conference in 2000, Durban, brought forth a new fight for freedom, when people started to fight for their rights to receive ARVs (Berry 2004). Justice Edwin Cameron said at the conference that the prospect of 25 million deaths in Africa is fundamentally unacceptable. He described how he nearly died of the disease three years before but was brought back to health by ARV drugs he was able to afford. 'I have the privilege of purchasing my health, for about $400 a month. Why should I have the privilege of purchasing my life, when 34 million people around the world are becoming ill and dying? It is a moral inequity of fundamental proportions. No one can look at it and not be spurred to action' (Berry 2004). It was as late as August 2003 when the Government ordered the health department to develop a detailed operational plan to provide ARV drugs to people living with HIV/AIDS.

Three years after and ARVs are still not reaching many pregnant women. Reasons are given as:

- Stigma associated of being known to be HIV positive deters many pregnant women from taking a test.
- Pregnant women not sharing their HIV positive status with midwives as they fear discrimination in the antenatal and delivery care.
- Lack of healthcare infrastructure, particularly in rural areas, means that many pregnant women may not come into contact with the medical services during their pregnancies.
- Shortages of drugs: medication is not getting to all of the areas in which it is needed.

## HIV/AIDS – burden for not only the client but the caregiver as well

A report using death certificate notification data showed that 13% of deaths among health workers were because of HIV/AIDS-related illnesses (Shisana et al 2003). However, using this method, it is difficult to estimate accurately the proportion of health workers who died from HIV/AIDS-related illnesses. This is because of the stigma associated with AIDS. Families and doctors fear that the insurance industry may not pay out benefits or that families may not take responsibility for the burial of the bodies if the deceased died of AIDS. The majority of health workers in the data were African and single. The occupations of those who died were mostly professional nurses and associated nursing staff members (Shisana et al 2003).

A further burden is the issue of absenteeism among health workers. HIV-related illness counts for 63.9% of absenteeism. Nurses experienced a feeling of low morale due to several factors such as stressful working conditions. These include high absenteeism of colleagues, heavy patient workload, staff shortages and low salaries. They stated that the patient loads are heavy as 46% of patients in public hospitals are HIV positive and need 'more' attention. A study done among healthcare workers showed that 43.9% of respondents felt that the prevalence of HIV/AIDS had a negative impact on their work. They reported experiencing stress, fear, frustration and depression due to their contact with patients living with AIDS (Shisana et al 2003).

Health workers are scared that they may become infected. Some respondents mentioned deliberate attempts by patients to infect health workers such as spitting and biting. They felt that it takes more time to care for HIV-infected patients. While performing their duties they have to take extra precautions against possible infection, such as wearing protective clothing. Many complained that the gloves available were uncomfortable, of poor quality and not the correct size and that this affected their working speed. In addition, some health workers stated that ill fitting gloves could increase the possibility of injuries. They pointed out that HIV/AIDS patients were usually very ill and needed a lot more attention and care and took more time to recover. Finally, healthcare givers felt that patients suffering from non-HIV diseases were being neglected because of the sheer volume of infected patients needing their constant attention. Half of all the health professionals were of the opinion that the stigma related to being HIV positive existed at work, while 81.5% believed that this was also the case in their direct community. From this study it is clear that the HIV/AIDS epidemic has a severe impact on midwives and that the burden of the disease is high (Shisana et al 2003).

# Conclusion

It is clear that the freedom to practise by South African midwives is curtailed by the culturally diverse and disease burdened environment within which they have to work. The maternal and neonatal morbidity stays high despite several strategies implemented to improve the outcomes for mothers and their babies. The Government needs to realise that midwives play a crucial role in saving the lives of mothers and babies.

More effort and resources should be directed to improving the working circumstances of midwives. This will go some way towards enabling them to enjoy the freedom to practise the profession for which they have studied and in which they are qualified. This is where their passion lies: total commitment to caring for women and their newborns.

> ## Reflective questions
>
> Unpleasant circumstances and difficult conditions contribute to a poor working environment and have an impact on midwives' freedom to practise. List the circumstances and conditions in your place of work which would affect your freedom to practise. What can you do about them?
>
> HIV/AIDS is a worldwide burden on pregnant women. Have you encountered this condition in your practice? Are women in your country receiving ARV drugs if necessary? If not, why not?

# References

Berry S 2004 HIV & AIDS in South Africa. Online. Available at: http://www.avert.org/aidssouthafrica.htm (accessed)

Brown HC 2004 Labour support and evidence based medicine – a randomised controlled trial of implementation. PhD thesis. Johannesburg: University of the Witwatersrand, Faculty of Health Sciences, Department of Obstetrics and Gynaecology

DoH 2003 Saving babies 2002 Third perinatal care survey of South Africa. DoH, Gauteng

Doherty T, Besser M, Donohue S et al 2003 Case Study Reports on Implementation and Expansion of the PMTCT Programme in the Nine Provinces of South Africa. Health Systems Trust, Cape Town

http://www.hst.org.za/publications/109

http://www.hsrcpublishers.ac.za

http://www.sanc.co.za/press403.htm (accessed 17 Nov 2006)

http://www.sanc.co.za/stats.htm

Matizirofa L 2006 Perceived quality and utilisation of maternal health services in peri-urban, commercial farming and rural areas in South Africa. University of the Western Cape, Bellville

Muller M 2003 Nursing Dynamics, 3rd edn. Heinemann, Sandown

National Committee for the Confidential Enquiry into Maternal Deaths 1998 Interim Report on the Confidential Enquiry into Maternal Deaths in South Africa. Online. Available at: http://www.doh.gov.za/docs/reports/1998/mat_deaths.html (accessed)

Noble R 2006 HIV and AIDS statistics for South Africa. Online. Available at: http://www.avert.org/safricastats.htm (accessed)

Nolte AGW 1998 A Textbook for Midwives. Van Schaik, Pretoria

Nursing Act 1978 Act No 50 (as amended)

Odendaal H 2004 Obstetric, Gynaecologic and Neonatal Services in the Western Cape: Situation Analysis. Cape Town, Provincial Government of the Western Cape

Patterson DK 1995 The Woman's Study Bible. The New King James Version. Thomas Nelson Nashville, Gen 35(17) p 71

Shisana O, Hall E, Maluleka KR et al 2003 The impact of HIV/AIDS on the Health Sector. National survey of health personnel, ambulatory and hospitalised patients and health facilities, 2002. Department of Health, Cape Town. Online. Available at: www.hsrcpublishers.ac.za (accessed 17 November 2006)

## Additional resource

Human Sciences Research Council (HSRC) website: http://www.hsrcpublishers.ac.za/

# CHAPTER TWELVE

# Birthing in Latvia: midwives serving lovingly

RUDĪTE BRŪVERE

## Prelude

Once upon a time in a far away country, where the sun rises early from the white summer night's bed and sets early into winter's ice green skies, a lonely log cabin stood on a hillside beside a pond. Small, yet solidly built, this bath-house of the homestead stood apart from the farmhouse and steading.

A crab-apple tree spread its late spring blossoms above the small roof. The early morning's sunlight glistened on the pond and on the small stream replenishing it. There was a warm smell of wood fire around this quiet place. Inside the bath-house piled stones formed an oven where the fire heated up the inside room and warmed the water in a big kettle between the stones of the hearth. Along three walls there were broad wooden benches, some built lower, some higher. In the corner beside the door were bunches of dried twigs of birch, oak, linden and remedy herbs hanging from the ceiling. The wooden walls were blackened by the smoke and heat of so many Saturday evenings when the bath-house was heated for hours.

The door was opened to let the smoke escape, the hearth was swept, ashes removed and the door closed. The place was now ready to enter and purify body and soul during the lengthy and calm routines of sweating, washing and resting.

A small white-haired woman, carrying some dried herbs and white linen sheets, approached and opened the door. She was met by a cloud of dense smoke. When it had cleared, a girl could be seen walking slowly from the farmhouse through the orchard. Her face was calm and yet there were fine lines of pain around her mouth and eyes. Her linen shirt showed signs of toil and sweat: her time for opening up and bringing her precious burden into the world had come. To encourage herself to become soft and wide, she had opened her braided hair, loosened her waistbands and untied the strings of her simple leather footwear. These had been tied to her ankles with leather strings; now she removed them and walked barefoot, drawing courage from her connection with the soil.

Near the bath-house a sudden force made her stop and cling to a young linden-tree. She closed her eyes, panted and let herself be carried away by the strong powerful wave surging through her body. As soon as the pain and strong bearing force subsided, she felt herself held by two strong arms. The old Wise Woman – Oldmother – led her into the warm cabin smelling of sweet old wood smoke and dried herbs. She had come in time to be with the girl in her hours of hardship and had prepared the place for her to give birth to her firstborn.

Now she closed the door and shut out the world. They were together in a narrow room with one little window letting in just enough light to tell the time of day. When she felt the next wave approaching, the young woman knelt on the warm wooden floor. 'My soul feels so small, like a wee kerchief bundle, hanging on the thinnest branch of a willow,' she whispered, and she thrust herself into the lap of the Oldmother. The young one sighed and wept and let herself be taken by the force that came like a fire now and went through all her body places it needed to touch and open. The Oldmother just held her, making low cooing sounds when she felt her need for comfort. After a while the girl stood and moved around, leaning on the upper bench for support. During a wave her fingers closed around the smooth darkened wood and she felt its firmness strengthening her body. These boards once had been a deeply rooted pine tree, steadfast in many storms. In the deep stillness of the place she heard it whispering to her, 'my dear, hold on to the roots, endure and be strong, take this from me,' So the young woman learned to ride the waves, following the ways of life under This Sun.

Sometimes both women chanted together, 'God, dear, is guarding, mother Earth is helping, I am bringing forth . . .'

When a birth wave subsided, they waited for the next one in patient silence, surrounded by mutual love and trust. When it came and almost took her breath away, the Wise Woman sang little encouraging sentences into the labouring woman's ear, like, 'Your mother has borne you, you can bear too', 'You go with this wave, it comes with this wave, your little child comes closer, your little child comes now . . .'

The sun had reached its zenith when the waves changed pattern. The young woman started to make little grunting sounds; suddenly there was a power that pushed, the next one pushed more strongly, the woman's accompanying sounds became louder and longer. She was now squatting over a small heap of dried herbs: Lady's mantle, St John's wort, linden leaves, hops, green ginger and ferns which Oldmother had wrapped in clean linen and warmed on the hot hearth stones. The herbal fragrance, the room's warmth and its sheltering calm helped the labouring woman to open, to trust and to give birth at last. In the soft light of the setting sun entering the room, she let a tiny girl slide out into the patiently waiting hands of the Oldmother. A small voice sounded for the first time. Both women smiled and wept at the same time, while the little girl tried to tell them what she felt about losing her home under her mother's heart. But soon she was stilled by the warmth at her mother's breast, her tender, happy well-known voice and wrapped in linen and a fine woollen blanket.

Earlier, the Wise mother had made an infusion of shepherd's purse and common motherwort in case of bleeding with the afterbirth. Now she saw, that as with most births, all was well. Soon the small girl was nursing happily, her mother rested, bedded comfortably on a padded bench. Joyfully she answered, when her husband knocked at the door.

He had offered to go with her when she left her bed at first light. Yet she knew she had to accomplish the task of giving birth to their child herself. Since early childhood she had learned to watch and trust the comings and goings of life around her. For everything and everyone under This Sun there was a time. Her time had started at sunset the day before with the first signs that her hour was near. So she had started to sweep the pathway to the bath-house, so as 'not to let Mara stumble'. Mara was the invisible mother, who would hasten to her aid, as would the Wise Woman now. She had known in time. Then the young woman had watched the moon rise and quietly joined her husband in their chamber.

As she knew she had God, kind and wise, Mother Earth, her child and Wise Mother to help her, she had let her man stay behind and hold out his hopes and prayers for her. Now it was time to rejoice together.

For eight days the young mother stayed in the bath-house's shelter, resting from this great work she had fulfilled and freed from the usual homestead workload. Just her husband and some women from the neighbourhood visited, bringing fresh food and welcoming gifts for the new child. On the eighth day after birth, the Oldmother continued the care for the new mother. She prepared a big wooden tub, filled with warm water and different kinds of remedy herbs. After a special massage for the baby, mother and child enjoyed the bath together as preparation to take up everyday life. Dressed in fresh clothing, with a calm smile on her face, the young woman walked the path to the main house to become part of the household again. In her arms she carried her newborn child and in her heart a new knowledge, a new strength. She had toiled and had endured, she had borne, she had done it. She had grown to be a mother.

Latvia, like nine other countries, joined the European Union (EU) in May 2004. This process of change taught Latvians about the idea and spirit of the EU and allowed comparisons to be made between our laws and practice and EU laws and directives. In addition, it revealed why different people and politicians thought it worthwhile to join the Big Community. Some thought of the relative safety of belonging to this Western Community rather than to the all-consuming Eastern Community: the remains of the former Soviet Union. Others looked for financial support for development into a 'real Western civilization' with its accompanying prosperity. A third, smaller group, welcomed the need not only to accept, but also to accede to EU laws. This for Latvia (and for other post-Soviet countries) was a way of regenerating human rights and ethics in all spheres of life, badly neglected during the Soviet time. But Latvia's restored democracy has not brought automatic change; there is still a long way to go.

Some, midwives included, yearn for radical change. (Radical: from *radix* (Latin): the root.) For healing to come from the roots, we must firstly examine ourselves for a diagnosis. We must look inwardly, back to examine from whence we have come, and what we have come through, and forwards to try to decide which is the best direction in which to go. Are we to be carried by the mainstream or do we have the powers to search and follow our own way? Where could these powers come from?

In Hebrew, 'holy' carries the meaning of being absolutely different, sacred, of God . . . Birth is HOLY, is special, is not belonging to anyone else, anyone from the outside, is pure, is spiritual. In Latvia and other post-Soviet and still Soviet countries, we still have a long way to go and many obstacles to overcome to return to humanised birth, the sacred beginning of each unique human.

## About Latvia and its birthing culture

Latvia is a rather small country – 64 600 km² are inhabited by 2.3 million people (Figure 12.1). Together with its neighbouring countries Lithuania and Estonia it is situated opposite Sweden and Finland on the eastern coast of the Baltic Sea. Latvia's ancient inhabitants are the Baltic peoples, a very old and very small branch of the Indo-European peoples. The language – Latvian, is similar only to Lithuanian.

The background of our country's birthing culture is well articulated in our ancient folk songs: short rhythmic four-line verses, uniquely telling the important truths of life on 'mother earth'. In these verses is expressed the people's loving respect of nature's beauty and of the harmonic rhythms of all life. Everything in nature is alive and personified and helps its human

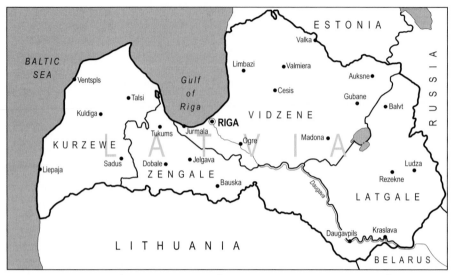

*Figure 12.1* Map of Latvia. Map ©: The Latvian Institute, 2004 (see also www.latvianinstitute.lv)

sisters and brothers. Within this loving attitude there is no reason to fear death, there is life afterwards 'under the other sun'. (There are about a million of these verses, going back to the tenth, eleventh century (Šmits 1928)).

Within these narrative folk songs is Mara, a goddess, or, even a personi-fication of the midwife. Mara is the one who hurries to help when the mother to be has her hard time: she is there to guard life. '*Radibas*' – the Latvian word used to express 'to give birth', literally translates as 'being creating', 'to let /out/ into the world'. Children come as gifts of life: here is an attempt to translate one of those verses (but almost impossible to do adequately and maintain the rhythm):

> A new bright star did rise
> And came to shine upon the mother's door
> Though no bright star this was
> The little child's soul had come to stay
> (*Spoža zvaigzne atteceja*
> *Virs ligavas namdurvim*
> *Ta nebija spoža zvaigzne*
> *Ta bernina dveselite*)

The Latvian word for midwife is '*vecmate*' or 'oldmother' ('old' means 'wise' here). In ancient times midwives were special women, known to the whole neighbourhood and beyond. Through long years of loving care for birthing women and their newborn and families they had achieved deep inner wisdom about the ways of life and were reliable and trustworthy. They watched and learned from life in nature and from respected older midwives. They had deep insight into what was going on and thus worked in harmony with soul and body. Our ancient midwives did not misuse their power by dominating. In accordance with the birthing woman, they calmly trusted nature's ways and the energies of life; they assisted with loving care, but became active only when there was a need to intercede (Brūvere 2003).

Birthing was always accomplished in a remote place – usually the so-called 'bath-house': *pirts*. Built of solid timber, the *pirts* was at a distance from the living facilities and the hustle of everyday life. It was small enough, very clean, dark and warm – almost like a mother's womb. A sheltered place to open and be ready to let go of the child and let him commence his own way. This chapter's Prelude has emerged from the spirit of this time.

## Midwifery in Latvia

The first Latvian midwifery training institute was founded in the western part of the country in 1804. Although life in Latvia was under permanent lordship of either the Germans, the Swedish, the Polish or Russians, the new institution was in keeping with the gradual modernisation of life in Latvia and indigenous Latvians' access to schools and institutions. Later there were three more midwifery schools and some private midwifery seminaries.

Education and the activities of midwives in Latvia improved significantly after the first Latvian independence in 1918 after World War I (Brūvere 2003). The Society of Latvia's Midwives was first founded in 1925; after five years the number of members had risen to 300. The society was a living body, with a journal, the *Latvian Midwives Messenger*, whose members exercised real care for each colleague, established a relief foundation to help the aged/ill midwives and discussed many work as well as personal issues. The Society also organised regular meetings, educational programmes, training and practice sessions in hospitals. Thus midwives could improve their skills and their ability to manage complications especially in the absence of timely medical help. Latvia's midwives were important providers of public health care at a time when most healthy women gave birth at home under the care of a district midwife: the Society's work was very valuable. In addition, by the late 1920s professional midwives in Latvia had organised a health supervision system for new babies and children, and cared for them together with the district nurses of the Red Cross.

As well as professional midwives, there were also traditional midwives. Here is the story of a country midwife as related by her granddaughter Aina.

## Wisdom that passed through the soul

Agata Senkane was born in 1898 in Latgale, the most eastern and also the poorest region of Latvia. There were many big families in this region: Agata herself had eight children. One died in early childhood; another son and her husband died working in the woods. Agata had to make a living for a family of seven by herself. The daily bread was hard to earn through hard toil on very small pieces of land. This led to many men taking to drinking although Agata herself did not succumb to this temptation.

In a neighbourhood village lived an old Wise Woman, the one who attended to births. Agata, an open minded and loving woman, learned from her and started to follow in her footsteps. She never locked her doors. Her philosophy was, 'You have come to my doorstep and need assistance? Then this is for me.' So she took the Wise Woman into their home. This old woman taught her old healer's knowledge and shared with her additional midwifery skills and wisdom.

Encouraged by her own life experience and this teaching, Agata started to attend births at home. She trusted God, she learned to trust the woman and to use her skills. She looked on giving birth as natural and expected no sudden disasters. She accepted women and situations she encountered and this attitude made up for the lack of formal education. When Aina, her granddaughter (who told this story) was studying midwifery at the First Medical School of Riga she related the many different risky situations that could happen during a birth to her grandmother. Agata mentioned that she had worked as a midwife too. Aina wanted to know how she had managed problems. Grandmother asked, 'What problems?' 'If the baby has a wrong lie, for example.' 'Then I would just bring him into a right position.' There seemed to be a way of meeting each need. And if a baby died just before or soon after birth, then these people knew that this sorrow belonged to life – that the small child had passed the same threshold twice. People in her region respected her, they called her often and, too poor to pay with cash, they showed their appreciation by paying in kind.

Aina's mother was killed when she was four; her father was lost. She was brought up by her mother's sister. Later Grandmother moved in with them for the last 10 years of her life: a cherished matriarch who spoke little but wisely. She died in 1983, aged 85, and was mourned by nearly 200 family members who, even today, follow her example.

Aina became a midwife at the suggestion of a friend. She came to love midwifery and worked faithfully for 20 years in a small hospital delivery department at the seaside by Riga. She attended to births with the same loving accepting attitude of her grandmother. But increasingly she felt that by being made to obey hospital laws and procedures she was doing harm rather than good. Chamberlain's work on the unborn and the newborn as a person (Chamberlain 1988) reinforced her opinion that babies are people already during pregnancy. They experience their birth, other people there and the way they are handled with perfect perception, and they will remember and learn from this experience. She felt that she was not in the right place any more. She studied psychology and engaged pregnant couples in counselling and was involved in establishing the Association of Perinatal Psychology of Latvia and is working there successfully and happily.

# Latvia: recent times

When World War II began and the period of the First Independency of Latvia ended, detrimental changes followed: the activities described above were stopped; organisations extinguished; most former national institutions closed. Rigorous changes took place almost from one day to the next. Many characteristic features of everyday life vanished. People just disappeared. It was forbidden to speak many words and names aloud. A time of terror, deep-rooted fears and unspeakable suffering began. This was to crush our heritage of an ancient birth culture and put an end to loving and personalised midwifery care. In 1940 Latvia was occupied, first by the Russian Soviet army, then by the German Nazi army, then again by the Soviet Red Army. This had a dramatic effect on the life and work of the people. The two million population of Latvia was diminished by nearly a third between 1939 and 1945 (Šmulders 1990).

The history of the processes of the Soviet totalitarian regime, upheld solely by terror and violence, is well known. The people of Latvia are a small part of mankind included in the suffering. Beginning in June 1941, the Russian occupants in one night forced more than 14400 of Latvia's inhabitants out of their beds and houses. More than 120000 Latvian inhabitants were imprisoned or deported to Soviet concentration (GULAG) camps. More than 140000 took refuge from the Soviet army by fleeing to the West. On 25 March 1949, more than 40000 rural residents were deported to Siberia in a sweeping repressive action. These included proud, hardworking farmers and their families, old and very young. All were forced from their homes and homeland into the state collective farms, the *kolkhozes*. The wounds of these destroyed lives have not yet healed, the evils not easily forgiven and forgotten. There are still problems between Latvians and Russians: there has been no acknowledgement of any misdeed and no plea for forgiveness by representatives and heirs of the evil-doers. The old fear is still very much alive.

Thus the Soviet occupant regime had secured safe grounds for obedience. The most effective means was the forceful application of militant atheism. This spread an atmosphere of hopelessness, absolute materialism and an utter empty coldness. Nevertheless, every force generates against itself a possibly stronger force. There was a great challenge to look for spiritual values. There was also the challenge to make a decision. For instance, if people wanted to have a career they had to sacrifice their conscience, or, at least bury it. The alternative decision of sticking to the truth and disobeying impossible orders led to personal suffering with the added responsibility of family suffering. So, fear of making things complicated and dangerous prevented many people, even within families, from communicating openly with each other about local or national issues. Churches were closed down and misused and all social work and charity was strictly forbidden: this was for 'the State' to deal with. As in the Soviet Union, the 'worker's paradise', there were no unmet needs – everybody was content and happy. And if not, then it was because of being unworthy. This applied the Marxian theory that human life is only valuable as long as the person is productive. So there is no need to care for those who are not of value. It was that simple. So they vanished from the public sight. Handicapped people never left their homes, or were put away in terrible institutions. Old people, if unable to stay in the family, were also put into institutions and forgotten by society. (Even in the early 1990s mothers feared to indicate the presence of their handicapped children by taking them outside their homes.) Many parents were persuaded to put their handicapped children into institutions in order to stay 'productive' themselves.

# Midwifery perspectives

## Zenta

The fate of midwives and changes of attitude and services can be illustrated by life stories of some old midwives I visited. One, Zenta, died of liver cancer shortly after I met her. She was 78 years old (born 1924) and had already lost her voice because of her illness. Although she was in pain and could only whisper, she was moved by my interest and keen to tell me her story. This is the experience she related:

The well functioning system of midwifery care that Latvian midwives had built up in the 25 years before 1941 was destroyed. Instead of individually working midwives, a centralised system was to be established to keep everybody under united control. Midwives were deprived of any independence; hospitals and polyclinics were now their only working places. No initiative was allowed: no dissonant opinions; no spontaneous actions; no independent thinking. This showed even in ridiculously small affairs: one morning, Zenta noticed that a famous Latvian artist's painting of *Mother with child*, usually hanging in the hospital's entrance hall, had been replaced by an ugly communist poster. She (being head midwife) replaced the painting. This resulted in the loss of her job at the hospital.

Zenta was made to work with timber cutting for a time (women in the Soviet system finally had the same 'rights' as men; they could and often were forced to do hard physical men's work). She met many medical staff there. Later she was able to resume her work as a midwife in Latgale. She was sent there to establish a delivery department and a nursing school which she did very successfully. Nevertheless, her main objective still remained: to help the young nurses and midwives to reconnect with themselves and with women; to accept midwifery as a serving profession and, be motivated by a feeling of empathy. When she finished her story, Zenta said, sighing a little sadly, 'How could I put love into them?'

## Occupation: its effects on midwifery

Formerly, an independently working district midwife took care of pregnant women, attended to their births at home and cared for the family. Now, every pregnant woman had to attend the town's polyclinics during pregnancy and then go to the hospital for the delivery. A number of smaller friendly hospitals were closed. The larger more impersonal ones remained. Wherever they worked, regardless of the size of hospital, all carers had to adopt to the last detail 'edicts' issued from Moscow regarding the one and only 'right' system of obstetric care (Chalmers 1997).

Midwives lost competencies and status. From now on 'higher authorities' regarded them as unable to carry the responsibility for their own work. Doctors controlled their every move. And doctors themselves were under the control and command of directives and directors, of the Party, and ultimately the powers in Moscow. In addition, in every working place there was always somebody to watch that the 'right things' were done and said, and to report if they were not. Statistical reports were invented for everything. However, as 'the plan' had always to be fulfilled, people in charge learned how to 'massage' the statistics, to make them look better than they really were. So it is still not possible to tell the numerical results of changes in the healthcare system, for instance, how many women suffered and in what way, and, how many infants died during the years until 1991. Midwives and mothers only remember many sad stories.

However, if something went wrong, it was always the midwife who was called to account and made the scapegoat, even after obeying a doctor's instructions. To speak out would mean severe punishment, loss of her job and worse. This was a communist characteristic: if there were sad outcomes and situations, then someone had to be guilty. There was a regular big staff meeting where the person involved was interrogated, blamed and accused, instead of the members looking objectively at cause and effect, and scientific evidence. This deep-rooted thinking of 'First of all – who is to blame now?' still dominates the way doctors and others, including midwives, treat problems occurring where healthcare is offered and babies are born.

Other difficulties in practice were evident. Twenty-four-hour working shifts started which would be against the law in many other countries; we still have these in most hospitals. Midwives were overworked and paid poorly; this is still the case today. Midwives were unable to establish real relationships with the women for whom they cared. This was because they worked in an impersonal organised way and often had to perform manipulations they knew to be futile and even harmful. The loss of trust and being 'with the women' was the worst. Under these living and working conditions midwives even missed the fulfilment and joy of seeing happy, healthy families. Postnatal contacts were abandoned, midwives could not give significant postnatal care any more. Today it is still the same.

Midwives' education suffered as well as their practice. Basic education was now standardised on the same low level as everywhere in the Soviet Union. Humanitarian subjects like psychology, ethics, the art of caring ceased to exist. A midwife did not need to be particularly good at midwifery skills provided she excelled in the obligatory Marxism-Leninism. A significant number of midwives chose midwifery because it was easy to access rather than anything else. The special love for our profession sometimes developed as time passed by, but very often it did not. All maternity care followed the so called 'scientifically based' methods (of Soviet origin only) to be applied regardless of their appropriateness. The result: disappointed and bitter midwives and disappointed and offended pregnant and childbearing women.

The impact of birth-medicalisation globally and system of Soviet medicine affected our birthing culture and midwifery care profoundly. As everybody had to be under control, births were confined to hospitals. On admission, women in labour had to leave all private clothing and possessions in the entrance room; they were routinely shaved, given an enema and showered. Then they were made to wear (often unclean) hospital slippers and clothes resembling prisoner uniforms. There was no individual assessment of the expected date of delivery; instead most often labours were induced, often violently done and badly controlled with little information to the mother and minimal care: bad outcomes, especially of the newborn were not uncommon.

No husbands (or other relatives) were allowed to be present. The father saw his newborn child eight days later, when the mother was finally released. As the mother often only saw her child for a short period of time only some days after birth, there was no opportunity for bonding. This also meant that breastfeeding suffered and most women believed that they 'just have not enough mother's milk'. Thus, at this time, both women and midwives felt that the communist system was telling them that they were nothing individually. They were worthless unless they earned praise by the potentates. It was safer not to want anything. Nobody was interested in what individuals wanted. This message was handed down to the next generation and seems in many families to have become part of the genetic makeup.

The unborn child was not 'the little child' anymore, as it had been called before, when its mother was 'walking in hope' (pregnant). The medical caregivers started to use a word that means, literally translated, 'fruit'. This term is originally Biblical, where Elizabeth says to Maria, who is carrying little unborn Jesus, 'blessed be the fruit of thy womb'. However, the emotionless technological Soviet medicine made it sound completely disconnected from its origins and from the pregnant woman. The state looked on the woman as a nobody; in addition, if the fruit might not be of top-quality or if it shows up at an inconvenient time, it can be thrown away. When a woman with one or two children obediently turned up at the gynaecologist's for confirmation of the next pregnancy, his first direct question after this was always, 'Which date would she come again for the abortion?' With no respect and no support, there is this 'simple solution' for unwanted human life. So the number of abortions increased greatly, even in the 1970s and 1980s. It exceeded by far the number of births in our sparsely inhabited country and still the abortion rate is more than two-thirds of the number of live births. Although the number of abortions has decreased by 50% since 1991, in 2003 there were 691 abortions for every 1000 births (Johnston 2005).

Under these spiritually void and physically hard living conditions many women were too exhausted to uphold respect for life; many pregnant women felt unable to build a mother–baby relationship during pregnancy. An increasing number of women secretly fled from the hospital and abandoned their newborns to be raised by the state in foster homes.

# Midwives in independent Latvia

In 1991 all the three Baltic States, Lithuania, Latvia and Estonia, regained their independence. Now (2006) we have had 15 years of new possibilities and open doors. How have we used this time to awaken and call forth changes of midwifery care and renew our birthing culture?

As the Iron Curtain fell and borders to other countries finally opened, different experiences and evidence*s* became accessible. Some of our colleagues used the new opportunities to meet, to watch and learn, and 'look over the brim of one's own plate'. An enthusiastic midwife, Astrida, working at the biggest maternity hospital in Latvia was one of the first to allow fathers to be present at the births of their babies. This was very brave on her part and she had to meet scornful resistance. She felt that midwives could attempt change better as a whole group and in 1993 she initiated the founding of the Association of Midwives of Latvia (AML): the successor to the earlier Society of Midwives of Latvia.

During the summer of 1993 Astrida spent 10 weeks visiting large hospitals in Munich and Bremen, Germany. There, she experienced rooming-in, breastfeeding, fathers taking part at births as close to natural as possible, even in those big hospitals, and midwives who cared, for 'their' women, for the babies, for one another. After that she attended a Conference for Natural Birth in Zurich, Switzerland. When Astrida returned to Riga she was even more eager for improvement. In addition, her experiences had reminded her that: women can give birth themselves and natural birth is the safest option for healthy women. So, when a couple asked her to attend the birth of their baby in their own home. it was natural for her to agree. News spread among pregnant women and the first home birth in Latvia was followed by a queue of others. For the next nine years Astrida worked 'under wraps'. Although everybody interested knew of her, the authorities were wise enough not to start an open discussion.

At last midwives arrived at a point where they could discuss these issues with groups of politicians. As evidence we used the EU directives (1980, art 4) and the Munich Declaration (2000) as well as the widely disseminated World Health Organization ((WHO) 2003) findings. Astrida had to attend a parliamentarian committee meeting where some members declared that there had never been home births attended by independent midwives in Latvia. Astrida contradicted this statement. She said openly that she had been in attendance at home births for 10 years (as those present very well knew). There was a storm of laments and accusations. However, she had supporters too: when this 'scandal' appeared in the newspapers, many of the home birth parents sent her encouraging and appreciative messages and phone calls. The lifting of the old insurmountable borders started a flow of exchange with practitioners of different beliefs from the early 1990s. All who were interested enough benefited from sources such as conferences, visits, books, the internet. The main benefit of this communication on so many different levels was renewed hope, faith and trust, a space to breathe spiritual sunshine, a space to grow and develop.

These benefits led to others – there are good things being achieved by midwives in Latvia for midwives:

- We are communicating again. Perhaps not sufficiently yet; however, we have made a vital beginning and, we are learning. We have bimonthly meetings, lectures, seminars, some contacts with colleagues in other countries.
- We have established a midwives' register (every working midwife has to be registered) and a certification examination. This is to secure an educational level that will meet the basic challenges of our profession.
- There is a lively and growing interest for more education, especially in subjects such as psychology and a need for deeper understanding of spiritual values.
- A few midwives are trying to regain lost competencies and widen the choices of midwifery care on offer. Some have started to work in independent practice.
- We have established a task group of approximately five midwives, to work with, for instance, legislative issues and expanded educational programmes.

There is a growing awareness that midwifery, when expressed in just two words, means 'serving lovingly': not judging, not dominating, not controlling. Consequently, in the past decade we have made some steps towards more humanised care for childbearing women and families:

- In most places the baby is not now taken away immediately after birth; bonding and early breastfeeding are encouraged.
- There is rooming in for all mothers who want this.
- The father of the baby (or some other trusted person) can be present during labour and delivery. This has significantly improved relationships within families.
- Breastfeeding is being practised again. Information and accessible help is offered at different places, and there is a growing number of midwives who have accepted that breastfeeding support is one of a midwife's duties. The president of the AML, Antra Kuprisa, undertook a wide-ranging project with the slogan – 'Breast milk for every baby'. She also became involved in the promotion of 'baby friendly' hospitals. There are now some hospitals who have earned this status.

- A programme for the 'education of parents-to be' was established with essential midwifery input. Now there is a growing number of midwives who offer antenatal classes for pregnant women and couples.
- Helpful educational literature on pregnancy, childbirth and childrearing is now available in Latvian.
- Psychotherapists are accessible.
- There are some places (mostly founded by non-governmental organisations) where special care is offered for children with special needs (and their parents).

Becoming a member state of the EU has been of immense support, and not only financially. Most importantly, there is now a well-established legal base with whom to engage and strong allies like the European Midwives Association (EMA) to contact when political efforts seem to lead nowhere.

Still, there are problems to solve and aims to achieve. We midwives in Latvia want to regain our special place, within the net of primary and secondary healthcare. This will involve an extensive process of change. The basis of legislation has been created formally in Latvia. This legislation respects midwives as independent professionals, competent to care for physiological pregnancies, deliveries and newborn on their own legal responsibility. But change needs to take place in the minds of practitioners and politicians who believe themselves to be, and act like an elite. Teamwork for many doctors in Latvia is still an unknown empty phrase. Fair payment for the work midwives do is also required. We need to be incorporated as separate caregivers into the healthcare net and thus earn salaries that would not make us look for other jobs. We have more than 800 educated midwives in Latvia; of those, only 530 are registered, that means working, as midwives. Most of all we need to let go of the deep inner fears still existing in many minds and souls. These fears withhold us from making creative and courageous decisions, from risking belonging to the group of first midwives in this country who will work in a different way, co-working but independently. This kind of practice is just at the very delicate beginnings. Nevertheless, there is evidence that progress is being made. Astrida is still attending home births, quite openly now and also gaining good media publicity.

Dina, a 30-year-old colleague, has also started attending home births and is ready to represent the wishes of women for undisturbed natural births without any medical intervention within their own homes whenever there is an option. She has been on a television talk show and on a well-known internet site. In addition, she rented a flat in central Riga, took a loan from the bank, renovated the flat and created a welcoming family health centre. This is really a midwifery practice. However, when she started three years ago, she did not want to create difficulties by calling it that. She is the first midwife in Latvia who is taking doctors (paediatricians and a gynaecologist) into service, to help care for the families coming to 'The Stork's Nest'.

I started to attend home births in 2000, when a pregnant woman told her gynaecologist she wanted a home birth. The gynaecologist referred her to me. This was my first experience of home birth, followed by many more. Those women and families who decide to birth at home are (almost without exception) those with university education, caring families with strong bonds. When working for a shelter house for neglected pregnant young women (mostly young girls, sometimes very young) and new mothers with a baby but no home, I became friends with the housemother there, Irēna. When her time there ended, she and I decided that we could work together more successfully, building a project together. Thus the society The Family Cradle was founded. Its aims and objectives are summarised in Figure 12.2.

A year later a Christian family bestowed on us a house in the country-side, including a piece of land. During the next year (2005) some midwives, some doctors and 12 couples who had joyfully borne their children at home, joined our society. So now we have about 35 members to build this project: there will be six shelter places for women in need, in order to offer help and thus avoid abortions; we will use the big family room for seminars and gatherings; and, closest to my midwife's heart, we will have two rooms for giving birth: warm and beautiful in a simple and welcoming way. There is still much building work to be done at this house. There is no private money coming from our membership and one of the most difficult tasks is that of seeking money. However, we believe that people need this place. That means: it will be, despite the obstacles. Many pregnant women have asked me when the Family Cradle's rooms will be available. For various reasons they feel their own homes are not suitable in which to give birth and are looking for a good alternative.

These women are typical of many women in Latvia. This country is still a place where most people feel connected with nature. They are longing to regain birth as their very own experience; to connect with their baby and with the midwife; and thus, to be the ones who have the authoritative knowledge (see also Davis-Floyd and Fishel Sargent 1997: 324–329).

Joining the international sisterhood of midwives, through formal organisations such as the International Confederation of Midwives and the European Midwives Association and informal meetings and friendships with colleagues in other countries who are struggling in similar ways, has

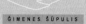

ĢIMENES ŠŪPULIS

public non—profit organisation Reg. No. 40008077466

## THE FAMILY CRADLE
### Education–Birth–Shelter

| | | |
|---|---|---|
| **Educational Centre** for midwives and other primary care staff | **Practical training of natural birth centre**<br>¥ natural childbirth<br>¥ family births<br>¥ promotion of family unity<br>¥ breastfeeding support<br>¥ postnatal activities for the promotion of regeneration | **Shelter** for abandoned expectant mothers —with attached subsistence farm |
| **Database and coordination centre** for primary care staff in birthing assistance —psychological support | | **Reproductive health education** for young people— prevention of abortions and STDs<br>**Support groups for new mothers** |
| **Education for expectant parents** | **Prenatal care** | **Massage and aromatherapy** | **Natural products** for infants and mothers |
| **Community of supporting friends** | **II part:** House of silence: recreation in peace and privacy | Preparation for natural childbirth— various courses | **Courses and seminars:**<br>¥ spiritual recreation<br>¥ humane and holistic health care |

The mission of the Family Cradle is to provide shelter, education and care for birthing women. It serves as the training and support centre for midwives, popularising a holistic and humane approach to birth and as an education centre for families and youth, it spreads knowledge on reproductive health, promotes spiritual health as well as family unity.

Project authors and implementers:
Rudīte Brūvere, **certified midwife**
 Kalna Dumpuri , Cēsu rajona Valves pagasts, p/n Rāmuļi, LV 4137
tel.  00371—41 56233 /mob. 9  11  95  93   e—pasts: ruditeb@apollo. lv

Irēna Bindemane, **teacher, artist**
 Vandadziņi  , Cēsu rajona Līgatnes pagasts, LV 4108
tel. mob. 00371—65 86 427

*Figure 12.2* The Family Cradle: a caring shelter.

strengthened and enlightened us. These contacts, visits, conferences, wonderful books written by midwives, have let us take part in lifelong learning, in being advocates for women again, in building up strength and self-esteem. Working in unity has supported us in developing 'birth models that work' ourselves (Davis-Floyd and Fishel Sargent 1997) instead of reluctantly applying 'birth models that don't work'.

As I write this chapter, we are about to start a special seminar for those midwives, who besides us three, want to start working outside hospitals. Eight certified midwives have registered. There would have been many more if, as they said, the 'legal atmosphere would be more relaxed and in order'. Three young home birth mothers have registered to listen in. They are still so impressed by their own experiences that they plan to become midwives in the future. The programme of this seminar holds different elements and issues to strengthen and encourage midwives to follow their midwife's vocation, their dream of true midwifery.

## Conclusion

This chapter has tried to demonstrate the progress of midwifery in Latvia. To do this I began by exploring the old history through the story of the Oldmother. To put the chapter into context, I described briefly the geography, demography and culture of Latvia and highlighted the old tradition of midwives' working in harmony with soul and body, demonstrated by Agata's story.

The old holistic ideas were set aside with the onset of the communist regime. Midwives became unhappy in their work; women were dissatisfied and frustrated by their birth experience; perinatal outcomes were poor: we yearned for change. Post-Soviet Latvia still suffered in mind, body and soul.

Change first has to come from within ourselves. Since 1991 midwives in Latvia have been going through the process of acceptance: of ourselves, of one another, and, that we are free to practise midwifery. Women can now once again give birth at home in Latvia. To begin with this was hidden; now it is open.

Believing that we have always been loved by God, we can love again. In Latvia now there are legal documents and directives for midwives which form a basis for some midwives to start to make professional decisions without being forced by someone holding more power. These include the EU directives and the human rights of women to choose their place for giving birth. This is just the beginning of freedom to practise midwifery in Latvia. The three midwives who have had the courage and energy to take a stand to work self-employed and out of hospital hope to be joined soon by other midwifery colleagues. Eight midwives attended our 'encouragement and preparation seminar' in March 2006.

From this beginning we hope to progress and to be able to decide freely: to serve and not to subdue; to work with women and not to control them; and, we can choose to love. This spiritual approach leads to many different ways and places of practising midwifery. It is the most powerful agent of change and epitomises midwives, who serve lovingly.

---

## Reflective questions

'Serving lovingly: not judging, not dominating, not controlling', a philosophy of midwifery evolving in Latvia, appears to go along with the midwifery/social model of childbirth. Are you able to achieve this where you work?

The chapter has emphasised that working through international organisations gives strength to midwives to progress. Given that not everyone can attend meetings in person, how would you go about communicating with and encouraging student midwives and midwives on an international scale?

---

## References

Brūvere R 2003 The effects of the Soviet Union occupation on the life and work of midwives in Latvia. RCM Midwives, 6(9):394–396

Chalmers B 1997 Changing Childbirth in Eastern Europe. In: Davis-Floyd R, Fishel Sargent C (eds) Childbirth and Authoritative Knowledge. University of California Press, Berkeley, 263–283

Chamberlain D 1988 Babies remember birth: and other extraordinary scientific discoveries about the mind and personality of your newborn. St Martins Press, New York

Council Directive of 21 January 1980 (80/155/EEC), Official Journal of the European Communities, No L 33/8, 11280

Davis-Floyd R, Fishel Sargent C 1997 Childbirth and Authoritative Knowledge. University of California Press, Berkeley

Johnston W 2005 Historical abortion Statistics Latvia http://www.johnsronesarchive.net/policy/abortion/ab-latvia.html (accessed 25 November 2006)

Latvian Midwives Messenger. Journal of the Society of Latvia's Midwives

Munich Declaration 2000 Nurses and Midwives: a Force for Health. The second WHO Ministerial Conference 15–17 June

Šmits P, 1928 Latvju tautas dainas, Riga Latviešu tautasdziesmas, 1993 6. sej., Latvijas Zinatnu Akademija, Riga, 'Zinatne'

Šmulders M, 1990, dr.oec. Who Owes Whom? Mutual economic accounts between Latvia and the USSR 1940–1990 Riga the Government of Latvia pp 24–25

WHO 2003 Profiling Midwifery in Newly Independent States and Countries of Central and Eastern Europe. WHO Regional office for Europe, Copenhagen

## Additional resources

Davis-Floyd R 1992 and 2003 Birth as an American Rite of Passage. University of California Press, Berkeley

Gaskin IM 2003 Ina May's Guide to Childbirth, Bantam Books, New York

Schmid V 2005 (translated by Manca Anna Lou) About Physiology in Pregnancy and Childbirth. Florence, Italy

WHO and World Bank 2003 High Level Forum on the Health Millennium Development Goals Improving health workforce performance. Issues for Discussion. WHO, Geneva

# CHAPTER THIRTEEN

# Normal birth in Scotland: the effects of policy, geography and culture

LINDSAY REID

The question 'Can we have normality in Scottish childbirth?' is closely linked with a social model of maternity care and freedom of midwives to practise.

Examination of the history of midwifery in Scotland has revealed that care of childbearing women became increasingly medicalised as the twentieth century progressed (Reid 2003). Any ideas of a social model of childbirth (although the term 'social model' was not widely used) became subsumed in the medical model of the day and normality in childbirth decreased sharply. Even before the 1915 Midwives (Scotland) Act was passed, the medical profession in Scotland held a dominant position in its relationship with midwives and childbearing women. As the twentieth century progressed events came together to make the position of midwives more subservient regardless of what the Act (and its successors) said about midwives working on their own responsibility. This chapter will put the discussion on normality in childbirth in Scotland in context by giving an overview of the historical narrative of twentieth century midwifery in Scotland regarding childbirth and intrapartum care.

Issues, both positive and negative, can be considered to influence normality in childbirth in Scotland today. This chapter will explore the question of normality through these issues: they appear to be particularly appropriate in this scrutiny of normality in childbirth in Scotland. For instance, policy, both local and governmental, covered change on a wide scale including the maternity services. Accordingly, policy has lately been influential in having a positive effect on the progress of normality in childbirth in Scotland. On the other hand, some aspects of the geography and demography of Scotland affect the possibility of normal childbirth and the ability of midwives to offer this to appropriate women because of where they live. In addition, the culture of medical dominance of maternity services in Scotland affected women's ability to achieve a normal birth. As stated above, midwives were also affected by medical dominance for many years. Now, multi-professional partnership and understanding is progressing with more midwives achieving greater freedom to practise. With this comes progress in the trend towards normality in childbirth for women in Scotland.

Place of birth is also an important factor influencing normality in childbirth. Today's choices appear to be wide. Yet, within the variations of where to give birth in Scotland are discussions, problems and different ideas. Can a woman really choose where she has her baby? Can she have a normal birth if all is well? Or do local policies and individual opinions prevail?

This chapter explores these issues, illustrates the problems and tries to come to a conclusion to answer the main question.

# Historical background

Knowledge of the background to a situation helps understanding why things happen the way they do. In 1915, 13 years after the first Midwives Act catering for midwives in England and Wales, the Midwives (Scotland) Act 1915 was passed. This Act established a Central Midwives Board for Scotland (CMBS) to oversee the registration (known at the time as 'enrolment'), training and practice of midwives. The CMBS remained in office until 1983. The Act brought the first formal recognition of midwives as a group throughout Scotland and gave them a legal identity. However, its provisions affected their freedom to practise. Throughout the twentieth century the identity and freedom of midwives were subject to negotiation and change, both through the institutional frameworks within which they trained and practised, and how they practised before, during and after birth (Reid 2003).

# Midwives and intranatal care

The shift from home to hospital as the place where most women give birth was one of the major changes in maternity care in the twentieth century. In Scotland, before the beginning of the twentieth century, nearly all mothers gave birth at home. The movement from home to hospital began slowly in the early decades of the twentieth century and reached a peak in

1981 when 99.5% of babies in Scotland were born in hospital (Reid 2003 App 5) (see Figure 13.1). This, along with increasing medicalisation of childbirth, took the normality out of many births and had a negative impact on normal midwifery.

Reasons for the change from home to hospital for birth particularly involved the growing medicalisation of childbirth through the twentieth century, including:

- Increasing use of medical forms of pain relief in labour (Moir 1986:1,5).
- Improved conditions in hospitals (Murray 1930, Johnstone 1939).
- Development in the 1920s of maternity nursing homes (Midwives and Maternity Homes (Scotland) Act, 1927:Part II 5–9).
- Advances in medicine, instrumental in reducing maternal mortality in the 1930s and 1940s, which also added to the increase in hospitalisation. These included the use of the first antibiotics for puerperal sepsis particularly prontosil, the development of blood transfusions, and, better education of doctors and midwives leading to greater awareness of problems and thus admission to hospital when necessary (Loudon 1992:258–261)
- As the profession of obstetrics developed through the twentieth century members of the profession had to deal with the threat that midwives posed to their control. By overseeing midwifery's regulatory process the obstetric profession was able to dictate midwives' area of practice and limits of what they were allowed to do (Walsh et al 2004). The concept of safety was also used by obstetricians as a powerful tool to keep midwifery subservient and, to further the development of obstetrics (Fleming 1998, Mander 2002).

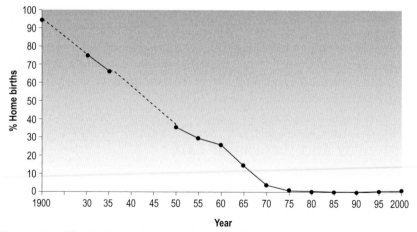

*Figure 13.1* The decline in home births in Scotland (1900–2000). – estimate: there are no data from the mid-1930s until 1946. Source: Reid (2003)

- The events of World War II exacerbated the trend towards hospitalisation. There was the problem of lack of help in the house with many women replacing men in jobs that were usually the male preserve. Emergency maternity hospitals were set up, often in suitable country houses. Some urban mothers were unhappy and returned home (Tait 1987:413–440). However many mothers found that they enjoyed the holiday, the fashion grew and this was seen as at least a contributory factor in the sharp post-war upturn in the institutional delivery rate (Sturrock, 1980:173–187, Oakley 1984:118, Reid 2003).
- Maternity beds, increased greatly due to wartime maternity policy, were inherited and developed by the regional hospital boards under the National Health Service (NHS) (Department of Health for Scotland (DHS) and Scottish Health Services Council 1959:7). Thus the implementation of the NHS Acts in 1948 and the resultant changes also contributed to the trend towards hospital births.
- The Queen's Institute of District Nursing gave other reasons in 1959 including excessive propaganda from hospital specialists stressing greater safety, lack of suitable housing in certain areas, insufficiently developed or insufficiently flexible home help services, economy to the mother, and encouragement by general practitioners (GPs) (to have a hospital birth), sometimes irrespective of medical, obstetric or social need (DHS 1959:14–16).

Thus, the change in the main location of childbirth in twentieth century Scotland coincided with, and was particularly involved with the growing medicalisation of childbirth. Whether the shift from home to hospital was good for mothers remains controversial, but there is general agreement that it has had a negative impact on midwives' freedom to practise and status thus posing challenges to midwives which remained as the century drew to a close (Reid 2003).

The phrase 'medicalisation of childbirth and midwifery' epitomises these challenges. van Teijlingen et al (2000:1) defined this term as:

> the increasing tendency of women to prefer a hospital delivery to a home delivery, the increasing trend toward the use of technology and clinical intervention in childbirth, and the determination of medical practitioners to confine the role played by midwives in pregnancy and childbirth, if any, to a purely subordinate one.

With the change in place of birth, midwives' relationships with mothers also underwent a change. At home, the mother retained a significant identity. When a woman came into hospital she was no longer in control of her environment. Circumstances dictated a weaker, more subservient role for her, and her significant identity was diminished. The midwife's identity in hospital was also lessened by the development of hospital policies to which she had to adhere. This meant that some midwives were no longer able to give mothers the complete care, emotional as well as physical, to which they were entitled. One midwife said:

> I always feel that women when they are pregnant, when they are in labour and just after, need to be mothered themselves in order to help them to mother, even if they have got a mother-figure in their own family. They need the caring that goes along with midwifery. There was no caring. The women were delivered – it was just like a sausage factory.
>
> *LR 85*

The change in place of birth affected the intranatal practice of domiciliary midwives. When the number of hospital deliveries was rising, midwives on the district became anxious about what would become of them.

> Towards the end of that five years [1952] – the home deliveries had just sort of imperceptibly started to decline . . . older midwives . . . were beginning to talk about . . . what was the future and what would they be used for . . . would they be maybe diversified into some other duties?
>
> *LR 27*

So, there was also the issue of lack of job satisfaction. Experienced district midwives expressed frustration at what they saw as a lack of domiciliary midwifery. Their remit had moved from giving full intranatal and postnatal care to some antenatal visits, and postnatal visits to women who had been confined in hospital. In addition there was concern that the lack of intranatal practice would result in a loss of skills for both midwives and GPs, and difficulties in arranging for intra-partum training for pupil midwives (DHS 1959:20). As the number of hospital births rose, few student midwives delivered a baby at home, although much depended on the area and the number of maternity beds there. Eventually home births were phased out as a compulsory part of the midwifery training syllabus. Wilma Coleman, midwife, said:

> Now, generally speaking, all community midwives have a hospital background. But they lose their intrapartum skills because once the [number of] home confinements went down and women came into hospital, the community midwives very quickly lost their intrapartum skills.
>
> *LR 74*

One solution to this issue was that 'domiciliary midwifery might become a hospital responsibility, which would allow some interchange of midwives between domiciliary and hospital services' (DHS 1959:20). This early suggestion on integration of the maternity services was to come to fruition in the years to come.

The move towards hospital births brought a change in the role of the midwife. In the home situation, the midwife's position was clearly defined. Within the hospital labour ward, even though midwives delivered most of the babies, there was a blurring of roles between midwives and doctors. Rosemary Mander (1993) writing about midwives' autonomy said, 'Whereas the midwives correctly saw themselves as autonomous in caring for mothers experiencing normal childbirth, the medical staff saw themselves as having overall responsibility and being able to exercise that responsibility as they saw fit'. Another midwife said:

> a great emphasis was put on what the doctor said, what the doctors wanted and how it was going to be. The women themselves were not considered and what they wanted wasn't considered. [For example] nobody said they did not want to be induced.

*LR 85*

As the effects of medicalisation of childbirth became more evident, midwives found themselves in the dilemma of obeying hospital policy and protocols rather than being free to practise as midwives, and be advocates to mothers (Reid 2003).

# Factors influencing normality in childbirth in Scotland

This section will explore some of the issues which influence normality in childbirth in Scotland. This question is inextricably linked with the social model of childbirth and freedom to practise for midwives. The issues discussed in this section include:

- obstetric policy, geography and culture
- the social movement for change backed-up by pressure from midwifery groups
- Government publications from Scotland, England and Wales and Northern Ireland advocating change in childbirth and woman-centred care
- other pro-active groups sponsored by the Scottish Executive and containing a broad spectrum of the professions working in maternity care

- the place of birth in Scotland
- recruitment and retention of midwives.

## Policy: local and governmental

The concept of normality linked with freedom to practise for midwives is influenced by factors such as obstetric policy, geography and culture (Mander 2002:182). The historical overview of childbirth in Scotland given earlier in this chapter has demonstrated how medicalisation of childbirth, dominant in Scotland since the nineteenth century, took off in the twentieth century and reached a peak in the post World War II decades. By the end of the twentieth century, women, the media and midwives slowly became stronger and more able to stand up for less medicalisation, fewer procedures performed routinely, and more woman-centred individualised care. In the meantime, procedures such as episiotomy and artificial rupture of membranes that originated as medical tasks or responsibilities became routine and part of hospital policy. As this happened, they were handed over to midwives and thus came into the realms of 'normal' because of the frequency with which they were employed. (See *Encarta* definitions in Chapter 2.)

Regarding episiotomies, Jan Fenton who practised in the postnatal ward in Dundee Royal Infirmary in the mid-1950s gave a very clear example of how midwives did not have freedom to practise. Many more mothers had episiotomy in hospital than at home and once the episiotomy was performed and sutured, it had to be cared for. With mothers still being kept in bed for about five days (and it was easier to enforce this rule in hospital than at home), an episiotomy nurtured in a warm moist atmosphere was an added potential source of infection. Jan Fenton observed that mothers with infected episiotomies were allowed up earlier than the usual day for a shower. She had what she thought was a good idea. She said,

> When they [the mothers] were in the wards they would be in for nine days. And . . . they were kept in bed for five days . . . If episiotomies went 'off', they used to let them get up for a shower, you see. And I said to the sister, 'I think it would be much better if we just got them all up for a shower. It would save these episiotomies going off.' And I was told I wasn't paid to think.
>
> *LR 116*

A further comment on this is that it was the senior midwife who stopped Jan Fenton from using her initiative. Although stories of conflict between medical staff and midwives abound (Mander 2002:183) there is also evidence of problems with midwifery management preventing midwives practising as they wished because of policy and rules. One senior midwife told of a time when she was much smaller fry:

> There was . . . an unwillingness at that time amongst the middle and senior managers in midwifery to accept that midwives could form judgements based on knowledge and experience which could lead to action which was perfectly acceptable. And . . . the doctor was the next thing to God. Well, I'm sorry it wasn't – I respected my medical colleagues absolutely and they had skills and experience I certainly didn't have and I didn't want to usurp them but I had skills too that I could – and not just me – the midwives round about me, but they were terrified to use them because somebody was going to come down on their head and say, 'You're not supposed to do that'.
>
> *LR 120*

In addition, even recently, midwives doing research have recorded problems where midwives have shown reluctance to allow research to occur, have been obstructive of, for instance randomised controlled trials, and, at senior and managerial midwifery level have appeared to be unwilling to take the responsibility of giving permission to undertake non-clinical research in midwifery practice (Fleming 2002:73).

Another example of habitual practice turning into 'normal' practice was routine induction of labour (IOL). This totally took away midwives' freedom to practise and normality in childbirth for women. One midwife practising in the 1970s said:

> I think when I saw the beginning of abnormal practices . . . was when I saw them starting this induction of labour and people knew that they were going to be put into labour. That for me was the beginning of abnormality. And including midwives as a part of it. In those days very very few mothers held their ground.
>
> *LR 9*

And midwives had to comply. Regarding routine IOL on the expected date of delivery, one Scottish midwife interviewed for oral history research purposes said that when she was a student in 1976 she nearly gave up midwifery altogether. She said:

> At this time all the women had . . . to have artificial rupture of membranes and Syntocinon on the day that they were due to have their baby . . . I remember women queuing up to go into a labour room to have their legs put up in stirrups, to have artificial rupture of

membranes done. I remember some women screaming because . . . the cervix was not ready . . . they were taken back to their four-bedded rooms and they were attached to a Syntocinon drip right away and it was turned up at regular intervals, so it was increasingly painful, with minimal pain relief . . . They were all on their beds. They were not allowed to walk around. [They were] all either crying quietly . . . moaning and groaning. We just had to do the clinical observations and move on to the next woman. You didn't have time to do the caring that is part of midwifery. It was awful . . .

*LR 85*

Now ideas about IOL have changed and it is no longer performed routinely but if it is appropriate, in consultation with the woman in question. But at the height of medicalisation of childbirth, what was usual became routine and therefore normal: a normal that does not comply with any of the theories of what is normal childbirth discussed in Chapter 2.

History, too, is constantly changing our ideas of what is normal. For instance, in the early decades of the twentieth century midwives had little input into the care of pregnant women; their main remit lay in the care of mothers during labour and the postnatal period along with the newly born infant (Reid 2003:301). Now it is normal for most midwives to play a large part in antenatal care although this too varies from place to place. Similarly, in the first half of the twentieth century when most mothers gave birth at home in the care of a midwife it was taken for granted that they would have a normal birth.

Schemes for integration of maternity services in Scotland marked the beginning of a positive response to consumer criticisms of the 1970s. This challenged the increasing medicalisation of birth and the apparent decreasing level of choice for women (Scottish Home and Health Department (SHHD) 1973:2, Hall et al 1985: 2, 8, 23). Thus, a breakdown of deference which began as early as the 1960s, gradually infiltrated into maternity care in general and midwifery in particular. The background to the need for change was UK-wide and sparked off UK-wide documents including *The Vision* (Association of Radical Midwives (ARM) 1986), *The Report on the Roles and Education of the Future Midwife in the United Kingdom* (Royal College of Midwives (RCM) 1987) and *Towards a Healthy Nation* (RCM 1991). Each of these documents, in its own way, indicated a need for change, for more informed choice for women and for more continuity in the way care is carried out. This led to a change in attitude which became particularly visible from the late 1980s onwards. In 1993 the consultative document *Maternity Services in Scotland: A Policy Review* was published by the SHHD at the same time as *Changing Childbirth* (Department of

Health (DoH) 1993), heralding the change which became known as 'woman-centred care'.

*A Framework for Maternity Services in Scotland* (Scottish Executive 2001) continued this aim and challenged the NHS in Scotland to provide an essentially community-based, midwife-managed service with easy access to specialist services wherever needed. The *Framework* set out a plan for the delivery of maternity care in Scotland with four broad themes:

- Safety and evidence-based care for mother and baby must remain the foundation of an effective maternity service.
- Pregnancy and childbirth are normal physiological processes in women's lives.
- Maternity services must deliver a woman and family-centred approach to care and support planned in partnership with the woman.
- Maternity services should be essentially community based and midwife managed, wherever possible, with an emphasis on community care.

The aim of the *Framework* is to deliver consistent, high-quality care that is locally accessible. At the same time, especially given the varied geography and demography of Scotland, there are occasions when, because of a woman's condition, she may have to travel further afield than what is considered to be local (see below). The idea of maternity care professionals working together as an inter-professional team with mutual respect for each other is vital to successful joint working between primary, secondary and tertiary services. The themes of the *Framework* taken together, reinforce the idea that the three thoughts – freedom to practise for midwives, a social/midwifery model of maternity care leading to normality in childbirth, with the benefit of evidence-based practice – are taking root in Scotland for the benefit of women, improved care in childbirth and midwives.

From the *Framework* evolved the Expert Group on Acute Maternity Services (EGAMS). This working group's role was to provide a mechanism to implement the recommendations of the *Framework*. EGAMS consulted, reported in 2002, concluding that because of the falling birth rate in Scotland at the time, the current organisation of maternity services could not be maintained as it was. EGAMS suggested the need to organise services so that appropriate care could be provided locally with tertiary services organised on a regional basis. This had implications for all professionals involved in maternity services and for their continuing professional development (Scottish Executive Health Department (SEHD) 2002). In addition, EGAMS comprised a cross-section of professionals working in maternity care who worked together to produce their report. This indicates a willingness for partnership working and a team approach in which no one group within EGAMS would dominate over another.

In a list of 13 important core principles in the report, two stand out as being particularly appropriate for this chapter. They are (SEHD 2002:77):

- Intrapartum care must be of high quality and clinically effective, consistent with the available evidence, woman-centred, seamless with a real multi-professional team approach.
- Promotion of normality of childbirth is integral to a quality maternity service, but it is essential that recognition of the ill mother and infant is paramount.

Thus, the Scottish Executive acknowledged the need for the promotion of normality in childbirth where appropriate. Using evidence-based practice, a woman-centred (social) model to offer women normal births would also go a long way towards providing an opportunity for midwives in Scotland to have freedom to practise.

The EGAMS report highlighted five main areas where education for health professionals involved in maternity care require to be focused:

- neonatal resuscitation
- maternal emergencies
- normality
- examination of the newborn
- history taking and risk assessment.

From this the Scottish Multi-professional Maternity Development Group (SMMDG) was born: a group drawn from all professionals who have a part to play in the maternity services for Scotland. Again, multi-professional team working prevails. The group is working on writing, producing and organising a continually evolving, evidence-based programme of courses validated by NHS Education for Scotland (SMMDG website). As far as women are concerned there is the hope that more mothers will be allowed to have real informed choice, and a greater chance of normal childbirth where it is appropriate. As far as midwives are concerned this initiative gives real hope that freedom to practise for midwives in Scotland will become a reality.

## Place of birth

As already discussed in this chapter the change in the place of birth in twentieth century Scotland had a significant impact on freedom to practise for midwives, the move towards medicalisation and therefore the use of a medical model of childbirth, and normality in childbirth. Currently, in the early twenty-first century, throughout Scotland there exists an informal network of different levels of provision of maternity care reflecting an evolved, tiered and geographical approach, encompassing morbidity, case mix and rurality (SEHD 2002:13). The levels are (SEHD 2002:13–14):

- Level III – consultant-led specialist maternal-fetal units.
- Level II – subdivided into
  - IIc – consultant-led but not specialist maternal-fetal tertiary centres
  - IIb – consultant-led with onsite neonatal facilities
  - IIa – consultant led but without onsite neonatal facilities.
- Level I – subdivided into
  - Ic – community maternity units (CMUs) adjacent to a non-obstetric district general hospital
  - Ib – stand-alone midwifery units
  - Ia – birth in the home setting.

Within these levels, there is real variation in provision of care. However, at all levels of care women should be allowed to maintain normality if that is appropriate. A senior midwife noted:

> From my perspective, we recognise that as a tertiary referral centre we are still the local maternity hospital for the women in our area so there has to be the full range of practices to suit individual need . . . I . . . get annoyed when there is an assumption that tertiary units are all about interventions and consultant control
>
> *Reid (2005:10)*

That this assumption still exists is sad but unsurprising given the long-term medicalisation of maternity care in Scotland. In a study comparing mothers' perceptions of birth centre versus hospital care, researchers observed how mothers noticed the apparent differences in philosophy of care between birth centres and hospitals and valued the normality of the birth centre approach. Also, women felt that individual practice of midwives as well as doctors was influenced by the philosophy of the institution: in hospitals, doctors adopted an invasive approach; the use of technology was an accepted part of the birth process; there was an assumption that women would want to use analgesia such as epidurals. Midwives also appeared to give control to the obstetricians. On the other hand, care in a birth centre was based on the attitude that birth was a normal life event and demonstrated mid-wifery care within the social model of care. Midwives appeared to be pre-pared to help the mother assume responsibility for decisions related to their care and make personal choices. Thus the behaviour of 'birth centre mothers' differed from that of the 'hospital mothers'. An important factor in women's perceptions of control was the nature of the relationship between the women and whoever was looking after them. Thus, women with a col-laborative relationship with their midwives indicated a sense of control over their experience. These findings have important implications for midwives' ability to help mothers have normal childbirth when appropriate and in their freedom to practise (Coyle et al 2001).

Tertiary maternity units in Scotland play a vital role in the care of mothers who require obstetric care and the use of high-tech equipment. However, given that there is an assumption that tertiary centres are all about 'interventions and consultant control', there is a need to strengthen the concept of individualised normal care of women. This could be achieved by, for instance, encouraging caseload midwives to work occasionally in a tertiary unit labour ward (Cooke 2004) and the other way around. In addition midwives and other professionals in maternity care should be encouraged to attend a normal labour and birth course as envisaged by the SMMDG (Reid 2005). The aim of this course is to give professionals in maternity care the opportunity to re-visit labour and childbirth in a manner that acknowledges the concept of normality in childbirth: that normal childbirth is a physiological rather than a pathological event. The long term objective is to explore and promote further the practice of normal labour and childbirth and empower each other while so doing. Tertiary maternity units are usually in larger centres of population but are, as the above quote indicates, the 'local maternity hospital'. Therefore, to fulfil the ethos of woman-centred care and to encourage normal childbirth where appropriate, a tertiary maternity unit, regardless of its high-tech environment, must offer what the individual woman requires, wherever her place is on the technological spectrum.

However there is a trend in Scotland towards accepting that encouraging individual normal care, often midwife-led, is becoming more usual and desirable. Within some consultant-led units there are midwife-led units, such as Forth Park Hospital in Kirkcaldy, with the aim of offering a social model of care and non-interventionist labour to women. There are also 23 CMUs in Scotland. Five of these are level Ic CMUs adjacent to a non-obstetric district general hospital, such as Balfour Hospital, Kirkwall, Orkney (SEHD 2002:15). Eighteen CMUs are level Ib stand-alone maternity units such as the North Angus Community Maternity Unit at Montrose Royal Infirmary (Leatherbarrow et al 2004). Like birth centres in England and Wales the philosophy of CMUs gives a focus for a social rather than a medical model of care (Kirkham 2003, RCM 2004). Thus, care in the CMU context is based on the philosophy that childbirth is a natural physiological process and largely a social event rather than a medical one (Matthews and Zadak 1991, Coyle et al 2001).

Practising midwifery in a CMU gives a midwife a greater opportunity for freedom to practise and direct her care towards the needs of the individual woman and promote normal childbirth. Women using CMUs have found an enhanced joint relationship with their midwives and therefore a greater sense of personal control over their experience of labour and child-birth. Thus, women find CMUs to be practical, safe and well-liked, offering a stress-free, supporting and well-equipped environment. At the same time working in this setting gives midwives the opportunity to enhance women's experiences by engaging with them in a more informal environment which includes empowering parent-craft sessions (Leatherbarrow et al 2004). Midwives are keen to work in CMUs and birth centres: these units offer the chance for midwives to practise and make decisions freely, give holistic care to women, provide excellent learning opportunities for students, and they could be the way forward to updating maternity services and enhanc-ing recruitment of midwives as job satisfaction increases (Walker 2000, Rosser 2001, Sandall 2001, Davies et al 2003). As another seal of approval, the RCM Position Statement on birth centres states: 'The RCM believes that birth centres offer a cost-effective, safe and satisfying alternative for women who are experiencing normal pregnancy and birth' (RCM 2004). Montrose CMU midwives also endorse this way of working: 'Although we are very busy, morale is high, the midwives are empowered and there is a buzz about the place' (Leatherbarrow et al 2004).

Birth at home is the traditional normal birth setting. Like CMUs, birth at home also uses the social model but offers the advantage of complete privacy (Robinson 2001, Kirkham 2003). Home birth can now once again be seen in Scotland and the rest of the UK as a realistic possibility for many women who choose this way of birthing. This is despite the doubts of one researcher who 'expresses concerns about whether a focus on "normality" may have a negative impact on the ability of caregivers and their clients to detect, act upon, and/or receive assistance with complications' (Murphy-Lawless 2003, Reid 2005:11). This reflects unfairly on the ability of mid-wives and women who wish a home birth, to think and act objectively in the desire for normality. This researcher also suggests increasing the 'sci-entific grip' on birth. But women and birth are not an exact science: scien-tific rationality and its need for predictability have helped to 'create distance, alienation, degradation and confusion around the deeply social act of giving birth' (Murphy-Lawless 2003).

Through the de-normalisation of childbirth both women and their primary caregivers – midwives – lost confidence. To enable childbearing women and midwives to loosen the scientific shackles will increase their opportunities and abilities to work together, not necessarily for a 'predict-able' labour and birth but for a safe satisfying experience (Murphy-Lawless 2003, Reid 2005). This includes the choice of giving birth at home. A number of studies have shown that home birth is a safe option for low-risk women. They have a moral and even a legal right to this if that is their informed choice (Campbell and Macfarlane 1994, Tew 1995, Chamberlain et al 1997, Jones 2003). In addition, midwives working with women giving birth at home are using their right of freedom to practise.

In any discussion on place of birth in Scotland, the geography of Scotland should be taken into account. This will have a bearing on where a mother has her baby and sometimes whether she is considered to be 'normal' or not and in the past, policy dictated how a midwife would practise. Real choice is hampered by distance, travelling time and geographical considerations. Take, for instance the Isle of Skye on the west coast of Scotland. In the early 1990s only a few mothers gave birth on the island even though there were practising midwives, GPs and a small maternity unit. There was no evidence to say that mothers on Skye were any less normal than anyone else. And yet, some mothers went to the nearest consultant unit in Inverness early to await the birth of their baby while some were transferred in labour. In December 1993, a labouring mother was being transported the 145 km (90 miles) from Skye to Inverness in snowy conditions with black ice on the sometimes single-track road. The ambulance crashed, killing the midwife and accompanying paramedic. Some time later, the mother gave birth to a stillborn baby. This tragic incident highlights the problem, not just of distance and weather, but also how the idea of normality shifts depending on the geography of the area and the thinking of the time. Now, with the trend developing towards normality and a social model of care, more mothers are giving birth on Skye, some in the CMU within the hospital where the facilities have been extended and some at home (H Bryars 2005, personal communication).

Similar progress is underway in Argyll and Bute. In wide geographical areas covering both island and mainland Scotland, women were frequently transferred to hospital before or in labour. Occasionally a baby was born on the lifeboat (Brown 2005). Midwives, some of whom undertook double and triple duties became quickly aware of rusting midwifery skills. This had an impact on how they interacted with women.

Now, the picture is changing. More midwives are practising as midwives only; they maintain their skills by focusing only on midwifery practice and working in the local CMUs. More women are giving birth on the islands, or in their local CMU, instead of having to travel to the bigger units. So far there has been an increase in the number of local births on the Isle of Islay both at home and in the small unit in Islay Hospital. While there is no birthing unit on the Isle of Mull, midwives anticipate that there the number of home births will increase. In addition, there is an acknowledgement of multi-professional practice and partnership with midwives, GPs, paramedics and accident and emergency staff working together on obstetric emergency courses. The main beneficiaries are women and their infants.

However, teamwork and forward, pro-active thinking is enabling midwives in the area to be free to practise and make decisions (P Tyrrell, J Lambert, personal communications, 2006).

However, the overall geography of Scotland with its mountains and wide open spaces on the one hand and lowland central belt on the other has an impact on how the maternity services are run and how midwives practise. Because of the terrain, the Highlands cover more than 50% of mainland Scotland but the majority of the population live in the narrow central belt that accounts for only 10% of the land area (SEHD 2001:27). This means that the distribution of midwives is also uneven; there are more tertiary maternity units in the greater centres of population. Thus, the senior midwife's plea for normality in tertiary centres (above) is an important one.

The number of midwives in practice is a further problem which could hinder the movement towards normality in childbirth in Scotland. Currently, NHS midwifery vacancy levels in Scotland are around 3.1% and this is exacerbated by the uneven distribution. A recent newspaper article indicated that the current shortage of midwives in Scotland has a direct bearing on the number of births occurring at home. The Scottish Executive through its *Framework for Maternity Services* and other reports and activities has demonstrated its recommendation for home births where appropriate and when the mother has made an informed choice for this. Yet some health boards appear to be rationing home births depending on their midwifery staffing levels. In maternity units although the ideal mother : midwife ratio is one to one, in reality, more mothers can be cared for by fewer staff if necessary. That in itself means that there is less midwifery support available for mothers in maternity units who are keen to have a normal labour. Home births are labour intensive, carrying a recommendation for two midwives at the birth. This may be a 'luxury' that some health boards have difficulty in supplying and some units have had to agree a ceiling on the number of home births they can accommodate. Thus, whatever the size of the place of birth, to encourage normal birth where appropriate, viable midwifery levels need to be maintained. There appears to be a developing demand for independent midwives in Scotland where currently there are two in practice (Gray 2005). However even if more independent midwives started practising it would not solve the overall problem. And, besides, the onus is on the State to provide adequate maternity services.

Wherever a birth is planned, the progress towards normality and normal birth needs to be an empowering force to create an environment away from the medicalised atmosphere. Midwives and women are part of this progress. Midwives can be a buffer against medicalisation by promoting planned home birth, the use of CMUs and birth centres, by questioning and 'shutting the door' on inappropriate interventions (Crabtree 2004). In a hospital situation the physical act of shutting the door is seen as symbolic: in creating privacy and safety it enables the woman to make the hospital room her own space. In this way a midwife can empower the woman by protecting her and by supporting her in her choices.

It is true that the stance taken by many obstetricians, both as individuals and as a group has changed towards a more moderate evidence-based approach to childbirth. However, stereotyping of the medical model is still very evident in information available to the public and there is evidence that women perceive levels of risk through their reading of the available literature and influence their choices accordingly (Mead 2004). Women should be informed of the benefits of a physiological approach to labour with 'normality' as the key word rather than 'intervention' or 'medicalisation'. Therefore, it is up to all maternity care professionals to update and inform specific literature and other media. If a woman is known to be healthy, today's evidence-based practice reflected in the media should encourage her to be normal and have normal midwifery care unless she manifests a change in her situation that requires referral to an obstetrician.

# Conclusion

This chapter has explored some of the factors that impinge on normality in childbirth in Scotland. This concept is closely linked with a social model of maternity care and freedom of midwives to practise.

A brief overview of the historical narrative of midwifery in Scotland with particular reference to intrapartum care gives a background to the question and puts the happenings of today into context. Normal childbirth was evident in Scotland at the beginning of the twentieth century. However, over the past 100 years the movement of maternity-world tectonic plates in Scotland could almost be heard as professionals clashed with each other, with women, with governments and their statutory bodies, as all strove for what they wanted in the name of 'best practice'. In the process, normality in childbirth largely disappeared until the latter part of the twentieth century when events conspired to return normality to the childbirth argument.

The largest section of the chapter is devoted to some issues which can be considered to influence normality in childbirth in Scotland today in one way or another. Policy, both local and governmental is instrumental in how women give birth and how midwives practise. Policy is driven by social change which was particularly evident from the 1960s and which did not leave the maternity services untouched. The movement for change was backed up by pressure from women's groups, midwifery groups,

Government publications advocating change in childbirth and woman-centred care from all the countries of the UK. In addition, the Scottish Executive sponsored and encouraged reports (SEHD 2001, 2002), and further pro-active work demonstrated by, for example, the Scottish Multi-professional Maternity Development Group (www.scottishmaternity.org). As a mark of progress these groups contain a broad spectrum of the professions working in maternity care demonstrating real partnership working. These initiatives have been influential in furthering the progress of normality in Scottish childbirth. On the other hand, other factors have affected normal childbirth in a less positive manner: these include the geography and demography of Scotland and how they can adversely affect maternity services; and the culture of medical dominance, evident in the Scottish childbearing scene for many years and epitomised by the medicalisation of childbirth. This fostered a lack of incentive for midwives 'to think' or use their initiative. However, multi-professional co-operation has gone a long way towards breaking down barriers and building midwives' confidence. This in turn will promote normality in childbirth in Scotland.

An important factor that influences midwives' freedom to practise and subsequently normality in childbirth, is the place of birth. Today there are many variations on the place of birth in Scotland, ranging from tertiary consultant units, which, because they are still the maternity unit for the area provide not only for women with problems but also look after those who are looking for a normal birth as well. This can sometimes be an issue: there is sometimes a mistaken assumption that a tertiary unit is only about obstetric care and interventions. From the tertiary level, the place of birth moves through wide variations of maternity care to birth at home which once again is becoming a real possibility in Scotland today. Statistics on place and type of birth vary. CMUs and other midwife-led units are gaining in popularity while a mother's request for a home birth, regardless of her legal and moral rights may be refused depending on the midwifery staffing levels in the area in question. However on the whole it is evident that the place of birth is much more of a choice for mothers today than it was 30 years ago. They are informed particularly by midwives as they develop ideas of how they would like to give birth. Thus, the trend towards normality in childbirth appears to be positive.

So there is a growing movement, interest and even passion, circling around the idea of exploring again normal, physiological childbirth (Anderson 2002). Midwives in their unique and privileged position, can consider and promote further, normality in childbirth, empower each other while so doing, take on board the concepts of freedom to practise along with evidence based practice and, in so doing, help mothers in Scotland to give birth with memories that are there for all the right reasons.

> ## Reflective questions
>
> 'Informed choice' is a much-used term now. Do you think the ideal of giving informed choice to mothers/parents could be improved, e.g. in terms of when and how it is given, who gives it, how much time is offered for discussion and, an opportunity provided to re-visit any issue under discussion?
>
> Many factors influence freedom to practise for midwives and normality in childbirth for mothers. The main section of this chapter has discussed some examples. What other examples can you list and discuss?

## References

Anderson T 2002 Peeling back the layers: a new look at midwifery interventions. MIDIRS Midwifery Digest 12:(2)207–210

Association of Radical Midwives 1985 The Vision. Association of Radical Midwives, Omskirk

Brown C 2005 A new life on ocean wave as baby girl is born on rescue boat. The Scotsman, 7 October, 7

Campbell R, Macfarlane A 1994 Where to be born? The debate and the evidence. National Perinatal Epidemiology Unit, Oxford

Chamberlain G, Wraight A, Crowley P 1997 Home births: The Report of the 1994 Confidential Inquiry by the National Birthday Trust Fund. Parthenon, London

Cooke P 2004 Promoting partnerships in Paddington: a consultant midwife's role. Midwives 7(7):310–311

Coyle K, Hauck Y, Percival P, Kristjanson L 2001 Normality and collaboration: mother's perceptions of birth centre versus hospital care. Midwifery 17(3):182–193

Crabtree S 2004 Midwives constructing 'normal birth'. In: Downe S (ed) Normal Childbirth: Evidence and Debate. Elsevier, London, 85–99

Davies M, McDonald S, Austin D 2003 Home from home: the key to success. The Practising Midwife 6(11):16–17

DoH 1993 Changing Childbirth. Part 1: Report of the Expert Maternity Group. HMSO, London

DHS and Scottish Health Services Council 1959 Maternity Services in Scotland (Montgomery Report). DHS and Scottish Health Services Council, Edinburgh

Fleming V 1998 Autonomous or Automatons? An exploration through history of the concept of autonomy in midwifery in Scotland and New Zealand. Nursing Ethics 5(1):43–51

Fleming V 2002 Statutory control. In: Mander R, Fleming V (eds) Failure to Progress: the Contraction of the Midwifery Profession. Routledge, London, 63–77

Gray R 2005 Labour pains prevent choice of home births. Scotland on Sunday 6:2, 6–7

Hall M, MacIntyre S, Porter M 1985 Antenatal care assessed. Aberdeen University Press, Aberdeen

Johnstone RW 1939 The Simpson Memorial Maternity Pavilion, Royal Infirmary, Edinburgh. Manchester. Reprinted from the Journal of Obstetrics and Gynaecology of the British Empire 46(6):1020–1028

Jones S 2003 Ethico-legal issues in home birth. Midwives 6(3):126–128

Kirkham M 2003 A 'cycle of empowerment': the enabling culture of birth centres. The Practising Midwife 6(11):12–15

Leatherbarrow B, Winters P, McLeod L, et al 2004 From vision to reality: the development of a community maternity unit. Midwives, 7(5): 212–215

Loudon I 1992 Death in Childbirth. Oxford University Press, Oxford

Mander R 1993 Autonomy in midwifery and maternity care. In: Midwives Chronicle, October:369–374

Mander R 2002 The midwife and the medical practitioner. In: Mander R, Fleming V, Failure to Progress: The Contraction of the Midwifery Profession. Routledge, London: 170–188

Matthews JJ, Zadak K 1991 The alternative birth movement in the United States: history and current status. Women and Health 17:39–56

Mead M 2004 Midwives' practices in 11 UK maternity units. In: Downe S (ed) Normal Childbirth: Evidence and Debate. Elsevier, London, 71–83

Midwives and Maternity Homes (Scotland) Act, 1927, [17 &18 Geo 5 Ch 17] Part II 5–9

Moir D 1986 Pain Relief in Labour, 5th edn. Churchill Livingstone, Edinburgh

Murphy-Lawless J 2003 Medical and social views of birth: the compromise with medical science. In: Lee B (ed) Forum on maternity and the newborn report: Session 1. Midwives 6(5):204–205

Murray EF 1930 Some observations on puerperal sepsis with special reference to its occurrence in maternity hospitals. In: Transactions of the Edinburgh Obstetrical Society, Session LXXXIX, Read 14 May 1930. Edinburgh Medical Journal, New Series, 27(10):145–153

Oakley A 1984 The Captured Womb. Basil Blackwell, Oxford

RCM 1987 The Role and Education of the Future Midwife in the United Kingdom. RCM, London

RCM 1991 Towards a Healthy Nation. RCM. London

Reid L 1997–2002 Archival collection of oral testimonies between these dates. Cited as LR 1–128

Reid L 2003 Scottish Midwives 1916–1983: The Central Midwives Board and practising midwives. Unpublished PhD thesis, University of Glasgow

Reid L 2005 Scottish normal labour and birth course manual. Scottish Multiprofessional Maternity Development Group, Edinburgh

Robinson J 2001 Privacy during labour and childbirth. British Journal of Midwifery, 9(9):553

Rosser J 2001 Birth centres – the key to modernising the maternity services. MIDIRS Midwifery Digest, 11(Suppl 2):S22–S26

Sandall J 2001 Birth centres could solve the midwifery crisis. In: Guardian Unlimited, Society Guardian.co.uk [comment]

SEHD, 2001 A framework for maternity services in Scotland. Scottish Executive, Edinburgh

SEHD 2002 Report of the Expert Group on Acute Maternity Services (EGAMS). Scottish Executive, Edinburgh

SHHD 1973 Maternity Services: Integration of Maternity Work, Tennent Report. HMSO, Edinburgh

SHHD 1993 Provision of Maternity Services in Scotland: A Policy Review. HMSO, Edinburgh

Scottish Multiprofessional Maternity Development Programme (SMMDG) website: www.scottishmaternity.org

Sturrock J 1979 Edinburgh Royal Maternity and Simpson Memorial Hospital. A Sir James Y Simpson memorial lecture delivered on 11 July. Reprinted from the Journal of the Royal College of Surgeons of Edinburgh, (May 1980), (25):173–187

Tait H 1987 Maternity and Child Welfare. In: McLachlan G (ed) Improving the Common Weal: Aspects of Scottish Health Services 1900–1984. Edinburgh University Press, Edinburgh, 413–440

Tew M 1995 Safer Childbirth? A Critical History of Maternity Care, 2nd edn. Chapman and Hall, London

van Teijlingen E, Lowis G, McCaffery P, et al 2000 Midwifery and the medicalization of childbirth: comparative perspectives. Nova Science Publishers, New York

Walker J 2000 Edgeware Birth Centre. Barnet and Chase Farm NHS Trust, North West London NHS Trust, Royal Free Hospital NHS Trust

Walsh D, El-Nemer A, Downe S 2004 Risk, safety and the study of physiological birth. In: Downe S (ed) Normal Childbirth: the Evidence and Debate. Elsevier, London, 103–119

# CHAPTER FOURTEEN

# Independence in practice:
# A New Zealand case study of
# midwives in partnership

REA DAELLENBACH AND JULIET THORPE

Midwifery in New Zealand has gone through a renaissance over the past 15 years. Midwives now have the choice of whether they work in the community providing continuity of care to women or take up employment within maternity facilities. Currently, about 40% of the registered midwives in New Zealand carry caseloads (New Zealand Health Information Service 2004) and more than 70% of women who are pregnant choose a caseloading midwife to provide their maternity care (Ministry of Health (MoH) 2004). These midwives are autonomous practitioners with all the professional and legal responsibilities this entails including being accountable to women and their families with whom they work.

The changes to midwifery were a consequence of legislation introduced in 1990 that enabled registered midwives to provide maternity care independently of medical practitioners (Nurses Amendment Act 1990). This entitled midwives to care for women during pregnancy, labour and birth and the postnatal period in hospital facilities or at home. Midwives also gained rights to prescribe the medicines and order the laboratory services that are commonly used throughout the childbirthing period. Independent midwives who took responsibility for the overall care of clients could claim the same maternity benefit fees from the Government as doctors and therefore offer midwifery services free of charge to women.

De Vries et al (2001) suggest that maternity services are characterised by more diversity across national boundaries than most other areas of healthcare. They argue that 'the design of care at birth varies widely and clearly bears the marks of the society in which it is found' (2001:xii). Thus, attention needs to be paid to the historical, political, and cultural contexts that shape the organisation of maternity services and women's ideas and aspirations within different countries. This chapter focuses on what 'freedom to practise' means for caseloading midwives. It traces the development of the contemporary social, professional and legal expectations of midwifery. At the same time, this chapter tells a story about how one group of midwives who offer home births in a major urban centre put autonomy into practice. It begins with a scenario of a group practice meeting in which the midwives discuss options to resolve a practical dilemma. The narrative illustrates that the way in which the midwives negotiate their relationships with each other reflects their shared commitment to partnership with each other in order to work in partnership with women. This scenario draws on the themes from Juliet Thorpe's (2005) research that investigated the collegial relationships within her own home birth group practice. To ensure confidentiality this story is a blend of a number of women's experiences. Pseudonyms are used for the midwives.

The home birth midwives' practice that is outlined in this chapter is not typical of midwifery in New Zealand. Most midwives attend their clients' births in hospital settings (MoH 2004). With the return of midwifery autonomy and greater birthing choices available to women, there was an expectation that home birth would become a more popular option, particularly as key players in the impetus for the legislative changes were home birthing consumers and their midwives (Donley 1992, Daellenbach 1999). Although accurate statistics have not been collected in New Zealand the planned home birth rate is thought to be around 5% of the total number of births annually (National Health Committee (NHC) 1999).

# The practice meeting scenario

It's been a good day. I have gone to meet with seven women. Four pregnant and waiting, three with new babies. All are healthy and well and all offering me food and cups of tea. Each visit has involved a stimulating hour of listening, talking, and learning from each other. The relationship built with these women over the course of their pregnancies has allowed me the privilege of being invited into the most intimate part of their lives. I have come to know them and their families and with the continuity of providing their midwifery care from early pregnancy, together we have made plans for each significant stage of their experience.

It can be lonely. Out there in the community there is a degree of invisibility about the work. Working with women in their homes means there is no one work setting and all that that entails. No colleague just outside the door to run things by, no one to talk over issues with at coffee break. As I drive from house to house I am thinking about whom I have seen and who will be next. I am processing each visit and being grateful for the evening catch up phone calls with my colleagues.

Tonight our group meets for its weekly get together. It is more than just a meeting. I get home and light the fire, heat the oven and grind the coffee. My head is full of the week's challenges and joys. Each of my four colleagues has had a similar week and coming together to talk is the highlight. One by one everyone arrives bearing soup, cheeses, bread, fruit and chocolate! Alison has brought a cake baked by one of her clients who birthed her tenth baby just a week ago. We are touched by the woman's generosity and wonder where she has found the time and energy! Karen and Madeleine have been at a birth in the small hours of the morning and are weary but full of the birthing story. We listen and they talk as coffee is made and the table is prepared. Each detail of the birth is discussed and reflected upon and finally they are done. Meanwhile spread out in front of us is our weekly feast. A ritual we never postpone, diaries open and plates laden, coffee cups filled, we begin.

Each midwife is given time to speak about her week, she recounts the meetings she has had with each of the women in her care and as issues arise we collectively contemplate and discuss each situation. This evening our main dialogue concerns Ann's client Lara, whose baby is in a breech position at 37 weeks' gestation. She has birthed her first baby at home with our midwifery practice and is keen to do the same with her second baby. With previous clients we have made a group choice not to support women birthing breech babies at home. Although we have had unexpected breech births at home, when the position is diagnosed in pregnancy we arrange for a booking at the local hospital. Lara and her husband are aware of our view on breech birth but want to continue with their decision to be at home.

There is a lot of deliberation about what to do next. First we talk of our usual practice of offering her a consultation with an obstetrician for another opinion and for an attempt at external cephalic version (ECV). If she chooses ECV and the baby turns her home birth plan continues. Acupuncture is mentioned and dietary advice and positional techniques are also discussed. The most recent research on breech birth is not encouraging for birthing at home (Hannah et al 2000). It is important, therefore, that Lara reads the New Zealand Ministry of Health guidelines for the care of women with a breech presentation which supports women being offered ECV and/or acupuncture, and information regarding her birthing choices including elective caesarean section (New Zealand Guidelines Group 2004). Ann would also lend her a text written by a New Zealand midwife supporting vaginal breech birth (Banks 1999). Everyone is sympathetic for her desire to birth at home. We are all hopeful that her baby turns to a cephalic position but if it remains in its present position how do we all feel about her determination to be at home? If Lara has read all of the available research and is aware of the risks of breech birth yet still wants to be at home, do we support her choice?

Tonight we discuss in detail the challenges of the midwife/woman partnership. We agree that she should be given all of the relevant information and be reminded of the group's views. Our preference if Lara opts for a vaginal birth is for her to spend her early labour at home and to come into hospital to birth with the support of two midwives from the practice, and obstetric back up if required. Ann, her midwife, has discussed this option with her but believes she will still want to birth at home.

When Ann visits with Lara next what information should she gather from her? What are the most important issues for her about being at home? What is it about being in hospital that she has difficulty with? What elements of Lara's home birth plan can we honour if she agrees to be in hospital? Are there any we can't honour? Around and around we go in an attempt to find options for Lara so she can formulate a plan that everyone will feel happy with.

If she chooses to have an obstetric consultation and is still sure about birthing at home what can we set up to protect Ann (her midwife), Lara herself, and the home birth community? It's going to be a long night. Fresh coffee is made, plates replenished with food, another log on the fire. Every one of us recounts the various decisions previous clients have made when in this predicament. Those choices have involved either having an elective caesarean section or going into spontaneous labour and birthing in hospital. We talk about situations in the past where clients have made choices we would not entirely support. In those circumstances we have liaised with the obstetric consultant on-call and discussed the situation so they were aware of our and the woman's views. By letting the hospital know what is happening in the community, should transfer to hospital be required, unhelpful criticisms are less likely. As a group, maintaining a collegial relationship with the obstetric team is important to us. It shows acknowledgement of the expertise of the secondary care staff and illustrates our understanding of the midwifery scope of practice. It also eases the transition from home to hospital making the experience less stressful for us as the referring midwife, and for the woman concerned.

As a group we need to be unwavering in our support of Ann as Lara's primary midwife. Should Ann be unavailable when Lara labours, Lara needs to know that she will have consistent care from whoever attends her. Madeleine is a new practitioner and feels that due to her inexperience with breech birth she should not be involved. We all agree but discuss the option of Madeleine's being present in a learning and observational capacity but only with Lara's consent. The rest of us are experienced in vaginal breech birth and support Ann unquestioningly. Alison tells the story of some years ago when we arranged for a woman to have a vaginal breech birth in hospital and on arriving at the hospital the obstetrician on call pressured the woman into having a caesarean section. We all agree that times have changed and that decisions made between a woman and her midwife are more likely to be respected as long as they are informed decisions. It comes down to Lara and her family having all the information and being enabled to make their own decisions without coercion. It is a challenging process.

It's getting late. We all have plenty of work to do over the next few days and everyone needs to get home to husbands and children. There is a feeling of lightness after this practice meeting. All week we carry the heavy responsibility of being accountable to our clients and the midwifery community around with us and at the meeting the load is lightened when we share that responsibility with each other. Ann has a plan for Lara to consider and we all wait in anticipation of next week's meeting to find out the next instalment.

# The framework for midwifery practice in New Zealand

The opportunities for midwives to organise their own practice are different in New Zealand from anywhere else in the world. The scenario of the practice meeting illustrates some of the strategies one group of midwives has crafted to meet the challenges of independent midwifery practice. Looking closely at what these midwives do provides a way into understanding what freedom to practise means for New Zealand midwives and birthing women. The autonomous nature of midwifery does not mean that midwives can practise any way they want. Midwifery practice is shaped by the organisation of maternity services, the midwives' own personal situations and the decisions made by their clients. The following section describes several of the most significant aspects of the professional and regulatory framework of midwifery in New Zealand. This framework enables and supports midwives to practise autonomously at the same time as it places limitations on midwives to protect the safety of the public. This framework includes:

- The New Zealand College of Midwives (NZCOM) which has established the Standards of Midwifery Practice and facilitates the professional development of midwives (NZCOM 1993, 2005). The College also represents midwives at a political level.

- The Code of Health and Disability Services Consumers' Rights which outlines consumers' legal rights when accessing health services (Health and Disabilities Commissioner 1997).
- The Maternity Service Notice (Section 88 of the New Zealand Public Health and Disability Act 2000) under which midwives are paid and which defines the service specifications for the maternity service. Midwifery care is provided free of charge to all women in New Zealand.
- The Midwifery Council of New Zealand which is responsible for the regulation of midwives.

# New Zealand College of Midwives

The most important guidance for all midwives is provided by the NZCOM Standards of Midwifery Practice (1993). They are based on the principles of partnership between women and midwives and continuity of midwifery care. The Standards also acknowledge the Treaty of Waitangi which was signed between Maori (the indigenous people of New Zealand) and the Crown in 1840. The Treaty is interpreted as a power sharing contract based on partnership, respect for difference and recognition of the right to self-determination (Royal Commission on Social Policy 1988, Tupara 2001). The development of the Standards was one of the first goals of the NZCOM when it was formed in 1989. They were drafted collaboratively by midwives and consumers and are an example of innovation born out of adversity.

The NZCOM was formed at a time when midwifery was on the verge of being subsumed by nursing. In the 1960s obstetricians argued that all births should take place in centralised, specialised hospitals (Donley 1998). Ironically for midwives, their union, the New Zealand Nurses Association (NZNA) supported this policy. Nursing leaders believed that these large maternity hospitals would give student midwives access to more clinical experience. The focus of midwifery education was changed from learning the skills to attend normal births to preparing midwives to become a member of an obstetric team (Donley 1998).

The obstetricians' moves to restructure maternity services politicised consumers and midwives. They fought against closures of birthing units, 'daylight obstetrics' – the routine use of interventions in childbirth – and the routine separation of mothers and babies after birth (Kedgley 1996). Over the next two decades, maternity consumer groups became increasingly well-organised and skilled at lobbying the Government. Maternity consumer groups pushed for more support for home birth, continuity of midwifery care and the establishment of three year direct-entry midwifery education (Daellenbach 1999).

The NZCOM was created at the conference of the Midwives Section of the NZNA in Auckland in August 1988 (NZNA 1989). Midwifery leaders decided to open the new college to consumer membership and include consumer representatives in decision-making processes. This was an acknowledgment of the contribution made by consumer groups in publicly and politically raising the profile of midwifery. Also, it was seen as important for midwives and consumers to continue working together as few of their political demands had been met. Karen Guilliland and Sally Pairman, the first national co-ordinator and president of NZCOM, recount that:

> Women's need to regain control over their childbirth experience and midwives' desire to regain independence in practice were complementary ... The achievements, discussion, information sharing and networking which occurred between women and midwives in the course of this political activity led to a greater understanding of the relationship between women and midwives. The interdependent nature of this relationship is personified in the catch phrase 'women need midwives need women' used by consumer groups and midwives alike to advertise their partnership.
>
> *Guilliland and Pairman (1994:9)*

Through NZCOM, midwives and consumer representatives have continued to work collaboratively for midwifery that places women, rather than institutions, at the centre of care (Tully et al 1998).

The NZCOM Standards of Practice are recognised by the profession as the foundation for midwifery practice and are used as a self reflection tool in the Midwifery Standards Review (NZCOM 2004). This is a professional process where a midwife presents her reflections on her practice, her practice statistics, client evaluations and examples of case notes to demonstrate documentation. She does this to a committee made up of two midwives and two consumer representatives who are elected by the NZCOM membership. The committee and the midwife then formulate a professional development plan which outlines goals for the coming year and her responsibilities with regard to maintaining her practising certificate (Midwifery Council of New Zealand 2005).

There are ten Standards of Practice. Standard One explores aspects of the partnership relationship between the woman and her midwife and recognises individual and shared responsibilities. Standards Two to Five focus on the processes of information sharing, decision making and the implementation of ongoing plans for midwifery care (NZCOM 2005). An example of the Standards informing the midwives in the scenario is the emphasis on developing 'a plan for midwifery care together with the woman . . . and colleagues as necessary'. In line with Standard Two Ann turned to her practice partners for opinions, advice and support to help her come up with creative options for Lara to consider 'in an effort to find mutually satisfying solutions' (NZCOM 2005:14). Being accountable to Lara, herself and the midwifery profession and recognition of the responsibilities of autonomous practice is also clearly described in Standard Seven (NZCOM 2005:19).

# The Commissioner and the Code

Informed choice is not just a professional standard but is also a legislative requirement in New Zealand through the Code of Health and Disability Services Consumers' Rights (Health and Disability Commissioner 1996). The Code specifies that consumers should be able to expect an appropriate standard of care, to be treated with respect and to be provided with the information and support needed to make informed choices about health care and about taking part in teaching and research.

The office of a Health and Disability Commissioner and the Code was established as a consequence of the findings from a Commission of Enquiry into a long-running experiment at the National Women's Hospital in Auckland. Treatment was withheld from some women with abnormal cervical lesions. This highlighted the degree to which obstetricians and gynaecologists placed their professional interests ahead of those of their patients. On the same day that the NZCOM was founded, Judge Silvia Cartwright's Report on the Cervical Cancer Enquiry was released. It recommended major changes to the delivery of health services, including more consumer participation on research ethics committees and in making informed decisions with respect to their health care (Cartwright 1988).

The Health and Disability Commissioner provides a forum for consumers to complain when they are unhappy with the healthcare received. The midwives in the practice scenario are aware that they have an obligation to provide an appropriate standard of care encompassing midwifery knowledge and skills which include facilitating Lara's right to informed decision making.

# The Maternity Services Notice – a contract for autonomy

The freedom to practise for caseloading midwives is circumscribed by the Maternity Contract, Section 88 of the Public Health and Disability Act 2000, signed between each midwife and the Ministry of Health (available online: http://www.moh.govt.nz/publications). The contract specifies the minimum service which every birthing woman can expect to receive rather than outline practice guidelines for how pregnancy, birth and postnatal care should be delivered. It sets out fixed payments for modules of care and the practitioner is paid the same per module irrespective of the needs of the client. This contract has developed out of the legacies of past struggles and current debates about the management of childbirth.

In 1938 the Labour Government passed legislation to finance hospital and primary health services through general taxation. Birthing women became entitled to free maternity care from a general practitioner (GP) of their choice, in hospital or at home. Government financing also covered the costs of home births attended by midwives. However, women who wanted to birth at home with a midwife had to go to a doctor or a hospital clinic for pregnancy care (Donley 1998). This effectively placed childbirth under medical control and home birth became increasingly marginalised (Donley 1998). At the same time, women became used to the concept of continuity of care from their GP and the idea that they had a right to choose their primary caregiver.

When the Nurses Amendment Act 1990 was passed the New Zealand Medical Association (NZMA) refused initially to enter into tripartite negotiations around the Maternity Benefit Schedule (MBS). In response the Minister of Health agreed that independent midwives who took responsibility for the overall care of clients should be allowed to claim off the MBS which was designed to pay GPs. In the long term this was untenable financially as many women chose to have both GP and midwifery care throughout their childbirth experience. Both practitioners then claimed fees from the MBS for providing care to the same woman (Guilliland 1996, Hendry 2001).

In 1993 the MoH initiated negotiations with the NZCOM and the NZMA to redefine the service specifications and payments for maternity care. The Ministry was interested in a capped primary maternity care budget and a standard of service that was acceptable to the women of New Zealand. The NZCOM and aligned consumer groups lobbied for women to be able to access continuity of care from a midwife or doctor of their choice (Pairman and Guilliland 2003). The Lead Maternity Carer (LMC) concept was introduced following protracted negotiations (MoH 1996). This enables each woman to nominate a practitioner who has the responsibility for coordinating if not providing all maternity care from 14 weeks of pregnancy, labour and birth until six weeks' postpartum. The LMC can be a midwife, a general practitioner or an obstetrician.

The vision of the LMC concept is that 'each woman and her whanau [extended family] and family will have every opportunity to have a fulfilling outcome to her pregnancy and childbirth, through the provision of services that are safe and based on partnership, information and choice' (MoH 2002:11). The Section 88 Maternity Services Notice outlines the LMC's responsibilities in relation to the care provided to the woman over the course of her childbirthing experience including attendance throughout the labour and birth and home visits for the first six weeks postpartum. The woman should be able to access care from her LMC 'twenty four hours a day, seven days a week' including 'phone advice . . . and attendance if required for urgent problems' (MoH 2002).

A main concern for the NZMA in the maternity contract negotiations was the interface between primary and secondary maternity services. They wanted the contract to include a clear and comprehensive list of conditions for which midwives would have to refer or transfer care to a medical practitioner. NZCOM and maternity services consumer groups opposed this as they viewed 'risk lists' as a way for doctors to retain control over childbirth (Daellenbach 1999). The final Notice includes a list of conditions and guidelines for referral to obstetric and related medical specialists. However a compromise was reached in the wording of the preface to the referral guidelines. This protects women's right to informed choice and midwives' right to be included in decisions about the maternity care plan. The guidelines list three levels of conditions. These are conditions for which an LMC:

- 'may recommend to the woman . . . that a consultation with a specialist may be warranted . . .'
- 'must recommend . . . that a consultation with a specialist may be warranted . . .'
- 'must recommend to the woman . . . that the responsibility for her care be transferred to a specialist . . .' [underlined in the original] (MoH 2002:31)

The guidelines define a breech presentation as a level two condition. Therefore, under the contract, the midwives in the scenario must provide Lara with the information that a consultation with an obstetrician is recommended but they do not necessarily need to hand over care to the obstetrician. The definition of each level of the guidelines for referral includes comment that: '*The decision regarding ongoing clinical roles and respon-sibilities must involve a three way discussion between the specialist, the lead Maternity Carer and the woman concerned.*' [italics in the original] (MoH 2002:31) While this has not put an end to obstetric coercion, it does empower women and midwives to retain some control in situations that may require medical support (Crabtree 2004).

The continuity of care defined under Section 88 Maternity Services Notice is compatible with the midwifery model involving obstetric consul-tation only as required. However GPs have found it difficult to meet the requirements of continuity without the assistance of midwives (Mein Smith 2002). Most GP LMCs need to provide their clients with midwifery care during labour and postnatally. There are a few midwives who have contin-ued to be involved in shared-care arrangements with GPs in which the GP is the registered LMC. The midwives are subcontracted to provide mid-wifery care for less remuneration, as the fees are divided between the two health providers. The introduction of the LMC model of care has prompted many GPs to cease offering maternity care services (Guilliland 1999, NHC 1999).

The majority of midwives who carry a caseload are self employed and work independently. A smaller number of midwives who act as LMCs are employed by a maternity facility who pay the midwives a salary and claim fees from the maternity contract on their behalf. For many independent midwives who were already practising, there was little change to the way they worked.

# Midwifery Council of New Zealand

In the wake of the massive changes that have occurred to midwifery in New Zealand since 1990, the Government, the profession and the public clearly see midwifery as distinct from nursing. This has been formalised in a new Act (Health Practitioners Competence Assurance Act 2003), which trans-ferred responsibility for maintaining the Register of Midwives from the Nursing Council of New Zealand to a newly established Midwifery Council of New Zealand. The intention of the legislation is to protect the safety of the public by requiring health professionals to demonstrate competency in order to be able to practise. Each health profession has its own designated registering authority that determines what counts as clinical and cultural competence and how practitioners maintain competency.

The Midwifery Council of New Zealand has defined the Scope of Mid-wifery Practice and Competencies guided by the essence of the NZCOM Standards of Practice (Midwifery Council of New Zealand 2005). The

Scope and Competencies are the same for all midwives irrespective of whether they carry a caseload or work shifts as an employee of a maternity facility. The expectation is that midwives have to find ways of working within the full Scope of Practice. This is in recognition that over the years midwives may move between working in hospitals and in the community. The programme that midwives have to engage in to be eligible for an annual practising certificate includes ongoing education and participation in the NZCOM Midwifery Standards Review process. For many midwives this will have a profound impact on how they work. As they reflect on whether their knowledge base and practice skills are current and appropriate, their understanding of autonomy and accountability will be enhanced.

## The 'business' of midwifery

Midwives who work as LMCs have the ability to design their own practice style and philosophy. Most find working with women deeply satisfying and enjoy the flexibility caseloading allows (Firkin 2003). At the same time it requires a considerable amount of stamina and resilience due to the unpredictable nature of the work. The day-to-day reality of providing this comprehensive yet time consuming service requires that midwives find ways of working that can be sustainable. Although there is no legal requirement, most caseloading midwives form partnerships or co-operative arrangements with other midwives (Guilliland 1998, Firkin 2003).

There is considerable variability in the ways that midwives organise their group practices. Some choose to work together with those who share a similar midwifery philosophy with recognition that the midwives' ways of working with women reflect those philosophies. Other midwives seek out colleagues who want to organise their business in a similar way, for example sharing the cost of rooms that can be used for appointments with women during pregnancy. They may put less emphasis on practice style. In sparsely populated areas, especially rural settings, midwives may often have very little choice of whom they work with. This can also be the case for employed caseloading midwives (Firkin 2003). Nonetheless most of these midwives feel that they need support from a midwifery group or colleague to be able to survive the demands of caseloading midwifery (Engel 2003).

The group practice in the scenario was formed more than 12 years ago and the midwives within it have developed their own support structures to enable their sustainability. As home birth midwives they work on the margins of the maternity service. In New Zealand as in many countries there is still the clear message from some medical practitioners and some midwives that home birth is a risky option (Edwards 2005, Thorpe 2005).

Home birth midwives are vulnerable to criticism and adverse outcomes following a planned home birth are far more likely to become news stories than those that occur within maternity facilities. When home birth is portrayed negatively in the media, the damaging impact on home birth rates can be considerable (Crabtree 2004). The strategies used by the group to deal with these challenges have involved working in ways that have created strong emotional and professional bonds. Their shared philosophy, weekly meetings, daily phone contact and preoccupation with talk has provided them with a virtual work setting where they do not have a physical one.

The midwives in the scenario have made home birth midwifery their destination through journeys of consciousness raising experiences. These experiences have included seeing the oppression of birthing women by the hospital environment, horizontal violence and unsupportive midwifery partnerships and emancipation through positive home birthing experiences and supportive collegial relationships. The realities of independent practice in a high stress profession have influenced these midwives to choose to work with like-minded others who share similar beliefs about the normality of the pregnancy and birth continuum (Thorpe 2005).

The home birth midwifery practice is not a formal business, nor is it a legal entity. When a new midwife joins the group, there is not a financial transaction. She is not expected to pay a fee in recognition of joining an established practice and having access to clients. The importance is placed on the philosophical approach and commitment to the collegial relationships with the other midwives in the group. Firkin in his study looking at midwifery as a non-standard work, uses the word 'generosity' to describe these kinds of midwifery practice relationships. He found that generosity is often more important within midwifery groups than any sense of a business partnership 'without it, independent practice would be even more demanding' (Firkin 2003:45; see also Cassie 2004). This expectation of generosity to each other is the cornerstone of the home birth midwives' collective identity and continued existence.

## Midwifery caseloads

Independent midwives in New Zealand determine for themselves the number of women for whom they provide LMC care. The NZCOM recommends booking four to six women per month as a full time caseload (http://www.nzcom.org.nz/index.cfm/Questions). Over the years there have been periodic discussions amongst midwifery and consumer organisations about whether this guideline should be made more prescriptive. There are concerns about caseloads greater than six births per month impacting on the quality of women's care and the health of the midwife. However, NZCOM has rejected more regulation of caseloads as it contradicts the principle of midwifery autonomy (Daellenbach 1999).

Just as there is no regulated maximum caseload there is no minimum caseload either. Some midwives choose to carry small caseloads so as to be able to meet both their home and work commitments. The Midwifery Council of New Zealand has also not set out a minimum number of women a midwife has to work with in order to maintain competency (Midwifery Council of New Zealand 2005). When a midwife's practice is reviewed during her annual Standards Review, her caseload management and the resulting statistics are discussed, for example the number of antenatal and postnatal visits for each woman, birth interventions and breastfeeding outcomes (NZCOM 2004, Midwifery Council of New Zealand 2005). Midwives are encouraged to review their caseloads continually and adjust the number of new bookings they accept according to their professional and personal needs.

# Time off and collegial support

Midwifery collegial partnerships provide the opportunity to have regular support, feedback, guidance and practical assistance from other midwives. Another key issue is how midwives manage planned time off and what arrangements they have for back up when they have more than one woman in labour at a time or when they are exhausted or sick. Firkin (2003) notes that there is great diversity in the ways that midwives organise time off call. Some midwives 'accept the lack of time off as part of the job' (Firkin 2003:83) and others have fixed rosters for scheduled time off and back up when cover is provided by other midwives in the practice. Because the labour and birth fee is the most lucrative module in the Section 88 contract, some midwives stay on call for labouring women, especially if they have a small caseload. The LMC has a contractual responsibility to ensure another practitioner is available to her clients when she has time off or is unavailable.

The home birth midwives in the scenario use their practice meeting to discuss the care each of their clients receives and negotiate who will provide cover and back up. The advantage of this is that when a midwife needs time off the practice knows what is happening for that midwife's clients and can take over her 'load'. The group's clients are aware that their personal details will be discussed weekly and therefore know that if their midwife is unavailable everyone else will be up to date with regard to what is happening for them. The knowledge that they share a similar practice style and philosophy means that each midwife can trust that her clients are in good hands when she takes time off.

Many midwives balk at the idea of meeting for four hours every week and question the value of such a commitment yet this group believes that what is gained from the meetings balances any interruption to their family or social lives. Studies looking at what is important to midwives in independent practice indicate that balancing work and home life and ensuring regular time off are paramount (Rolston 1999, McLardy 2002, Firkin 2003, Engel 2003). Although social/family support is an important part of managing the lifestyle of independent midwifery practice the midwives in this practice have an awareness that the practice meeting, and the support from that, is an integral part of keeping work at work and assists in protecting their personal and family lives.

# Inter-professional relationships

It is not uncommon for independent midwives at times to feel isolated and pressured with the responsibilities associated with their midwifery practice. There is clear evidence that the most effectual strategy to deal with this stress is the establishment of open, flexible and supportive collegial relationships (Sandall 1997, Shallow 2001, Baston and Green 2002, Stevens and McCourt 2002). One of the negative consequences of the rapid and far-reaching changes to maternity services in New Zealand has been the exacerbation of inter-professional tensions. Independent midwives, midwives employed within facilities and obstetricians often have differing views of their respective roles and styles of practice (Campbell 2000, 2004). This can vary greatly between individuals, localities and over time (Firkin 2003). Some caseloading midwives feel watched and judged when they enter a maternity facility with the women for whom they provide care. Midwives employed on shifts in maternity facilities sometimes feel that their skills are not valued and that they are excluded by the LMC midwives (Campbell 2004, Isa et al 2002, Wynn-Williams 2004). Acceptance of independent midwifery is improving slowly as more midwives over time shift between hospital employment and caseloading to suit their personal circumstances. However, midwives still often find themselves negotiating relationships with other health professionals on a case by case basis (Firkin 2003). This depends on a variety of factors such as the culture of the hospital, the particular staff on duty, the reputation and skill of the midwife and the personality and needs of the individual woman and her support people (Firkin 2003).

The Midwifery Scope of Practice and the standards of practice clearly outline that midwives need to know and refer appropriately when they reach the limits of their expertise (Midwifery Council of New Zealand 2004, NZCOM 2005). There is a professional expectation that midwives work collaboratively with other health professionals in the interests of the woman. When there is a lack of mutual trust and respect between health professionals it can be challenging for independent midwives to facilitate integration of care for women and their babies across primary and secondary/tertiary services. Midwives sometimes find it difficult to be advocates for women in situations where medical assistance needs to be considered. This in turn can undermine the partnership between women and midwives and lead to defensive practice and inappropriate intervention in childbirth (Crabtree 2004).

The home birth midwives from the scenario always have two midwives at every birth whether they are at home or in hospital. The second midwife arrives at home when the birth is imminent or the first midwife needs a break or a second opinion. In this practice, the expectation of the second midwife if they transfer into hospital is that she comes in no matter what stage the woman is at in her labour. Her role then is to provide that buffer between the woman and her midwife, and the hospital staff and their philosophies and protocols. Having at least two midwives to present a united front has become the expected norm and accepted by hospital staff as the way that 'they' do it. Although judgments made may not always be complementary there are many times when the home birth identity assigned to the group and their clients means that allowances are made for choices made which may not be mainstream. The desire to maintain a home birth philosophy around the woman's experience even though she is in hospital means that by having two midwives present there is a strong advocacy service for both the woman and each other and this is, in the main, recognised by hospital staff. This understanding has evolved over time (Thorpe 2005).

## Conclusion

This chapter has investigated New Zealand independent midwives' freedom to practise within a regulatory framework which positions partnership between midwives and women at its centre. The details of that framework have been explored by outlining the historical background to legislative changes and the subsequent development of New Zealand midwifery as a flourishing profession. There has been an acknowledgment that despite these developments midwives still have to work hard at sustaining their professional commitments without compromising other parts of their lives. The challenges of autonomous independent midwifery practice are many. The practice meeting scenario has illustrated one midwifery group's way of supporting each other and their clients within an environment that can at times confront the essence of the midwife/woman relationship.

For independent midwives to demonstrate freedom to practise they also need to provide opportunities for the women they care for to have a freedom of their own. The mission for the future is for midwives to continue to strive towards working effectively within a framework that allows them to facilitate women to make their own decisions throughout every aspect of their childbirthing experience.

# Postscript

Lara's baby remained persistently in a breech position despite an attempted ECV and acupuncture treatments. She read the available research, met with an obstetrician for another opinion and discussed her options with her midwife and family. The decision she eventually came to was to plan for a vaginal breech birth in hospital with the support of her LMC, a second midwife from the home birth practice, her family and the watchful eye of the on call obstetric team. She went into spontaneous labour and after assessment at home with her midwife Ann, transferred into the hospital. Waiting there on her arrival was Alison, the second midwife, who had paved the way for their arrival to be as seamless and non-interfering as possible. Alison's negotiation with the hospital staff involved an agreed compromise, asked for by Lara, that an obstetrician would be in the room for the birth but that she would not be restricted by constant monitoring or epidural anaesthesia. Madeleine was a quiet background presence listening and learning, whilst assisting with documentation.

Lara laboured beautifully and proceeded to give birth in a standing position, her baby daughter gently caught by her midwife, Ann. Three hours later, following the birth of her placenta and time for the family to enjoy their new baby, they were at home tucked up in their own bed. Other than the place of birth, Lara's original birth plan was able to be honoured and respected. For this to be possible her midwives needed to have clarity with regard to their roles, professional responsibilities and legal requirements. To be able to confront the potentially conflicting philosophies of the on-call obstetric team Lara's birth plan needed to exhibit informed decision making and choices. This process involved constant discussion and negotiation between all parties.

## Reflective questions

The Midwifery Council of New Zealand's Scope of Midwifery Practice and Competencies, the NZCOM Standards of Practice and NZCOM Midwifery Standards Review process will all: have an impact on midwives' way of working; help them to reflect on their knowledge base and practice skills; and, enhance their understanding and accountability. How are these factors handled in your country? Please take some time to find this out so that you are up to date with this.

The scenario and chapter describing midwives in partnership give a picture of midwives working closely together. Would you like to work like this? Would you be prepared to make the commitment?

## References

Banks M 1999 Breech Birth Woman-Wise. Birthspirit Books, Hamilton

Baston H, Green J 2002 Community midwives' role perceptions. British Journal of Midwifery, 10(1):35–40

Campbell N 2000 Core Midwives – The Challenge. Proceedings NZCOM 6th Biennial Conference Proceedings, Hamilton, 29–30 September

Campbell N 2004 Maintaining professional competence as an employed midwife in Aotearoa, New Zealand. A thesis submitted in partial fulfilment of the degree of Master of Midwifery at Otago Polytechnic, Dunedin

Cartwright SR 1988 The Report of the Committee of Inquiry into allegations concerning the treatment of cervical cancer at National Women's Hospital and into other related matters. Committee of Inquiry, Auckland

Cassie F 2004 Cruising collective. Midwifery News 33:13–15

Crabtree S 2004 Midwives constructing 'normal birth'. In: Downe S (ed) Normal Childbirth Evidence and Debate. Churchill Livingstone, Edinburgh

Daellenbach R 1999 The paradox of success and the challenge of change: home birth associations of Aotearoa/New Zealand. Unpublished PhD thesis, University of Canterbury, Christchurch

De Vries R, Benoit C, van Teijlingen E et al (eds) 2001 Introduction. Birth by design: pregnancy, maternity care, and midwifery in North America and Europe. Routledge, New York

Donley J 1992 The influence of the home birth movement on midwifery in New Zealand. Proceedings NZCOM 2nd National Conference, Wellington, 29–30 August

Donley J 1998 Birthrites. Natural versus unnatural childbirth in New Zealand. The Full Court Press, Auckland

Edwards N 2005 Birthing Autonomy: Women's Experiences of Planning Home Births. Routledge, London

Engel C 2003 Towards a sustainable model of midwifery practice in a continuity of carer setting: the experience of New Zealand midwives. New Zealand College of Midwives Journal, 28:12–15

Firkin P 2003 Midwifery as non-standard work- rebirth of a profession. Research Report Series 2003/1. Labour Market Dynamic research programme, Albany & Palmerston North

Guilliland K 1996 Section 51, contract for autonomy. Proceedings NZCOM 4th Biennial Conference, Christchurch, 28–31 August

Guilliland K 1998 A demographic profile of independent (self-employed) midwives in New Zealand Aotearoa. Unpublished MA thesis, Victoria University of Wellington, Wellington

Guilliland K 1999 Shared care in maternity services; with whom and how? New Zealand College of Midwives National Newsletter 14:1–4

Guilliland K, Pairman S 1994 The Midwifery Partnership – A Model for Practice. Proceedings of the NZCOM 3rd Biennial National Conference, Rotorua, 12–13 August

Hannah ME, Hannah WJ, Hewson SA et al 2000 Planned caesarean section versus planned vaginal birth for breech presentation at term: a randomised controlled trial. Lancet 356:1375–1383

Health and Disability Commissioner 1996 Code of Health and Disability Services Consumers' Rights. Health and Disability Commissioner, Wellington

Health Practitioners Competence Assurance Act 2003 New Zealand Government, Wellington

Hendry C 2001 Riding the waves of change: the development of modern midwifery within the New Zealand health sector. New Zealand College of Midwives Journal 25:10–15

Isa T, Thwaites H, McGregor B et al 2002 Core Midwifery – the challenge continues. Proceedings of the NZCOM 7th Biennial National Conference, Dunedin, 4–6 July

Kedgley S 1996 Mum's the Word, The Untold Story of Motherhood in New Zealand. Random House, Auckland

McLardy E 2002 Boundaries: work and home. New Zealand College of Midwives Journal 27:33–34

Mein Smith P 2002 Midwifery re-innovation in New Zealand. In: Stanton J (ed) Innovations in Health and Medicine. Routledge, London

Midwifery Council of New Zealand 2004 Competencies for entry to the register of midwives. Online. Available at: http://www.midwiferycouncil.org.nz/main/Publications/ (accessed 30 October 2005)

Midwifery Council of New Zealand 2005 Recertification programme. Online. Available at: http://www.midwiferycouncil.org.nz/main/ Publications/ (accessed 30 October 2005)

MoH 1996 Maternity Benefit Schedule under Section 51 of the Health and Disability Services Act 1993. MoH, Wellington

MoH 2002 Maternity Services Notice pursuant under Section 88 of the Public Health and Disability Act 2000. MoH, Wellington

MoH 2004 New Zealand Health Information Service Report on Maternity 2001–2002. MoH, Wellington

NHC 1999 Review of Maternity Services in New Zealand, Wellington

NZCOM 1993, 2005 Midwives Handbook for Practice. NZCOM (Inc), Christchurch

NZCOM 2004 Midwifery Standards Review Handbook. NZCOM, Christchurch

NZCOM. Questions to ask your midwife. Online. Available at: http://www.nzcom.org.nz/index.cfm/Questions (accessed 30 October 2005)

New Zealand Guidelines Group 2004 Care of women with breech presentation or previous caesarean birth. Evidence-based best practice guideline summary. MoH, Wellington

New Zealand Health Information Service 2004 The New Zealand Workforce Statistics Nurses and Midwives. Online. Available: http://www. nzhis.govt.nz/stats/nursestats.html#03 (accessed 30 October 2005)

New Zealand Public Health and Disability Act 2000. New Zealand Government, Wellington

NZNA 1989 Midwifery Policy Statement. NZNA, Wellington

Nurses Amendment Act 1990 New Zealand Government, Wellington

Pairman S, Guilliland K 2003 The New Zealand experience. In: Kirkham M (ed) Birth Centres: A Social Model for Maternity Care. Butterworth-Heinemann, Oxford

Rolston L 1999 The issue of midwife self preservation. New Zealand College of Midwives Journal 20:25–26

Royal Commission on Social Policy 1988 The April Report. Royal Commission on Social Policy, Wellington

Sandall J 1997 Midwives' burnout and continuity of care. British Journal of Midwifery 5(2):106–111

Shallow H 2001 Teams and the marginalisation of midwifery knowledge. British Journal of Midwifery 9(3):167–171

Stevens T, McCourt C 2002 One-to-one midwifery practice: sustaining the model. British Journal of Midwifery 10(3):174–179

Thorpe J 2005 A feminist case study of the collegial relationships within a home birth midwifery practice in New Zealand. A thesis submitted to the Otago Polytechnic Dunedin, in partial fulfilment of the degree of Master of Midwifery, Dunedin

Tully L, Daellenbach R, Guilliland K 1998 Feminism, partnership and midwifery. In: Du Plessis R, Alice L (eds) Feminist Thought in Aotearoa New Zealand. Oxford University Press, Auckland

Tupara H 2001 Meeting the needs of Maori women: The challenge for midwifery education. New Zealand College of Midwives Journal 25:6–9

Wynn-Williams B 2004 Defining and delivering core midwifery care. Kai Tiaki Nursing, New Zealand, 14–16 April

## Additional resources

Health and Disability Commissioner Act 1994 New Zealand Government, Wellington

Health and Disability Services Act 1993 New Zealand Government, Wellington

# Women supporting midwifery: the influence of consumer organisations on best practice

MARY NOLAN

This chapter looks at the ways in which childbirth organisations the world over have contributed to the understanding and development of best practice in midwifery. It explains how the voices of childbearing women have been heard in different countries, and how consumer organisations have worked alongside midwives to shape services that are truly responsive to the physical, emotional, social and spiritual needs of women.

## Women and freedom to birth: a brief historical overview

Midwives' 'freedom to practise', historically and today, in the context of both East and West, in affluent and impoverished communities, has been and is still inextricably linked with the respect and freedom accorded to women. The value placed on the unique contribution of women, on the female, and on feminine values, is reflected in the way in which society allocates resources to pregnancy, labouring and newly delivered women. To control birth is to control the start of every new citizen's life. The way in which a society organises birth and the importance which it attaches to it, is strongly indicative of the way in which it handles relationships between the weak and the strong, the dependent and the powerful, women and men, nature and technology.

The debate around who 'controls' childbirth has been ongoing – at least in the UK – since the invention of forceps in the late sixteenth century by Dr Chamberlen. The Chamberlen medical dynasty (a family of doctors spanning 150 years) soon realised that their invention would guarantee them professional supremacy and personal wealth, and used to transport their forceps from case to case in a locked box to avoid anyone stealing their design (Towler and Bramall 1986). Doctors now had something to offer women (but only women who could pay for maternity care) over and above midwifery skills and wisdom as summarised in this extract from Jane Sharpe's *The Midwives Book*, published in London in 1671:

> When the patient feels the throws coming, she should walk easily in her Chamber and then again lie down, keep her self warm, rest her self and then stir again, till she feels the Waters coming down and the Womb to open. Let her not lie long a Bed, yet she may lie sometimes and sleep to strengthen her, and to abate pain
>
> *In: Smith (2005)*

The way in which labour and birth were seen in European countries began to change as the primary caregivers shifted from being 'wise' women known to the labouring woman, to wise women plus a doctor (if the labouring woman could afford him), to just a doctor as the English-speaking colonies came to the fore and America became the world's role model. The professional turf-war has gradually redefined the role of women in childbearing, a role defined and redefined by the terms used to describe the act of giving birth. To begin with, women 'gave birth'; then they were 'delivered' and in the twenty-first century, they are often 'sectioned'.

# The twentieth century: women and freedom of information

For centuries, the people most concerned in all of this, namely mothers and their babies, were silent. In the twentieth century, however, the world both shrank in terms of how quickly it was possible to travel from one country to another and communicate with far-away places, and expanded in terms of the amount of information available to everybody with access to the internet. Women who had traditionally been denied information in every country in the world, whether affluent or poor, suddenly became – at least in some countries – information-rich. They found out:

- That 525 000 women die each year from maternal causes
- That maternal health complications contribute to the deaths of at least 1.5 million infants in the first week of life and 1.4 million still-born babies

- That each year over 15 million women experience severe pregnancy-related complications which lead to long-term illness or disability (Mirsky 2001:3).

In the 1970s, Eddie Cochrane instigated the Cochrane Collaboration which took the sacred bull of research firmly by the horns and demonstrated to an unnerved medical profession and an initially astounded and subsequently angry child-bearing population that the majority of rituals around contemporary childbirth were either not based on research at all, or were based on poor research. From 1989, women in Britain could buy *A Guide to Effective Care in Pregnancy and Childbirth* (Enkin et al 1989) and discover that there were 60 forms of care – many of which they had experienced at first hand – which the authors described as needing to be 'abandoned in the light of the available evidence' (363–365). These included areas which touched fundamentally on women's freedom and dignity, such as:

- insisting on universal institutional confinement
- restricting maternal position during labour and delivery
- separating healthy mothers and babies routinely.

In America, the 'Maternity Center Association' (now Childbirth Connection, http://www.childbirthconnection.org) informed the women of the most powerful and richest nation on earth that 'A large body of scientific research shows that many widely used maternity care practices that involve risk and discomfort are of no benefit to low-risk women and infants. On the other hand, some practices that clearly offer important benefits are not widely available in U.S. hospitals.' Childbirth groups in many parts of the world found a fresh impetus for the campaigns they had been conducting for 30 years and more. They now had powerful weapons to combat what the members of such groups saw as unwanted interventions in labour. They also discovered that research supported a model of care with a far longer history than the medical model and many groups shifted their attention away from attacking doctors to supporting midwives. New groups were formed with the principal aim of securing midwifery care for all women.

It was zealously recalled by such groups that the word 'midwife' means 'with woman' whereas the Latin verb 'obstare' from which 'obstetrics' is derived means 'to stand in front of'. The question posed to women by the campaigning organisations was whether mothers wanted professionals to stand alongside them or in front of them? Greene (2000) describing cultural change in American birthing practices, wrote about how medical technology stands between a woman's child and her body, to protect the child from her body, and to control women:

American society uses routine obstetric ritual procedures to mold all childbearing women into conformity.

Of course, after 400 years of indoctrination into the dangers of childbirth, many women were not sure that they minded. Having someone to stand in front of you to protect you from the terrors and dangers of giving birth and to take responsibility for your baby remained extremely reassuring. However the days of ceding responsibility to healthcare professionals appear to be numbered: there is an ever-increasing access to information; all medical procedures require informed consent; and some governments are insisting on users being more involved in healthcare policy.

# Valuing women's experience of childbirth

Childbirth groups have always insisted on the value and authenticity of women's first-hand experience. This is what Baggott et al (2005:114) define as a 'core value' of voluntary organisations, namely 'a belief in the validity of personal experience and of a "lay" knowledge':

> Experience was seen to provide a unique insight that was accepted as valid and as representing a form of 'truth'. It was the basis of a claim to be heard.
>
> *Baggott et al (2005:116)*

The pooling of the experiences of a large number of people with the same 'condition' enables organisations to build up 'intellectual capital' from which they draw when making their case for greater recognition and more resources. Examples of this include: The Australian Multiple Birth Association Inc which has as its motto 'support from "those who know"'; the Group B Strep Association which has members in the United States, Canada and England, and educates local communities and health professionals by 'sharing their own experiences with GBS' (Group B Strep Association, http://www.groupbstrep.org/about.html).

The mission statement of the UK National Childbirth Trust (NCT) is that all parents should 'have an experience of pregnancy, birth and early parenthood that enriches their lives'. This emphasis on the value of every woman's unique experience of giving birth has led childbirth organisations to seek moral and political support from, and offer them to midwives as the health professionals whom they see as most committed to helping women have a positive experience of birth. As Lindsay Reid explains in the first chapter of this book, midwives have defined best practice as being 'woman-centred'. Van Teijlingen (1994) describes midwifery best practice in terms of seeing the experience of childbirth as valuable in its own right, and speaks about choice and women's active involvement in the process of childbearing. This coincides perfectly with the childbirth movement's insistence on the profound psychological impact that the birth act has on a woman's lifelong mental health. The work of Penny Simkin (1991, 1992) has provided a credible evidence base for this belief. Simkin explored women's long-term recollections of giving birth, concluding:

> It is clear that the birth experience has a powerful effect on women with a potential for permanent or long-term positive or negative impact.
>
> *Simkin (1991:210)*

Interviewing women in 1988 who had given birth between 1968 and 1974, she records how one woman vividly recalled her feelings at her class reunion:

> I can remember . . . one woman was talking about her experience and how the nurses had told her that she did such a good job and she was so proud of that.
>
> [How did you feel when you heard that, do you recall?]
>
> Pretty bad, because no one told me I was doing a good job and in fact I probably thought I didn't do a good job.
>
> *Simkin (1992:69)*

In the United Kingdom, the Natural Childbirth Association, founded in 1956 and renamed the National Childbirth Trust (NCT) in 1957, laid claim to expertise because its volunteers were themselves mothers. Thus, by virtue of having personally experienced childbirth, they felt they could legitimately provide education and support to other mothers. From the inception of the organisation, the only criterion for admission to its antenatal teacher training programme (now a validated University course) has been that the applicant must have given birth at least once. Claims of discrimination and prejudice down the years against women wanting to train but who have not had a baby have been resisted. The requirement to have given birth stands today.

Childbirth organisations the world over have defined their intellectual capital in terms of what women know from first hand experience about giving birth. They have then made it their mission to spread this understanding in order to assist enactment of 'best practice'. One of the founding mothers of the NCT, Sheila Kitzinger, wrote in the 1960s about *The Experience of Childbirth* (1967) (author's underlining). Her aim was to broaden understanding of and sensitivity towards childbearing women's feelings and needs. In *The Parents' Emotions in Childbirth* (1971) she presented women's first hand accounts of different kinds of labour:

- a long labour with the baby in an awkward position
- coping without her husband to help
- a caesarean section
- an 'elderly' primip of 38.

Contractions were described in the imagery chosen by women rather than in medical terminology: they were 'like a huge Atlantic wave rising to a crest and subsiding'; the sensation of crowning was described as: 'one of extreme stretching and a tingling, burning feeling . . . not at all unpleasant'. Kitzinger annotated her text for the benefit of mothers and midwives, for example:

> By 6.00 a.m. they [the contractions] were coming about every 4 minutes and lasting anything up to a minute and a half, so we went to the hospital – whereupon nothing happened for about 20 minutes.[1]
>
> NOTE
>
> [1]This quite often happens, and the woman can feel guilty because she 'ought' to be having contractions.
>
> *Kitzinger (1967:156–157)*

It is hard now to appreciate just how radical Kitzinger's work was at the time; since then, the childbirth movement has provided ever more sophisticated (although not necessarily more vivid) information for midwives about how to make birth better. Surveys of large numbers of women have been undertaken, and childbirth organisations publish audit toolkits which are advertised in professional journals and used in all types of maternity care settings. In 2003, the NCT published its *Creating a Better Birth Environment* detailing what women most value about the environment of maternity units:

- clean room
- able to walk around
- not be in sight of or overlooked by others.

Childbirth organisations may run meetings for mothers to discuss particular aspects of childbirth, and invite midwives to attend in order to raise their awareness of what the key issues are for women. Birthrites: Healing after Caesarean (Western Australia) provides monthly 'get-togethers where women can be around other like-minded women, have a chance to talk about their experience and hear other women's stories.

Often a midwife attends the meeting' (Birthrites, www.birthrites.org). In poorer parts of the world where women's rights are still largely unrecognised, women's groups try to raise their profile by organising events which they hope will be noticed by policy makers and health professionals. In May 2004, the 'Women's Access to Health' campaign of the Women's Global Network for Reproductive Rights ran a wide range of events. In India, Grameena Vikas Samithi (GVS) organised an activity on 'Healing with Herbs' at a women's university campus to educate staff and students on women's sexual and reproductive health. In Nepal, the Women's Development Society ran an event to raise awareness of women's health in conflict situations, and in Peru, the Movimiento Amplio de Mujeres – Ayacucho (MAM-A) publicly launched their movement to promote women's access to healthcare. In seeking to increase the knowledge of women and about women, the childbirth movement's work is akin to midwifery best practice:

> The midwife will provide information to women and their families that promotes the understanding of birth as a normal life process and enables women to make informed choices during health care.
>
> *Appropriate Intervention in Childbirth (International*
> *Confederation of Midwives (ICM) 1999)*

## Childbirth organisations and the midwifery model in the New World

Women in many parts of the world where they have a voice have become more insistent that the quality of maternity care, both in terms of safety and satisfaction, is unacceptable. They have examined their aspirations, drawn up their agendas, and found that they are similar if not identical to those of activists within the midwifery profession. In Chapter 2, Lindsay Reid explores a social model of midwifery which places the woman and her family at the centre of care. The 'freedoms' encapsulated in this model include:

- seeing women as the 'main players' in birth
- considering psychological well-being as important as physical
- encouraging the woman to have a sense of power and active involvement.

The ICM's position statement on Appropriate Maternity Services for Normal Pregnancy, Childbirth and the Postnatal Period, adopted at the Manila International Council meeting in May 1999, stated:

In each country, services that seek to serve and meet the needs of women as they give birth to future generations must be designed and planned in partnership with women.

In America, Maternity Wise (www.maternitywise.org/mw/aboutmw), drawing credibility from the Cochrane Collaboration, described its goals for women as:

- envisioning a positive childbearing experience that is consistent with the best current scientific evidence
- gaining access to accurate information and supportive resources
- understanding and exercising maternity care rights
- navigating the complex healthcare systems and making informed decisions that will influence the quality and impact of their care.

Another American organisation sees these goals as inextricably linked to a stronger and more accessible midwifery profession. Citizens for Midwifery, a non-profit, volunteer, grassroots organisation, demands care that is 'safe, respectful, family centered, health promoting and cost effective' and defines its vision as:

> To see that the Midwives' Model of care is available to all childbearing women and universally recognised as the best kind of care for pregnancy and birth.
>
> *www.maternitywise.org/mw/aboutmw*

Its four principal goals are:

- To promote the Midwives' Model of care.
- To provide information about midwifery, the Midwives' Model of care and related childbirth issues.
- To encourage and provide practical guidance for effective grassroots action for midwifery.
- To represent consumer interests regarding midwifery and maternity care.

Supporting midwifery is the basis on which the Association for Safe Alternatives in Childbirth (www.asac.ab.ca) in Canada campaigns on behalf of birth choices for parents in the community. Through lobbying political parties, it has helped in the struggle to win recognition and legal rights for midwives in various provinces including Ontario, British Columbia, Alberta, Quebec and Manitoba.

In New Zealand, midwifery practice is now an integral part of the country's maternity care; this is a relatively recent development, achieved through women's groups and midwives working in partnership (Guilliland

1999). In the 1970s, maternity services in New Zealand reflected an entrenched medical model with services being provided almost exclusively in hospitals. As in other English-speaking and wealthy countries, a new feminist agenda (arguably launched by the Boston Women's Health Collective's publication *Our Bodies Ourselves* in 1970) which aimed to reclaim birth for women, joined forces with a politically reinvigorated nursing workforce to assert its unique contribution to the care of women. In 1990, the Nurses Amendment Act was introduced by Helen Clark, Minister for Health, enabling a registered midwife to care for women in pregnancy and birth without having to be supervised by a medical practitioner. Today, midwives are firmly established as the mainstream carers in New Zealand's maternity services.

In Australia, the Maternity Coalition (www.maternitycoalition.org.au/midcamp/vision.html) has supported midwifery by aiming:

> To achieve for all women the right to choose a midwife as their primary caregiver during pregnancy and birth within the health system (public and private) whether in the community or hospital

A small but powerful organisation supporting home birth, Home Birth Australia, has had an influence on mainstream childbirth out of proportion to the numbers of its members. Its campaigns have led to many maternity units making some effort to provide a more homely environment for birth and have paved the way for a few domiciliary programmes. While obstetrics remains institutionally strong, Home Birth Australia's propaganda has changed to some extent the way in which childbirth and maternity services are talked about, with a greater emphasis on and understanding of birth as a social rather than as a medical event (Gosden and Noble 2001).

## Women and midwives in the developing world

A brief look at global statistics for maternal mortality and morbidity makes clear the need for women's and midwives' voices to be heard conjointly in the least privileged parts of the world (Table 15.1). When mothers die, their babies are likely to die, and this is especially true if the babies are female. If they are motherless, older girls are less likely than boys to complete their schooling as they are required to stay at home to look after their smaller brothers and sisters (Strong, 1992).

Maternal mortality is linked to the undervaluing of the contribution women make to society. When women are considered as equal citizens with men, resources become available to ensure their health and social care. The former President of the World Bank, James Wolfensohn, has said:

| Table 15.1 Lifetime risk of maternal death by country | |
|---|---|
| **Country** | **Probability of death over a woman's reproductive life** |
| Afghanistan | 1 in 7 women |
| Nepal | 1 in 10 women |
| Kenya | 1 in 21 women |
| Philippines | 1 in 75 women |
| Brazil | 1 in 130 women |
| Mexico | 1 in 220 women |
| China | 1 in 400 women |
| US | 1 in 3500 women |
| UK | 1 in 5100 women |
| Canada | 1 in 7700 women |
| Hong Kong | 1 in 9200 women |

Source: WHO 2000 The State of the World's Mothers 2000: Report by *Save the Children, US* 'Maternal Health around the World' (wall chart). WHO, Geneva

I do not believe for one minute that if men were dying in their prime in these numbers, so little would be done.

*Mirsky (2001:14)*

I remember being at a user group conference almost 20 years ago when a consultant obstetrician commented querulously that he thought it was a pity so many intelligent young women found it necessary to devote their time to organisations arguing for a reduction in the number of episiotomies (episiotomy rates were then one – among many – concerns of UK childbirth groups). Why did they not choose to do something worthwhile with their energy and intellect? At the time, this comment encapsulated for me exactly why I was so committed to the work I was doing in the NCT. Episiotomy was in the 1980s and remains today, a common surgical intervention in the UK (12%) (Department of Health (DoH) 2005); in the United States, 30% of women having a vaginal birth experience episiotomy (Hartmann et al 2005). It is a procedure to which only women are subjected. It involves short-term pain, and sometimes long-term physical and mental distress. It is often unnecessary. What do these combined facts say about the way in which women's bodies are viewed by some health professionals, and perhaps by society at large? If well educated, privileged Western women tolerate these attitudes, what hope is there for ill educated, impoverished women in the developing nations of the world? When affluent women allow such abuses to continue, it is unlikely that far more serious anti-women practices common in other parts of the world – practices such as early marriage leading to childbearing before physical development is complete, high levels of coercion at first intercourse and denying women access to contraception – will cease.

Western governments exert enormous influence on the economic, social and healthcare policies of the struggling nations of the world. For example, in the USA, the access of many poor women to safe abortion is severely limited by the 'gag' rule which applies to organisations receiving family planning funds from the US government. The aid is given subject to the proviso that these organisations will not campaign for changes in harsh abortion laws or provide abortion information, even if they use their own monies for such campaigning, and not the US gift-aid. This law was introduced in 1984 under the Presidency of Ronald Reagan and remains in force, having been reaffirmed by George Bush in his first term of office.

Childbirth groups have a responsibility to speak loudly and clearly about what women want and to base their demands on the best available current evidence. This responsibility is particularly onerous regarding the way in which often outdated or non-evidence-based Western birthing practices are exported to the poorer, developing nations of the world. In China, in 1999, 73% of women received a pubic shave during labour and 99% gave birth lying flat on their backs (Xu et al 2000). Yet in 1989, the first edition of *Effective Care in Pregnancy and Childbirth* (Enkin et al) included in its list of 'Forms of care that should be abandoned in the light of the available evidence':

- shaving the perineum routinely prior to delivery (363)
- restricting maternal position during labour and delivery (364).

In the Lebanon, Khayat and Campbell (2000) found that very little information was given to women before birth or during birth about what to expect; yet Enkin et al (1989:363) condemn:

- failing to involve women in decisions about their care.

Knowledge is power. The childbearing organisations of the affluent world have fought for women to be well informed so that they can make their own choices in pregnancy and labour based on application of accurate facts to their personal circumstances. When the dissemination of healthcare information based on high quality research is limited, the losers are often women.

In the poor countries of the world, women need to understand how midwives can help them, what role doctors play in maternity care, and then to have access firstly to midwifery care and, if needed, to secondary and tertiary level services. Ensuring that midwives are free to practise is vital. The Safe Motherhood Initiative (launched 1987) believes that:

> The keys to success in dealing with complications in labour are professionally trained front-line midwives or other health professionals with midwifery skills.
>
> *Mirsky (2001:17)*

Graham et al (2001) note that effective and appropriate management of *normal* labour and birth, the preserve of the midwife, would have a significant effect on maternal mortality and morbidity in developing nations. For this reason, the developed nations of the world have to demonstrate that they have confidence in and prefer the Midwives' Model of Care for the vast majority of childbearing women, and that they support and properly remunerate midwives.

Supporting midwives means supporting women. When maternity services disrespect women, women may not feel able to challenge them. This is either because it is not the role of women to challenge any aspect of the management of their lives, or, because the power of the medical profession leads women to feel intimidated. They may not challenge, but they may vote with their feet, and fail to present themselves for antenatal clinic visits (a common occurrence with marginalised groups in this country); or, they may choose to stay at home as long as possible before going to the hospital in labour (Kabakian-Khasholian et al 2000). Such a situation means that complications of pregnancy such as pre-eclampsia may go unnoticed and babies may be born without professionals in attendance to help if problems arise.

The need to get women involved in advocating for other women as happens in the rich nations of the globe has been recognised in some of the poorest. In West and Central Africa, UNICEF and local health officials tried some years ago to interest the countries' leading ladies in speaking out about childbirth. First ladies from Benin, Burkina Faso, Gabon, Ghana, Guinea, Mali, Nigeria and Senegal were asked to speak out in an effort to cut maternal and neonatal deaths in the region by half by the year 2010. The idea proved controversial with some journalists commenting that these women were out of touch with what the majority of their sisters were experiencing in their lives. However, a UNICEF spokesperson justified the attempt, saying:

Our idea was to get the first ladies to plead the cause. They are important role models for African women.

*BBC News (2001)*

## Supporting best practice environments

Childbirth organisations have worked for some years now to ensure that
childbearing women, their families and their communities understand that
women and their babies enjoy outcomes at least as good as those they can
expect under medical care, when they are cared for during pregnancy and
labour by a midwife. The Australian Maternity Coalition is committed
'to seeing women have the choice of a known midwife to care for
them throughout pregnancy, birth and the first weeks after the birth'
(http://www.maternitycoalition.org.au/). This is a choice that is not currently available in Australia. In the USA, the Georgia Friends of Midwives
(Midwifery Task Force 1996–2001) group advocates for 'the preservation
of safe, accessible and affordable childcare alternatives as exemplified by
the Midwives' Model of care, including midwife-attended birth at home
and in birth centers' (Midwifery Task Force 1996–2001).

In Europe and America, increasing interest in homebirths and birth
centres reflects women's search for an environment where the likelihood of
experiencing a normal birth is enhanced, and the aspirations of at least some
members of the midwifery profession for opportunities to be practitioners
in their own right, exercising their skills to the full. The birth centre project
is a fairly new one, resisted by vested medical and political interests in many
countries. It is heartening, however, to observe how childbirth groups and
midwives have come together once more to attempt to break down the barriers to women taking control of childbirth. In Italy, a birth centre opened
in Milan in 1990, only to be closed shortly after; however, a group of
mothers and midwives has since found new premises and the money required
to open another centre. Verena Schmid (2003:170) concludes that 'Italians
are nearly ready, socially and culturally, for the advent of birth centres'.

The German Network of Birth Centres has grown out of the work of
local women's groups, families and organisations such as the Gesellschaft
für Geburtsvorbereitung (Association of Childbirth Preparation). It actively
promotes the idea of birth centres and supports them when established
(Groh 2003:186). In the UK, the Edgeware and Crowborough Birth Centres
have made national headlines and women in other parts of the country
have campaigned vigorously to keep their own local centres open. Boulton
et al's evaluation (2003) of Edgeware presents women's experiences in their
own words:

The midwives were excellent and very informative. They allowed me to feel relaxed and be in complete control of my labour. Also, I would emphasise how natural they made my baby's birth seem.

*127*

The Centre was an amazingly warm and relaxed atmosphere. The midwives were wonderful, both in experience and attitude.

*127*

In the United States, McGlyn (2003) has declared that:

The birth centre movement is the only large-scale response to the barriers to midwifery practice throughout the USA and to the demands of consumers seeking alternatives to routine obstetric care.

*196*

It would seem that here is an environment where midwives can realise what their profession sees as its core value. The midwife will: Promote childbirth practices that enhance the normal physiological processes of labour and birth as well as the psychological, spiritual and cultural aspects (ICM 1999).

In Australia, childbirth organisations seeking to support midwifery and the midwife model of care have focused their campaigning recently on stand-alone midwife-led units and some state governments, led by New South Wales, are increasing the number of these. In 2002, 97.2% of the country's 250 758 births took place in hospital wards. Only 2.1%, or 5379 births, happened in midwife-run birthing centres attached to hospitals, and almost none – just 522 or 0.2% of the total – were home births (Cresswell 2005). The medical dominance of childbirth in Australia is driven, at least in part, by the large proportion of women whose care is managed in the private sector where doctors are paid on a fee-for-service basis for each consultation and procedure. In contrast, public hospital staff are paid a salary and have nothing to gain by maximising the number of interventions women have in labour.

# Future challenges

In her excellent commentary *On Changing the Social Relations of Australian Childbirth*, Taylor (2002) discusses the problem of 'organising the midwifery/obstetrics boundary'. This is an ongoing challenge for the midwifery profession and one in which women's and childbirth organisa-tions are keenly interested. Recently, in the UK, a professional and a childbirth organisation (Association for Improvement in the Maternity Services (AIMS)/Association of Radical Midwives (ARM), came together to run a conference in Birmingham in 2005 entitled: 'Do women want midwives or obstetric nurses?' Edwards (2005) explored the political dimensions of this question, noting how midwives adopt a holistic approach to care, associate themselves closely with women's triumphs and their deepest unhappiness, and respond through the kind of care they provide to the complexity of women's lives. She saw obstetric nurses as representatives of a patriarchal, technological system of care, aligned with capitalist values and ignorant of the social, emotional and spiritual dimensions of the ideology women express around birth.

At the same conference, Kirkham (2005) discussed her research into why midwives leave the profession and concluded that midwives' job satisfaction is almost exclusively linked to the relationships they form with clients. She pointed to the considerable accumulation of evidence which demonstrates how outcomes for women and their babies are better when women are well supported, and invited childbirth organisations to encourage their members not to tolerate task-focused, non-individualised care from midwives whose employment circumstances prevent them from adhering to a social model of midwifery.

Midwives and women spoke one after the other to affirm certain 'inalienable rights':

- not to have the normal made abnormal
- to have both a healthy baby *and* a good birth (a healthy mother and baby being the *minimum* standard of acceptable care)
- not to be corrupted by powerlessness
- to have strong midwives to make women strong (and strong women to make midwives strong).

As part of my research for this chapter, I contacted representatives of childbirth organisations in many parts of the world and was fascinated to find that the midwife/obstetric nurse debate is very much the key one for many of these consumer activists. Thus, a respondent from Spain commented:

> Midwives are becoming more respected and Spain is working hard to replace the obstetric nurses with trained midwives. The Asociacion Andaluza de Matronas (AAM) campaigns for training and development for midwives and defining the role that midwives have in public and private institutions.
>
> *C Kennell (personal communication, 2005)*

And from France, I was informed:

Midwifery is well established – they are called sage-femmes (wise women). Within the public hospital system, they are the birth attendants, only calling upon the Dr if there is a problem. However, there are many Cliniques here, a combination of private/public concerns, and in these, all births are attended by the obstetrician, assisted by the midwife on duty. I would say sage-femmes are respected, but subservient to the doctors.

*H Thorpe (personal communication, 2005)*

In America, midwives are still not recognised in many States, let alone allowed to practise autonomously:

Midwifery is still illegal in some States. Most parents go straight to an obstetrician. Midwives are very subservient to doctors in general.

*R Bee (personal communication, 2005)*

If the comment of one Australian mother about her midwife-supported birth is indicative, childbirth groups and midwives in Australia have still much work to do in raising women's understanding of what midwives have to offer:

The surprise for me was that I just didn't realise the level of skill that midwives had . . . but the midwife who was with me throughout the whole birth . . . left me feeling secure and safe. I think it's easy to underestimate the skill and knowledge that they have.

*Cresswell, 2005*

In the UK, a debate arose recently over the desirability or otherwise of midwives becoming ventouse practitioners. While some argued that this would make midwife led units more attractive to women who wanted to feel that their carers were trained in such skills, others expressed great concern at this erosion of the boundary between what midwives do and what doctors do. The question put to midwives was whether they wanted to be midwives – with woman – or whether they wanted to be 'mini-obstetricians'. If midwives go down the second path, they are likely to find that the support they have traditionally enjoyed from women's organisations may start to be withdrawn and that women will look elsewhere for people who can help them realise their aspirations for a straightforward vaginal delivery. Childbirth Connection (www.childbirthconnection.org) in the United States says clearly in its Charter for The Rights of Childbearing Women that:

Both caregivers skilled in normal childbearing and caregivers skilled in complications are needed to ensure quality care for all.

The key word is 'and', emphasising that women need carers who understand and practise solely around normality in order to protect their experience of normal childbearing. Best practice as defined by Childbirth Connection is 'maternity care that identifies and addresses social and behavioural factors that affect [the mother's] health and that of her baby' (The Rights of Childbearing Women). It is quite possible that other carers could carry out this work if midwives prefer to extend their role within the medical rather than the social model of childbirth.

A story is told of an obstetrician out for a walk who picks up an interesting-looking golden lamp. She gives it a rub to remove some of the filth and a genie appears. The genie grants her three wishes. After some thought, the obstetrician says that she would like to be able to make women feel good about themselves and confident in their ability to give birth, reduce the caesarean section rate, and minimise the number of painful and humiliating interventions that women receive during labour. 'Easy', says the genie and with a puff of smoke, turned the obstetrician into a midwife. The serious moral of this humorous (and rather prejudiced) tale is that women need midwives to have freedom to practise as midwives. *Partnership with women* is what defines midwives' professional status and the unique and precious contribution that midwives make to women's experience of having a baby.

Women need midwives to give them confidence to accept and welcome new evidence which undermines what they have been persuaded over many years to believe. Hence, the research recently published in the *BMJ* (Johnson and Davis 2005) demonstrating the safety of home birth should be explained by midwives to the women in their care. If the guardians of normal birth do not shout about the evidence that supports normal birth environments, technological hospital birth will, by default, continue to be preferred by women. In the UK, the Royal College of Obstetricians (2003) has been more than happy to issue a press release stating that:

> Pregnant women are not sick. Midwives should look after women who have no complications.

This proclamation is representative of a group of health professionals who are extremely confident about their own remit, about their freedom to practise and about what constitutes best practice in their field. The College is happy to cede normal childbirth to midwives. Midwives have only to pick up the baton and run with it. That is what women want and need.

Midwives' freedom to practise will, in many parts of the world, equate with women having increased power over their own lives. Greene (2000) describes how midwives and women are at their strongest in every country when the emphasis is on valuing women. Women have traditionally been denied information and remain uneducated or ill-educated in most parts of the globe. One aspect of best practice in midwifery is the sharing of information with women in language that women can understand so that they can apply it to their personal circumstances. Even in the most powerful nation on earth, the aspiration of women to receive sufficient information to be able to make their own choices remains a dream. Childbirth Connection (www.childbirthconnection.org) campaigns for:

> The right to full and clear information about benefits, risks and costs of the procedures, drugs, tests and treatments offered to her, and of all other reasonable options, including no intervention. She should receive this information about all interventions that are likely to be offered during labor and birth well before the onset of labor. (The Rights of Childbearing Women)

Childbirth organisations see midwives as the professionals with a commitment to sharing information with women. The information women want may vary from country to country – in some parts of the world, women need first and foremost to know that services exist and how to access them. The struggle to be informed is part of a world-wide struggle for the rights of women. Casas (quoted in Frasca 2001) notes that the suppression of free speech in many parts of South America contributes to the strength of conservative, anti-feminist forces and keeps governments in power that are either not interested in, or positively hostile to women's emancipation.

# Conclusion: past successes and future challenges

How successful have childbirth organisations been? Do midwives want their support? Do the majority of women want a midwifery, as opposed to a medical, model of childbirth? These are the kind of questions that all campaigning groups have to confront. I am in no doubt at all that maternity services improve when women and midwives work together. In addition, strong, vocal childbirth organisations keep maternity services on the agenda along with the rights of women to a childbirth experience that leaves their physical and mental health intact. Across the world, my respondents inform me that childbirth organisations are making a difference, sometimes a huge difference although often, the pace of change is slow:

> It was the birthing women of New Zealand who campaigned strongly to have independent midwives to uphold their right to birth where they wanted. The Home Birth Movement paved the way to the inde-

pendence of the midwifery profession which is now fully recognised.

*K Boalch, New Zealand (personal communication, 2005)*

From mothers requesting certain choices, there have been small changes in facilities and services e.g. most hospitals now have a 'nature room' with birth balls and cushions for those women who do not want an epidural.

*K Cram, Belgium (personal communication, 2005)*

Campaigning organisations are successful. More and more midwives who believe in normal birth are infiltrating the hospitals. Women are becoming aware that they have choices in childbirth and are starting to ask questions.

*C Kennell, Spain (personal communication, 2005)*

There have been some changes such as an increase in neonatal units being attached to the clinic or hospital rather than across town so mother and baby can stay together.

*J Fagan, France (personal communication, 2005)*

The economies of perhaps all the nations of the world can no longer afford a medical model of childbirth: the richer countries because they are struggling with citizens' heightened expectations of health care which take little account of the funding available; and, the poorer countries because they have insufficient money to feed their people let alone pay for unnecessary medical attention. The UK Audit Commission (1997) noted that:

Increasing caesarean section rates have cost implications for the NHS. A caesarean section was costed in the mid-1990s at an estimated £760 more than a vaginal delivery. By this calculation, every 1% increase in the national rate costs the NHS £5 million.

Midwives and childbirth organisations must work together to help women understand that surgical birth is appropriate only for a few mothers and babies and that in order to ensure their own safety and the safety of their babies, most women's goal should be normal birth.

The confidence that women in the affluent world demonstrate in their midwives, and their efforts to support midwives as autonomous practitioners, will influence the development of services in the struggling parts of the world. This will help to ensure that the least privileged of women receive front-line care from trained midwives. Midwives' freedom to practise and their understanding of what constitutes best practice can only be enhanced by working closely with childbirth organisations. Dr Marsden Wagner, an immense champion of the childbearing rights of women the world over has said on many occasions that in every country where he has seen real progress in maternity care, it has been as a result of women's groups working together with midwives (e.g. *Pursuing the Birth Machine* 1994). The achievement of autonomy and freedom to practise for the midwifery profession has been and still is intrinsically interwoven with the women's movement and women's right to self-determination (Guilliland 1999).

---

## Reflective questions

Here we have a strong case for consumer organisations working with and for women and midwives and, their influence on best practice. Please list ways and discuss with your colleagues how you see consumer organisations helping midwives across the world achieve freedom to practise.

As a midwife or student midwife, how would you find out about different relevant groups, make contact with them and encourage midwives and organisations/groups to work together?

---

# References

Audit Commission 1997 First Class Delivery: Improving Maternity Services in England and Wales. London: HMSO

Baggott R, Allsop J, Jones K 2005 Speaking for Patients and Carers: Health Consumer Groups and the Policy Process. Basingstoke, Palgrave

BBC News 2001 Fighting for life in birth. 11 May Online. Available at: http://news.bbc.co.uk/1/hi/world/africa/1325293.stm (accessed Nov. 13th, 2005)

Boulton M, Chapple J, Saunders D 2003 Evaluating a new service: clinical outcomes and women's assessments of the Edgware birth centre. In: Kirkham M (ed) Birth Centres: A Social Model for Maternity Care. Books for Midwives, London, 115–130

Childbirth Connection 2006 The Rights of Childbearing Women http://www.childbirthconnection.org/article.asp?ck=10080 (accessed Sep. 20, 2006)

Cresswell A 2005 Birthing sweet http://theaustralian.com.au report 10 September

DoH 2005 NHS Maternity Statistics. 2003–2004 Online. Available at: http://www.dh.gov.uk/assetRoot/04/10/70/61/04107061.pdf (accessed Nov. 13th, 2005)

Edwards N 2005 Do women want midwives or obstetric nurses? Presentation at AIMS/ARM conference, 1 October, Birmingham UK

Enkin M, Keirse MJNC, Chalmers I 1989 A Guide to Effective Care in Pregnancy and Childbirth. Oxford University Press, Oxford

Frasca T 2001 US wrongs and women's rights. Panos Features. The Panos Institute (April), London

Graham WJ, Bell JS, Bullough CHW 2001 Can skilled attendance at delivery reduce maternal mortality in developing countries? In: Van Lerberghe W, De Brouwere V (eds) Safe Motherhood Strategies: a Review of the Evidence. Studies in Health Services Organisation and Policy, 17

Gosden D, Noble C 2001 Social mobilisation around the act of childbirth: subjectivity and politics. Annual Review of Health Social Sciences 10:69–79

Greene M 2000 Cultural change as seen in U.S. birth practice. Online. Available at: www.midwifery2000.com/culture.html (accessed Nov. 13th, 2005)

Groh E 2003 Birth centres in Germany. In: Kirkham M (ed) Birth Centres: A Social Model for Maternity Care. Books for Midwives, London, 183–190

Guilliland K 1999 Autonomous Practice in New Zealand: The Highs and Lows. Birth Issues 8(1):14–20

Hartmann K, Viswanathan M, Palmieri R et al 2005 Outcomes of routine episiotomy: a systematic review. Journal of the American Medical Association 293:2141–2148

ICM 1999 Appropriate intervention in childbirth. Manila. Online. Available at: http://www.internationalmidwives.org/Statements/Appropriate%20intervention%20in%20childbirth.pdf (accessed Nov. 13th, 2005)

International Confederation of Midwives 1999 Position statement: Appropriate intervention in childbirth. Adopted at the Manila International Council meeting, May 1999

Johnson KC, Davis BA 2005 Outcomes of planned home births with certified professional midwives: large prospective study in North America. BMJ 330:1416

Kabakian-Khasholian T et al 2000 Women's experiences of maternity care: satisfaction or passivity? Social Science and Medicine 51:103–113

Khayat R, Campbell O 2000 Hospital Policies and Practices for Normal Childbirth in Lebanon. Health Policy and Planning 15(3): 270–278

Kirkham M 2005 Should I stay or should I go? Presentation at AIMS/ARM conference, 1 October, Birmingham UK

Kitzinger S 1967 The experience of childbirth. Penguin, London

McGlyn A 2003 Birth centres and the American spirit. In: Kirkham M (ed) Birth Centres: A Social Model for Maternity Care. Books for Midwives, London, 191–200

Midwifery Task Force 1996–2001 About Georgia Friends of Midwives. Online. Available at: http://www.gamidwifery.org/about.html (accessed Nov. 13th, 2005)

Mirsky J 2001 New approaches to safe motherhood. Online. Available at: http://www.panos.org.uk/resources/reportdetails.asp?id=1026 (accessed Nov. 13th, 2005)

NCT 2003 Creating a better birth environment. London: NCT

Royal College of Obstetricians 2003 Press Release 22 Oct http://www.rcog. org.uk/index.asp?PageID=880&PressReleaseID=74 (accessed Nov. 13, 2005)

Schmid V 2003 Birth centres in Italy. In: Kirkham M (ed) Birth Centres: A Social Model for Maternity Care. Books for Midwives, London, 161–172

Simkin P 1991 Just another day in a woman's life? Part I Women's long-term perceptions of their first birth experience. Birth 18(4):203–210

Simkin P 1992 Just another day in a woman's life? Part II Nature and consistency of women's long-term memories of their first birth experience. Birth 19(2):64–81

Smith A 2005 Why education for birth is important. In: Nolan M, Foster J (eds) Birth and Parenting: New Directions in Antenatal Education. Churchill Livingstone, Edinburgh, 33–49

Strong M A 1992 The health of adults in the Developing World: the view from Bangladesh. Health Transition Review 2(2):215–224

Taylor A 2002 On changing the social relations of Australian childbirth: a cautionary note. Health Sociology Review 11(1&2):87–95

The Maternity Coalition Inc. Title Page: The Maternity Coalition Inc. http://www.maternitycoalition.org.au/ (accessed Sep. 21, 2006)

Towler J, Bramall J 1986 Midwives in history and society. Croom Helm, New Hampshire

Van Teijlingen E 1994 A social or medical model of childbirth? Comparing the arguments in Grampian (Scotland) and the Netherlands. Unpublished PhD Thesis. University of Aberdeen

Wagner M 1994 Pursuing the Birth Machine: the Search for Appropriate Birth Technology. Camperdown, ACE Graphics, Australia

WHO 2000 (press release) Nursing and midwifery services facing crisis, experts say. 20 December

Xu Q, Smith H, Li Z et al cited by Dr Jose Villar at the WHO International Conference on the Humanization of Childbirth, 2–4 November 2000, Fortaleza, Brazil

## Additional resources

Association for Safe Alternatives in Childbirth (www.asac.ab.ca)
Birthrites: Healing After Caesarean Inc (www.birthrites.org)
Georgia Friends of Midwives (www.gamidwifery.org)
Group B Strep Association (www.groupbstrep.org)
International Confederation of Midwives (www.internationalmidwives. org)
The Maternity Coalition Inc (www.maternitycoalition.org.au)
Childbirth Connection (www.childbirthconnection.org/)
Midwifery 2000 (www.midwifery2000.com)
PANOS London (www.panos.org.uk)
SafeMotherhood.org (www.safemotherhood.org)

# INDEX

NB: Page numbers in italics refer to figures and tables

05597859